Conceptual Bases of Professional Nursing

Contributors

Marie G. Finamore, R.N., Ed.D.,
Mercy College, Dobbs Ferry, New York

Susan E. Gordon, R.N., Ed.D.,
Pace University, Pleasantville, New York

Eleanor Rudick, R.N., Ed.D.,
Mercy College, Dobbs Ferry, New York

Conceptual Bases of Professional Nursing

Susan Leddy, R.N., Ph.D.

Professor of Nursing and Dean, College of Health Sciences
University of Wyoming, Laramie, Wyoming

J. Mae Pepper, R.N., Ph.D.

Professor and Chairperson, Department of Nursing,
and Director of the Graduate Program
Mercy College, Dobbs Ferry, New York

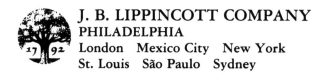

J. B. LIPPINCOTT COMPANY
PHILADELPHIA
London   Mexico City   New York
St. Louis   São Paulo   Sydney

Sponsoring Editor: Paul R. Hill
Manuscript Editor: Lauren D. McKinney
Indexer: Carol Kosik
Design Director: Tracy Baldwin
Design Coordinator: Earl Gerhart
Designer: Carol Bleistine
Production Supervisor: N. Carolyn Kerr
Production Coordinator: George V. Gordon
Compositor: International Computaprint Corporation
Printer/Binder: R. R. Donnelley & Sons Company

5 6 4

Library of Congress Cataloging in Publication Data

Leddy, Susan.
    Conceptual bases of professional nursing.

    Includes bibliographies and index.
    1. Nursing. I. Pepper, J. Mae. II. Title.
[DNLM: 1. Nursing. WY 16 L472c]
RT41.L53 1984   610.73   84-7903
ISBN 0-397-54396-4

To the memories of two people whose beliefs and values helped to shape my professional identity: my father, Dr. Bert B. Kun, and my baccalaureate program chairperson at Skidmore College, Miss Agnes Gelinas

S.L.

To Janis H. David, a mentor who taught me the essence of professional nursing, helped me develop as a nurse educator, demonstrated what it means to be an advocate for patients, served as a guide throughout my professional growth, and remains a friend

J.M.P.

Preface

In the last quarter century, nursing has moved decisively toward becoming a scientific discipline. It has begun to develop and test its own theoretical bases, to promote scholarly development of its professional practitioners, and to apply its own theory to its practice. Although progress in attaining control of its own practice has been slow and is still not completely accomplished, a clearer picture of the special service offered to society by the profession is emerging. As the autonomous body of knowledge that is called nursing is developed and disseminated, and as the profession assumes accountability to the public it services by requiring excellence in the education of its practitioners and the delivery of its services, control of its practice is more likely to be completely accomplished. Acknowledging the absolute necessity for the profession to practice from its own body of knowledge, we have recognized the need to emphasize the conceptual bases from which professional nursing is practiced.

Conceptual Bases of Professional Nursing represents our efforts to present an overview and synthesis of professional concepts that we believe to be basic to the development of professional practitioners. This book was originally conceived to assist the registered nurse engaged in baccalaureate nursing education to become resocialized into the full professional role. In the process of writing, however, it seemed to us that the contents of this book could serve as a useful resource to all professional nursing education programs; to facilitate resocialization in "second step" programs, to serve as a resource at multiple points in the educational development of students in first professional degree programs, and to provide a professional review with a consistent framework in the early part of the education of graduate students from diverse baccalaureate nursing programs.

The book is organized into four sections. Section 1 addresses the nature of the profession through exploration of historical influences, philosophical perspectives, factors that influence socialization into the profession, and the development of a professional self concept by the practitioner. Section 2 focuses on theoretical bases of professional nursing, with separate chapters related to scientific thought and theory development, the research process, theories applicable to nursing, and models of nursing. Section 3 addresses concepts relevant to the delivery of professional nursing, the health process, the health care delivery system, and accountability. Finally, in Section 4 the components and roles of professional nursing are considered. These include nursing process; communication and helping relationships; leadership; and the roles of change agent, client advocate, and contributor to the profession. Future perspectives are then projected briefly.

The book has been written as an integrated text with a common framework and liberal use of cross references; however, each chapter can "stand alone," and thus the content can be read in any order. If the contents are assigned in a different sequence from that presented, however, we would encourage an early review of our conceptual framework for nursing, which is found at the end of Chapter 2.

We have been fortunate to have received feedback from a number of our professional colleagues. Special appreciation is expressed to Sharron Humenick, Donea Shane, Roanne Dahlen, Carolyn Lansberry, Hanna Jacobson, and Carol Lofstedt, who all critiqued parts of the manuscript; however, we take full responsibility for the philosophical and conceptual views expressed.

We could not have completed this book without the support and tangible assistance provided by Ed and Carol, to whom we express our heartfelt appreciation and love.

The contents of this book reflect the current synthesis of ideas, knowledge, and values that we began to articulate seven years ago, as we struggled with the development of a new curriculum. Our conceptions are continuing to evolve. We eagerly anticipate the debate and dialogue we hope this book will engender, in order to further the development and refinement of nursing science.

Susan Leddy, R.N., Ph.D.

J. Mae Pepper, R.N., Ph.D.

Contents

Conceptual Bases of Professional Nursing

Section 1

Nature of
the Profession

Chapter 1

Dynamics in the Development of Professional Nursing

THOUGHT QUESTIONS

1. What factors led to the establishment of nursing education within a service dominated model? Why was this pattern of education perpetuated for 80 years?
2. What factors led to the establishment of levels of nursing practice and education?
3. What is the relationship between factors inherent in the formation of the ANA and the NLN and in their competition today?
4. What factors led to the dominant position of the hospital as an employer of nurses?
5. What can nursing learn from medicine about how to achieve professional status?

Nurse, nourish, and nurture are all words that are derived from the same Latin source. These words have been so closely associated through the years that some people have labeled any caregiver as a nurse. Thus, some historians have identified the roots of modern nursing in the care given to the sick by military camp followers or religious sisters, or even the nurturance of children by their mothers. The assumption that nursing is an art possessed automatically by any female has hindered the development of a concept of nursing as a profession with an organized body of knowledge and specialized skills of its own.

Nursing as an organized occupation began in the United States in 1873 with the formation of educational programs based on the British Florence Nightingale model. However, because of enormous social and technologic changes taking place at that time in history, nursing was rapidly manipulated for the profit and advantage of other groups. Given the dependent position of women in Victorian society, and the lack of a conceptual base for practice, nursing education was vulnerable to control by hospital administrators and physicians. These same forces have continued to influence the development of nursing so that it is only now, after more than 110

3

years, that modern nursing is finally emerging into professional status. This chapter presents a historical perspective on the forces that are currently influencing the growth and development of the nursing profession.

THE INFLUENCE OF THE ROLE OF WOMEN

During the mid-19th century women led very circumscribed lives. Legally, a woman was considered a ward of her father or husband. She had no independent rights, since common law stated, "the husband and wife are one, and that one is the husband" (Kalisch and Kalisch, 1978, p. 71).

The "Victorian age" also produced an exaggerated chivalry and etiquette. The "lady" was considered fragile and physically weak. "Smaller and weaker than man, she was obviously mentally and physically inferior as well" (Kalisch and Kalisch, 1978, p. 49). The American woman was expected to be modest, humble, pious, and chaste. The "cultured, educated and 'womanly woman' intuitively discovered and appreciated her limitations and did not venture beyond them" (Kalisch and Kalisch, 1978, p. 184).

The woman's role was in the home. Her prime duty was fulfilled in motherhood. It was not considered proper for respectable women to have careers or even to be educated. In fact, there was some concern that education would interfere with childbearing by focusing energy on the brain instead of the reproductive organs! Even working as a governess in a socially acceptable home was suspect. Few women ever went beyond grammer school, although a few exceptions may have attended a "finishing school" where they learned social graces and the art of piano playing and singing.

Thus, in the 1870s women who had to work were in a very difficult position. The choices for untrained lower-class women outside of the home were "virtually limited to retail clerking, factory labor, domestic service or prostitution" (Bullough and Bullough, 1978, p. 118), since teaching or even office work required some education. For these reasons, nursing training seemed to be a reasonable alternative for women of modest means who wanted or needed a career.

However, until that time nursing had been considered an inferior, undesirable occupation. Much of the care of the sick in hospitals was provided by women paupers from the workhouses who had neither the experience nor the desire to be good "nurses." In New York, female criminals who had been arrested for drunkenness or vagrancy were required to work in Bellevue Hospital for 10 days instead of serving a jail term. Sairey Gamp and Betsy Prig, both sloppy, careless, and slovenly old women, were immortalized by Dickens (1910) in *Martin Chuzzlewit* as a "fair representation of the hired attendant on the poor in sickness." Certainly no respectable woman would have stooped to hospital "nursing" had it not been for the example of Florence Nightingale.

The example of Florence Nightingale during the Crimean War began the change in the public's image of nursing. "She made public opinion perceive, and act upon the perception, that nursing was an art, and must be raised to the status of a trained profession" (Kjervik and Martinson, 1979, p. 22). As a product of an upper-class English Victorian upbringing, Florence Nightingale saw nursing as being closely related to mothering, since both used the "natural feminine characteristics of nurturance, compassion, and submissiveness" (Kjervik and Martinson, 1979, p. 38). Although she developed a theoretical model for nursing (in which the environment influenced health outcomes), she believed that the nurses' role should be to follow protocol rather than use independent decision-making. She thus believed that the emphasis of nurses' training should be on the carrying out of orders. This belief set a crucial precedent in defining nurses as subordinate to physicians, even in giving basic nursing care, an area in which physicians lacked any semblance of expertise.

Florence Nightingale's determination to improve the dismal reputation of nursing led her to propose stringent policies that were appropriate at that time, but were perpetuated to the detriment of the professional development of nursing. Good character was emphasized in the selection of student applicants, but intellectual characteristics were ignored. The nursing "residence" was installed to protect and monitor morality, but it also promoted the dependence and isolation of the students, and gave the hospital control over all aspects of their lives. The strict nursing service hierarchy, which was installed to maintain discipline, promoted an emphasis in nursing on deference to authority rather than on the development of an individual's leadership qualities. But, because of Florence Nightingale's example, the popular image of the nurse became the "lady with the lamp" with saintlike qualities of selfless compassion and endless toiling to ease suffering. Almost singlehandedly, Florence Nightingale had made nursing respectable, and women were attracted in droves.

In the United States the nurse training system was instituted at the very time that college education was becoming available for upper-class women. By the end of the 1870s, most of the state universities were admitting women. Vassar opened in 1865, and both Smith (1871) and Wellesley (1875) were established in the 1870s. Since these colleges were just in the process of establishing themselves, they did not want to be associated with an occupation of questionable reputation. They were also financially out of reach for the lower-class women who were attracted to nursing as a way to improve their status. It remains an irony of time that at the same time that medical education moved into the postgraduate university, nursing education became established as apprenticeship training under the control of physicians and hospitals.

THE INFLUENCE OF THE HEALTH CARE DELIVERY SYSTEM

The Home as a Setting for Care

Nurses were first trained in the United States in the 1870s. At that time medical care was provided in the home for paying patients, with nursing care provided primarily by females of the patient's family. As nurses began to graduate from the training schools, they were hired to provide nursing care in the home, under the supervision of the physician.

The only alternative for those too poor to afford a physician and nurse in the home was to go to a hospital, with "care" provided by untrained medical students and slovenly attendants. It was not until 1886 that the first organized district nursing organizations were formed in Boston and Philadelphia, to provide care to all who were sick regardless of ability to pay. Nurses followed the physician's orders, gave treatments, recorded temperature and pulse, and taught hygiene to the patient and his family (Moore, 1900, pp. 18–20).

Lillian Wald and Mary Brewster opened the Henry Street Settlement House in New York in 1893, and used the term "public health nurse" for the first time to describe their trained nurses. By 1900 there were 20 district nursing organizations in the country that employed 200 nurses (Roberts, 1954, p. 14).

> Some of the basic principles of public health nursing were becoming apparent. It was increasingly evident that nursing should be available to all who were sick, regardless of ability to pay or religious affiliation; a definite distinction was being made between nursing and almsgiving; nurses were beginning to recognize the importance of keeping records; professional relationships between the doctor and nurse were carefully guarded and maintained; and the importance of cooperation with other groups in the community was being stressed in order to provide the best care to the patient. It was recognized that district nurses needed more preparation than they received in hospital programs. (Tinkham and Voorhies, 1972, p. 22)

Public health nursing continued to prosper from 1900 until the time of World War I. Social consciousness was widespread, and social and legislative reform were encouraged. Voluntary agencies developed rapidly in this climate. The National Organization for Public Health Nursing was established in 1912, with membership open to public health nurses, public health agencies, and interested citizens. At this time (1910), the Department of Nursing and Health was established at Teachers College in New York, the first nursing department in a college. Post-basic nursing courses for the preparation of teachers, administrators, and public health nurses were offered.

As hospitals and the medical profession developed, the home lessened in importance as the setting for care. Hospitals became respected institutions in the community for all classes of patients. However, trained nurses were not employed in hospitals in any significant numbers until the early 1930s. Until then, care by trained private duty nurses and public health nurses continued to be provided in patients' homes.

The Hospital as Employer

At the beginning of the last quarter of the 19th century when nursing education in the United States began, hospitals were institutions for the "accomodation of strangers and the sick poor" (Kalisch and Kalisch, 1978, p. 24). Most hospitals were dirty, unventilated, and contaminated by infection. The causes for infectious diseases such as typhoid fever, cholera, and diptheria would not be discovered for another 10 years. Rubber gloves for use in surgical operations were not invented until 1891. Even the thermometer and the hypodermic syringe were not commonly used until the 1880s. The major treatment for most illnesses was bloodletting, which certainly killed more patients than it helped.

Hospital conditions were so miserable that people began to demand reform. During the Crimean War in Europe 20 years earlier (1854–1856), Florence Nightingale and her small group of self-proclaimed nurses had reduced mortality in one army hospital from 42% to just over 2% (Goodnow, 1938, pp. 95 and 97). Several years later, during the American Civil War (1861–1865), women volunteers demonstrated their ability to handle the hard work and improve the conditions in military hospitals. Thus, after the war, the movement to establish nurse training schools was seen as a way to bring an improvement in hospital conditions while, at the same time, provide a respectable occupation for women.

Hospital growth was promoted by the tremendous scientific discoveries and social change that occurred during the last quarter of the 19th century. The discovery of radiography, anesthetics, and the value of aseptic procedure, led to the development of aseptic surgery, requiring specialized equipment that could seldom be found outside of the hospital. Because of the industrial revolution there was an influx of people to the cities, thus increasing the demand for medical care. Previously, physicians had cared for paying patients at home, and only those too poor to pay for a private physician went to a hospital. The improving conditions in hospitals, combined with the need to centralize medical care led to rapid growth of hospitals. From 1873 to 1923, the number of hospitals in the United States grew from 149 to 6,762 (Bullough and Bullough, 1978, p. 132); many were under the proprietary ownership of physicians. That enormous growth could not have taken place without the cheap, efficient service provided by nursing students in the hospital training schools.

The hospital training school remained the primary educational source of nurses until the 1960s when associate degree programs began their spectacular growth (Table 1-1). Since hospitals have also been the primary employer of nurses since the 1940s, they continue to exert an important influence on nursing practice today.

Development of the Medical Profession

The current status of medical education and the medical profession seems incredible when compared with the situation just after the American Civil War. In the United States as a rule, a medical school conferred a degree on completion of "annual courses of four months' duration over a two year period. Both first and second year students attended the same lectures each year" (Kalisch and Kalisch, 1978, p. 25). It was hoped that in between the two courses of lectures the students would spend some time observing patients with a physician preceptor, but there was no systematic hospital teaching.

Medical schools of that period were proprietary schools, not associated with a university or a hospital. The best medical schools finally began to strengthen their links with hospitals in the 1870s and 1880s. Regular attendance at classes was not required and examinations generally were cursory. Admissions standards varied

TABLE 1-1.   Graduations From Baccalaureate, Associate Degree, and Diploma Programs of Nursing

Year	Baccalaureate (No.)	(% of total)	Associate Degree (No.)	(% of total)	Diploma (No.)	(%)	Total (No.)
1960–1961	4031	13	917	3	25071	84	30019
1965–1966	5488	16	3349	10	26072	74	34909
1970–1971	9856	21	14534	31	22065	48	46455
1975–1976	22579	29	34625	45	19861	26	77065
1981–1982	24523	33	38770	52	11682	15	74975

(Data modified from Nursing Data Book, pp. 39, 56. New York, National League for Nursing, 1982, and Vaughn J: Educational preparation for nursing—1982. Nurs Health Care, October 1983)

from some high school to college graduation. A common saying of the time was that "a boy who is unfit for anything else must become a doctor" (Kalisch and Kalisch, 1978, p. 25).

During the last quarter of the 19th century and the beginning of the 20th century, the focus of medical education reform was on upgrading the standards of entry, "to level the whole profession above a recognized base rather than create an educational elite" (Stevens, 1971, p. 38). (As we will see later that is exactly the emphasis in nursing education 100 years later!) The reforms at Harvard in the 1870s that led to a graded curriculum, lengthening of the curriculum to 3 years, administration of regular examinations, and the requirement of a college degree for entry, marked the beginning of a new movement toward a genuine university medical education (Stevens, 1971, p. 41). Between 1900 and 1926 the number of medical schools decreased from 160 to 79 and the number of yearly graduates from 5,214 to 3,962 (Burgess, 1928, p. 35). The rapid increase in the knowledge base for medical practice mandated an increase in standards for admission and graduation and an increased emphasis on quality.

Thus, through a coincidence of history, the late 1800s were a crossroads for both nursing and medicine. The establishment of hospital-based nurse training programs provided nursing students with constant access to patients. This was threatening to physicians, most of whom had little practical training. All efforts to increase the education in nurse training was resisted strenuously by physicians and organized medicine. Domination effectively prevented competition. At the same time the exploding scientific and technologic revolution as well as rapid urbanization and immigration "sparked the development of hospitals and medicine" (Stevens, 1971, p. 34). Medical education moved into the postgraduate university, which led to true professional education. Nursing education remained apprenticeship training that maintained the subservient relationship with hospitals and physicians.

Why didn't nurses break out of the apprenticeship mold? Why didn't nursing education move into the university as had medical education? The simple answer is that nursing was comprised almost solely by women. And in the 19th century United States, women had very limited opportunities. In the absence of nursing theory to provide a power base separate from medicine, nursing was easily controlled by hospitals and physicians.

Growth of the "Nursing Team"

By the time the United States entered World War II, graduate registered nurses had become accepted as part of the hospital staff. Many hospitals had closed their schools of nursing when they discovered that they could hire graduate nurses more cheaply than the cost of staffing with students. Thus, when large numbers of graduate registered nurses joined the armed forces, a serious shortage of nurses developed in civilian hospitals. Nursing schools received federal monies to increase student nurse enrollment, and, at the request of the Office for Civilian Defense, trained volunteer nurses' aides who were hired to assist nurses. In addition, certificate holders from the Red Cross home nursing classes first volunteered for nonprofessional duties and later were paid as auxillary workers.

Early federal concern for production of adequate numbers of nurses led to the Nurse Training Act of 1964 (P.L. 88-581). "Adding Title VIII to the Public Health Service Act, it authorized (1) grants to assist in the construction of teaching facilities, (2) grants to defray the costs of special projects to strengthen nurse education programs, (3) formula payments to schools of nursing, and (4) extension of professional nurse traineeships. Subsequent enactments in 1966, 1968, 1971, 1975, and 1981 reauthorized and revised provisions of the nurse training program. Between 1965 and 1982 almost $1.6 billion was appropriated under the Nurse Training Act" (IOM Study, 1983, p. 231).

After World War II the shortage of nurses intensified as demand for hospital beds increased. Many nurses retired from nursing because of marriage or better paying employment, or retired from hospital nursing for a nursing position in industry or public health, which offered more autonomy. Hospitals had found that a number of duties could be performed by aides and auxillary workers, at a perceived lower cost! In addition, many hospital administrators and physicians were angered by the aggressive push by the professional nursing association, the American Nurses' Association (ANA), for an 8-hour day and 40-hour week, improved salaries, and a voice in the planning and administration of hospital nursing services.

One way to obtain relatively low-cost service and maintain control over the worker was to establish schools for practical nurses. In 1947, there were 36 practical nurse training schools. Between 1948 and 1954, 260 were established, mostly in hospitals. Local public schools also established programs that affiliated with hospitals, to take advantage of federal vocational education funds. By 1950 to 1952 there were more than 144,000 practical nurses, forming 52% of the nursing service personnel. Only about 12,000 were trained (Bridgman, 1953, p. 182). Aides trained in a 6-week course had replaced the wartime auxillary workers. With graduate registered nurses, graduate practical nurses, students, and aides all giving nursing service in the same setting, hospitals began to use a "team" plan for the efficient care of a group of patients. This approach is still used in many hospitals today.

The proliferation of workers giving "nursing care" made it possible for hospitals to increase their operating profit. The graduate registered nurse was increasingly assigned managerial roles that took her away from the bedside. The public, confronted with an array of caregivers, confused the aide with the professional nurse. The image of nursing held by nurses and the public became increasingly blurred. Adding to the confusion of levels of health workers was the development of levels of registered nurses.

THE DEVELOPMENT OF DIVERSE PATTERNS FOR NURSING EDUCATION

The Development of Hospital Training Programs

The first four nursing training programs were established in the United States in 1872 through 1873 in Boston, New Haven, and New York City (at Bellevue, Massachusetts General, New Haven, and New England Hospital for Women and Children). Their growth was phenomenal. In 1880 there were 15 programs, and by 1900 there were 432 programs with 3,456 graduates (Burgess, 1928, p. 35).

The early training "schools" were semiautonomous in relation to their affiliated hospital. However, they lacked financial endowments and independent budgets, and rapidly became dependent on the hospital for support. What had begun as separate and relatively autonomous programs became nursing service departments in their respective hospitals. Since the hospital controlled service and "education," the students worked 7 days a week, 50 weeks a year for 1 to 2 years, in exchange for on-the-job training, a few lectures, and a small allowance. It is not surprising that a "training school" became essential to the financial success of a hospital.

The "old order" of untrained attendants giving hospital care was rapidly replaced by the nursing students. However, there were few opportunities for hospital work for the trained graduates. After graduation a few nurses were retained to fill head nurse positions, but practically all graduates worked in homes as private duty nurses. In addition, many hospitals sent their students into patients' homes, keeping the student's pay for hospital income. The nurse moved in with the family and was on duty 24 hours a day, for an average of 3 weeks. By 1920 the average pay was $120 a month, but while the nurse was overworked for some months, she was often idle while waiting for a new case. When nurses began to get older, many found that they were unable to cope with all-night vigils and the hard work (Goldmark, 1923, pp. 168–169).

For the next 50 years most trained nurses were employed in private duty. However, by the end of the 1920s many private duty nurses were in desperate financial straits. Because of the development of specialized equipment and services, an increasing number of people were being treated in the hospital rather than in the physician's office or at home. The number of hospitals increased dramatically, and, of course, there was an increase in the number of training programs. The number of student nurses to staff the hospitals increased steadily, despite the lack of jobs for the nurses when they completed their training. By the time of the depression, some trained nurses were willing to work for a hospital just for room and board. Despite resistance by some hospitals, graduate nurses were "allowed" to remain in the hospital, often with little more pay than they had received as students. Those hospitals without training schools could hire graduate nurses for lower wages than they had been paying untrained "attendants." "The typical hospital connected with a school of nursing during 1938 employed an average of ten graduate nurses for general duty or bedside nursing" (National League for Nursing Education, 1939, p. 898). The movement toward hospital employment for graduate nurses accelerated as the post-World War II scientific discoveries increased medical care specialization.

Although the hospital diploma program was the dominant educational pattern for registered nursing from its inception in 1873 until the mid-1960s, the variety in the quality of the programs caused widespread concern about the care of the public and the future of nursing.

The Influence of Studies of Nursing

From the time the Flexner report on medical education (1910) revolutionized that profession, nursing leaders have encouraged studies that would hopefully lead to improvement in the quality of nursing education. Between the Goldmark Report of 1923, and the 1949 "Nursing Schools at the Mid-Century," a number of studies and surveys indicated that the root of most difficulties was the dual service and education purpose of nursing schools. However, the studies resulted in limited reform.

Around 1950 a number of studies were published that finally resulted in action. Brown's *Nursing for the Future* (1948) recommended placing the preparation of professional nurses in the mainstream of higher education; the Ginsberg report (1949) recommended the preparation of professional nurses in baccalaureate programs, the preparation of technical nurses in community colleges, and the eventual discontinuation of practical nurse education (Abdellah *et al.,*1973, pp. 145–155); and Bridgman's *Collegiate Education in Nursing* (1953) warned that superimposing a liberal education on a diploma base was not the solution. She argued that nursing should have an upper division major like other academic disciplines. The emphasis on the placement of nursing education within higher education continues in the National Commission on Nursing study (1983) and the National Institute of Medicine study of nursing and nursing education (1983). The issues related to educational preparation, its financing, and educational mobility are discussed in Chapter 17, "The Contributor to the Profession Role", in relation to the recommendations of these latest national studies.

The Associate Degree Program

In 1951 Montag published her doctoral dissertation, "The Education of Nursing Technicians," which proposed education for the technician registered nurse in the community college. The program was to be complete in itself (terminal) to prepare the nurse for immediate employment. The concept was researched for 10 years after which community college nursing flourished in the growing societal emphasis on educational accessibility and mobility. "In 1962, students from associate degree programs constituted 3.7 percent of the graduating registered nurses. By 1972 they were 37 percent of the graduating class" (Facts About Nursing 1972–73, p. 78), and by 1982 they constituted over 50% of graduations (Vaughn, 1983, p. 463). (See Table 1-1.)

However, in the intervening years, the original conceptualization of the associate degree as both technical and terminal has to all intents and purposes been abandoned. An increasing number of students have begun their education in an associate degree nursing program with the intention of continuing on to the baccalaureate level. Between 1971 and 1980 total baccalaureate enrollment nearly doubled, but registered nurse enrollment in baccalaureate programs increased 338% (data derived from NLN Data Book, 1981). In the fall of 1982 over 35,000 registered nurses (graduates of associate degree and diploma programs) were enrolled in baccalaureate nursing education programs, an increase of nearly 7% over the previous year (Vaughn, 1983 p. 463).

The Brown and Ginsberg reports had stressed movement of professional registered nursing education into the college, with the eventual end of technical practical nursing education. Instead, Montag simply replaced the technical hospital registered nurse with a technical college prepared nurse. With the vision of hindsight we could wish that the associate degree program had been suggested to prepare the practical nurse. This would have upgraded practical nursing, and with the hospital program obsolete, all nursing education would have been at the college level. Instead, registered nursing was splintered into three modes of educational preparation, while practical nursing continued to flourish in vocational and hospital settings.

The rapid growth of associate degree nursing programs has intensified concern with issues such as differentiation of levels of registered nurse licensure, appropriate education for professional (registered) nursing, differentiation of expectations of graduates of various levels of education, increasing the supply of professional rather than technical nurses, and how best to facilitate professional education for the registered nurse. These issues are discussed in Chapter 17, "The Contributor to the Profession Role".

The Position Paper

In 1965 the ANA published "Educational Preparation for Nurse Practitioners and Assistants to Nurses: A Position Paper." This report concluded that:

> The education for all of those who are licensed to practice nursing should take place in institutions of higher education; minimum preparation for beginning professional nursing practice should be a baccalaureate degree; minimum preparation for beginning technical nursing practice should be an associate degree in nursing; education for assistants in health service occupations should be short, intensive preservice programs in vocational education rather than on-the-job training. (American Nurses Association)

This report intensified the conflict over the future role of hospital diploma programs and widened the schism in nursing education.

Baccalaureate Nursing Education

In 1909 the University of Minnesota established a 3-year diploma program in nursing within the College of Medicine. In the years that followed, a frequent pattern in colleges was a combined academic and professional course of 4 or 5 years, leading to a nursing diploma and a bachelor of science degree. The college liberal arts and hospital nursing studies were completely separate, a pattern that has again recently surfaced and is being promoted as "innovative."

"The first university school to be established on an independent basis with its own dean, a substantial endowment, and all students entered in the degree program, was opened in Yale University in 1923" (Dock and Stewart, 1938, p. 179). By 1929 a bachelor's degree was required for admission. Although truly collegiate schools were established at Western Reserve University (1923), Vanderbilt University (1930), and the University of Chicago (1925), there was opposition from physicians who argued that "intelligence and sound knowledge of theory were unnecessary and might handicap the prospective nurse" (Kalisch and Kalisch, 1978, p. 340). Nursing education remained associated with the hospital diploma school in the minds of the public, and the number of nurses who graduated from baccalaureate programs remained a small percentage of total graduations.

The real growth and development of baccalaureate nursing education has taken place since 1950, with a dramatic increase after 1967 with the development of nursing as a scientific discipline. The Brown report and Bridgman's study, accreditation standards formulated by the National League for Nursing (NLN), and federal monies to increase the pool of nurses eligible for graduate study, all contributed to growth in the baccalaureate sector of nursing education. The ANA position paper and societal acceptance of community college education are two factors that have led to an accelerating decline in diploma schools.

THE DEVELOPMENT OF ORGANIZATIONAL INFLUENCES

There were no national women's organizations of any type in the United States before the Civil War. The nursing associations were the first professional groups to be organized and controlled by women (Bullough and Bullough, 1978, p. 135).

In 1894 an organization called the Society of Superintendents of Training Schools for Nurses of the United States and Canada (which became the National League of Nursing Education [NLNE] in 1912) was established. Two years later this organization sponsored a conference of representatives of nursing school alumnae associations. They organized the Nurses' Associated Alumnae of the United States and Canada, which was to become the American Nurses' Association (ANA) in 1912 (Bullough and Bullough, 1978, p. 136). Thus, from the very start of organized nursing, nurses were separated into two national nursing organizations: one for the graduate nurses and the other for the leadership group. The following section briefly describes the structure and purposes of the ANA and the NLN as they are today. The national honor society in nursing, Sigma Theta Tau, is also discussed briefly.

The National League for Nursing

The Superintendents Society concentrated on the improvement of nursing education. Through their efforts a course in hospital economics was offered by Teachers College, Columbia University, "to prepare potential teachers and administrators." The course was later (1905) lengthened to a 2-year program, which for many years was the only source of advanced education available to nurses.

Improvement of the hospital training programs focused on requirements for admission (high school graduation), limitation of work hours of students (first to 12 and then to 8 hours a day), and efforts to close the wide gap between good schools and poor ones. However, as late as 1949, only about 25% of state approved schools met or approached standards set 12 years earlier, while 50% were nearer to standards set 22 years earlier, and 25% were still struggling to meet these earlier standards (NLN, 1963, pp. 3-4).

In 1949 the National Nursing Accrediting Service, established by the National League for Nursing Education (NLNE) in association with the Association of Collegiate Schools of Nursing (ACSN) and the National Organization of Public Health Nursing (NOPHN), ranked schools based on 1937 and 1942 criteria. No programs were accredited however, until 1952, when an accrediting service became part of the new NLN, which was formed by combining the NLNE, ACSN, NOPHN, Joint Committee on Practical Nurses and Auxiliary Workers in Nursing Service, Joint Committee on Careers in Nursing, National Committee for the Improvement of Nursing Services, and the National Nursing Accrediting Service. The accreditation process was influential in improving educational quality. It is still a major function of the NLN.

The NLN is recognized in the United States as the national accrediting body for all basic nursing education programs, as well as for master's level nursing programs. In addition the NLN co-sponsors, with the American Public Health Association, a voluntary peer-review accreditation program for home health agencies and community nursing services. In addition to its accreditation activites, the NLN provides consultation services, continuing education programs, analysis of statistical data related to nursing education and manpower resources, various examination and test services, and a variety of information packages to affect recruitment, image, and legislative affairs. Agency membership in the NLN is open to nursing education institutions and providers of nursing and other health care services. Individual membership is open to anyone who is interested in nursing and the improvement of health care.

The American Nurses' Association

The Associated Alumnae concentrated their early efforts on obtaining state registration of nurses in an effort to differentiate trained nurses from those who had no formal training. Separate drives for registration were mounted in each state, and the first registration acts were passed in 1903 in North Carolina, New Jersey, New York, and Virginia. A "registered nurse" was defined as someone who had attended an approved or registered nursing program (although most states placed absolutely no restrictions on the scope or quality, and some nurses were "grandfathered" in with no formal training) and, in some states, had passed a board examination. None of the original registration acts defined the scope of professional nursing practice (Am J Nurs, 1903, pp. 562–564).

In 1938 New York State began a new phase by mandating the licensure of all who sought to give nursing care. This act made it illegal for any others to practice nursing, and was the first nurse practice act to define the practice of nursing (Hicks, 1938, p. 563). Unfortunately, the new practice acts specified rigid hour and subject requirements that had to be completed. The apprenticeship system of education was legally mandated, and the rigidity made curriculum experimentation practically impossible.

Many states incorporated into their nurse practice acts the language of a 1955 ANA "model definition of nursing," which included the disclaimer: "The foregoing shall not be deemed to include acts of diagnosis or prescription of therapeutic or corrective measures" (ANA, 1955, p. 1474). This created many problems as nursing responsibilities began to expand. The third phase in nursing licensure began in 1971 when Idaho revised its nurse practice act to provide legal protection for nursing diagnostic and therapeutic responsibility. Currently, many states are revising their nurse practice acts to conform with the model nurse practice act developed by the National Council of State Boards of Nursing in 1982. The practice of nursing was defined as "assisting individuals or groups to maintain or attain optimal health throughout the life process by assessing their health status, establishing a diagnosis, planning and implementing a strategy of care to accomplish defined goals, and evaluating responses to care and treatment" (National Council of State Boards of Nursing: Model Practice Act, 1983, p. 4). This type of definition differentiates nursing diagnoses from medical diagnoses and provides clear guidance for the development of nursing practice and nursing science.

The ANA is a federation of constituent nurses' associations in each of the 50 states and in the District of Columbia, Guam, and the Virgin Islands. The ANA is the professional organization for registered nurses in the United States. Individual registered nurses join at the state level. The purposes of the ANA are to "work for the improvement of health standards and the availability of health care services for all people, to foster high standards of nursing, and to stimulate and promote the professional development of nurses and advance their economic and general welfare" (ANA, 1984, p. 366).

The ANA accredits continuing education programs, provides for certification for individual registered nurses, supplies data for research and analysis, provides public policy analysis and political education and maintains government relations, implements an economic and general welfare program, publishes a variety of publications including *The American Nurse*, and holds conferences and a biannual convention. Through its six cabinets, standards are developed for nursing education, nursing practice, research, organized nursing services, economic security and employment, and priorities for human rights. Through its fourteen councils, members of constituent state nurses' associations can participate at the national level to discuss and communicate issues and concerns relevant to specialized areas within nursing (*e.g.*, nurse researchers, nursing administration, clinical nurse specialists, medical-surgical nursing practice, and so forth).

Sigma Theta Tau

Nursing as a specialty discipline was recognized as equal to other disciplines with a scholarship base when Sigma Theta Tau was founded in 1922 by six students at the Indiana University Training School for Nurses. The name was chosen using the initials of the Greek words storga, tharos, and tima, meaning love, courage, and honor. From a beginning of six members and one chapter in 1922, the organization has grown to more than 65,000 members and 161 chapters (in 1983), and is now a member of the Association of College Honor Societies.

Sigma Theta Tau was organized to encourage and recognize superior scholarship and leadership achievement at the undergraduate and graduate levels in nursing. Membership is available by invitation through active chapters based on demonstrated superior scholastic achievement, evidence of professional leadership potential, and/or marked achievement in the field of nursing. Students in baccalaureate or higher degree programs in nursing or nurse leaders in the community with a minimum of a baccalaureate degree are eligible. The national organization contributes to the advancement of nursing through research by way of small grants, conferences, and publication of reports in the professional journal *Image: The Journal of Nursing Scholarship*. In addition, the national organization sponsors writer's seminars, a media development program, and awards in recognition of outstanding contributions to nursing practice, research, education, creativity, leadership, professional goals, and chapter programming. Individual chapters present educational programs and award scholarships.

SUMMARY

A number of the forces that have affected the development of professional nursing still continue to affect significant issues that are discussed throughout this book. These forces include societal images and expectations of nurses, degree of control by the profession of quantity and quality of practitioners, impact of technology and theory on practice roles and settings, financing of health care services, and the self-image of nurses.

Modern nursing has been developing in the United States for more than 110 years. The factors that shaped its early formation also limited the development of nursing as a profession for more than 80 years. However, in the past 30 years there has been demonstrable progress that can be related to an improving self-image and the emergence of a theoretical base for practice. Although there are still residual problems associated with factors in nursing's roots, there are numerous indications that nursing is finally emerging into true professional status.

REFERENCES

Abdellah FG, Beland IL, Martin A et al: New Directions in Patient Centered Nursing. New York, Macmillan, 1973
Am J Nurs 3:562–564, April 1903
ANA Board Approves a Definition of Nursing Practice. Am J Nurs 55, 1955

American Nurses' Association's First Position on Education for Nursing. Am J Nurs 66, March 1966

Bridgman M: Collegiate Education for Nursing. New York, Russell Sage Foundation, 1953

Brown EL: Nursing for the Future. New York, Russell Sage Foundation, 1948

Bullough V, Bullough B: The Care of the Sick: The Emergence of Modern Nursing, ed 3. New York, Prodist, 1978

Burgess MA: Committee on the Grading of Nursing Schools: Nurses, Patients and Pocketbooks. New York, Commonwealth Fund, 1928

Dickens C: Martin Chuzzlewit. New York, Macmillan, 1910

Dock LL, Stewart IM: A Short History of Nursing, ed 4. New York, GP Putnam's Sons, 1938

Education Preparation for Nurse Practitioners and Assistants to Nurses: A Position Paper. New York, American Nurses' Association, 1965

Facts About Nursing 1972-73. Kansas City, American Nurses' Association, 1974

Facts About Nursing 1982-83. Kansas City, American Nurses' Association, 1984

Flexner A: Medical Education in the United States and Canada. New York, Carnegie Foundation for the Advancement of Teaching, 1910

Ginsberg M: Committee on the Function of Nursing: A Program for the Nursing Profession. New York, Macmillan, 1949

Goldmark J (Secretary): Nursing and Nursing Education in the United States. New York, Macmillan, 1923

Goodnow M: Outlines of Nursing History. Philadelphia, WB Saunders, 1938

Hicks EJ: A crusade for safer nursing. Am J Nurs 38:563–566, May 1938

Institute of Medicine: Nursing and Nursing Education: Public Policies and Private Actions. Washington, DC, National Academy Press, 1983

Kalisch PA, Kalisch BJ: The Advance of American Nursing. Boston, Little, Brown, 1978

Kjervik DK, Martinson IM: Women in Stress: A Nursing Perspective. New York, Appleton-Century-Crofts, 1979

Montag ML: The Education of Nursing Technicians. New York, GP Putnam's Sons, 1951

Moore EJ: Visiting nursing. Am J Nurs 1:17–21, October 1900

National Council of State Boards of Nursing: Model Nurse Practice Act, 1983

National League for Nursing Education: More graduate general duty nurses. Am J Nurs 39:898, August 1939

Nursing Data Book. New York, National League for Nursing, 1982

Roberts MM: American Nursing: History and Interpretation. New York, Macmillan, 1954

The School Improvement Program of the National League for Nursing 1951–1960. New York, National League for Nursing, 1963

Stevens R: American Medicine and the Public Interest. New Haven, Yale University Press, 1971

Tinkham CW, Voorhies EF: Community Health Nursing: Evolution and Process. New York, Appleton-Century-Crofts, 1972

Vaughn J: Educational preparation for nursing—1982. Nurs Health Care: 460–464, October 1983

Chapter 2

Philosophical Perspectives in Nursing Education and Practice

THOUGHT QUESTIONS

1. Explain how the nursing process incorporates the three basic areas of philosophy—knowledge, values, and existence.
2. Why is a personal philosophy of nursing significant to the individual nurse?
3. What are three criteria for logic in nursing?
4. What is the significance of sentience in the nurse-client relationship? What gives sentience power?
5. How can it be argued that nursing is a moral art?
6. What is the relationship between well-being and the perceived sense of balance?
7. What is one justification for the belief that nursing is a process?

The nurse's philosophy of nursing is critical to the practice of professional nursing. Philosophy encompasses the belief system of the professional nurse as well as a quest for knowledge. One's belief system and understanding are strong determinants of the way one thinks about a phenomenon or a situation. The way one thinks is a strong determinant of one's actions. Since professional nursing can be defined as a process of purposeful actions between the nurse and the client, the nurse needs to understand the definition, purposes, significance, and elements of philosophy in order to thoughtfully evolve a personal philosophy of nursing. Thus, this chapter presents a discussion of the essential elements of philosophy, examines the questions of philosophy that are essential to the practice of nursing, and presents a brief statement of the philosophical beliefs underlying this book.

WHAT IS PHILOSOPHY?

It is generally accepted that philosophy encompasses three areas: concern with knowledge, values, and being, or one's beliefs about existence. In all three areas, intellectual enterprises are the methods of philosophy. The concern with knowledge is important to nursing because nursing is a science and the nursing process is based on logic and scientific method. The emphasis on values is important to nursing because nurses continuously make attitudinal, preferential, and/or value statements as they commit themselves to nurse-client relationships. Since nursing has been intensively involved with its theory development in the last two decades, it is evident that nursing is committed to its own beliefs about its professional existence. The three areas of philosophy can be related to the nursing process as follows:

Areas of Philosophy	*The Nursing Process*
Knowledge	Based on logical thinking and the scientific method
Values	Governed by a code of ethics
Existence (metaphysics)	Concerned with the nurse and client as humans and the evolution of theory-based practice

The integration of philosophy in the nursing process and the assumption that one's philosophy is a determinant of one's actions support the need for professional nurses to develop and reflect on their own philosophies of nursing.

Philosophy Defined

The literal definition of philosophy is "love of wisdom," derived from the combination of the Greek nouns "philia," meaning love, and "sophia," meaning wisdom (Webster, 1949, and Glenn, 1947, p. 1). Webster says that in actual usage, philosophy means "the science which investigates the facts and principles of reality and of human nature and conduct" (Webster, 1949, p. 632). Defined in this manner, philosophy is a science that comprises logic, ethics, aesthetics, metaphysics, and the theory of knowledge.

Given the definitions of philosophy and the assumption that humans have an endless thirst for knowledge, we define "Philosophy of Nursing" as the intellectual and affective outcomes of the professional nurse's efforts to (1) understand the ultimate reasons and relationships of humans and environment, (2) approach nursing as a scientific discipline, and (3) articulate a personal belief system about humans, environment, health, and nursing as a process.

The Purposes of Philosophy

It has been suggested that philosophy is distinguished from all other sciences by its purpose—the quest for ultimate reasons for all that is knowable. Silva (1977) suggests that this formal purpose really was possible from the time of its Greek origins until the industrial revolution. She states: "To designate all knowledge as philosophy was possible because our body of knowledge was relatively small and no real distinctions were made between different kinds of knowledge" (Silva, 1977, p. 59). Since the industrial revolution, however, there has been an explosion of knowledge. Specific sciences have emerged, each asking their specific questions. Silva further concludes that each discipline provides enlightenment about specific aspects of humans while at the same time leading to a new problem—the problem of compartmentalizing humans. As discrete sciences have developed, the need to "unify scientific findings so that man as a holistic being might emerge" (Silva, 1977, p. 60) has become apparent. Questions of nature and purpose have substantiated the following purposes of philosophy: to be concerned with the theory and limits of knowledge, to study the purpose of life, specifically human life, and to be concerned about the nature of being and reality (Silva, 1977, p. 60).

The Significance of Philosophy to Human Systems

To achieve intellectual enlightenment is considered better protection against calamitous mistakes than ignorance. Thus, the study of philosophy over time has accrued great benefits for individuals, societies, and particularly the specific sciences. Pursuing the objectives of philosophy, the individual is afforded the opportunity to exercise both understanding and value judgements. Understanding is developed by the quest for reasons. Value judgements are developed by the quest for ethical and aesthetic decisions. Society is improved when members grow in their knowledge of "truths." Sciences benefit from philosophy essentially because philosophy governs their methods through logic and ethics. Although the specific purposes of philosophy and discrete sciences differ, both philosophy and science share a "common goal of increasing mankind's knowledge" (Silva, 1977, p. 60). For a developing young discipline like nursing, the active participation in evolving a "philosophy of nursing" serves to remind the profession of its belief systems, guide the profession in the pursuit of ethical goals in nursing education, practice and research, and govern the development of the theoretical basis for nursing practice. All of these consequences undoubtedly lead to improvement in the quality of health and health care available to all humans.

Basis for Ethical Decision-Making

There are two theoretical systems that form the basis for most ethical decisions. *Teleological theory* is concerned solely with the end product of actions. The claim is that "the rightness and wrongness of human action is *exclusively* a function of the goodness and badness of the consequences resulting directly or indirectly from that action" (Mappas and Zembaty, 1981, p. 4). In other words, "the end justifies the means." Judgements about moral decisions based on this theoretical rationale are usually made by "consensus agreement on which questions are important and which reasons are acceptable" (Thompson and Thompson, 1981, p. 9).

An alternative theoretical system is *deontology*, which "establishes the right or wrong (rule) without regard to anyone, or their personal situation, or time, and without regard to the circumstances" (Thompson and Thompson, 1981, p. 8). Some people believe that there are some absolute right or wrong moral decisions, in which case judgements about those decisions are clear-cut. In practice however, moral decisions often require a balance between principles of right and wrong, which is derived from deontological theory, and considerations of utility and efficiency, which is derived from teleological theory.

The Significance of Philosophy for Nursing

Nursing needs leaders who are philosophers of nursing. In a document entitled "A Brave New Nursing World—Exercising Options for the Future," Schlotfeldt states:

In our rapidly changing, increasingly complex, pluralistic society, there is an unprecedented and pervasive need for each of the groups that comprise it to

work toward the common good; and to fulfill that need there is an unprecedented and pervasive requirement for leadership of a particular kind. The
need is for leadership from visionaries who can judge the social significance
of discoveries in science, who can determine how technologic developments
can and indeed must be used to achieve human purposes and to make social
progress, and who can translate advances in their own fields of specialized
knowledge and work to the betterment of human kind (Schlotfeldt, 1982,
p. 2).

More than 15 years ago, Kahn and Weiner stated: "Technology is changing and
population increasing so rapidly that the fundamentals of social life and the human
adjustments to material and social environment will, by the twenty-first century,
have many aspects starkly different from anything we know today . . . the evolution of society may produce the devolution of man" (Kahn and Wiener, 1967, pp.
345–347). At best human value systems will be challenged.

We believe that nursing must prepare nurse practitioners who have a vision for
nursing as a scientific discipline, a concern for the ultimate good of humankind,
and a belief system reflecting ethical soundness. These practitioners need to have
developed a personal philosophy of nursing that reflects a belief in leadership "as
the recurrent interplay between private personality and public performance"
(Rustow, 1968, p. 683). Such leaders are more concerned about recasting the
health care institutions for the benefit of humankind than ruling the institutions.
They are more concerned with creating new systems of thought than developing
dogmas to direct nursing practice, research, and education. An important step in
the development of this kind of nursing leader is the understanding of and participation in all essential components of a "philosophy of nursing."

Elements of a Philosophy of Nursing

To develop a "philosophy of nursing" the professional nurse must show concern
about the nature of humans and the science of being. From the perspective of nursing, each nurse must attempt to answer the following questions, which reflect the
fundamental elements of nursing:

1. What is society—of whom is it composed and what is the nature of the relationship among its components?
2. What is your central belief about the individual person and that individual's potential?
3. What constitutes the environment?
4. How does society, the individual person, and the environment interact?
5. What is your view of health—is it a continuum? a unidirectional phenomenon?
6. How does illness relate to health?
7. What is the central reason for the existence of nursing?
8. Who is the recipient of nursing?

From the perspective of a philosopher's concern with knowledge, the nurse must
attempt to answer the following questions that reflect the essential elements of the
scientific discipline:

1. What is the process of nursing?
2. What is the cognitive base from which the professional nurse operates?

3. How is the nursing process implemented? What is necessary in the application of knowledge?
4. How is the theory base for nursing derived?
5. What is the theoretical framework for the profession?
6. What are the essential concepts for the practice of professional nursing?
7. What are the purposes and process of nursing research?

From the philosopher's concern with ethics and aesthetics, the professional nurse must attempt to answer the following questions that reflect the valuation elements of nursing:

1. What are the essential rights and responsibilities of the professional nurse?
2. What are the essential rights and responsibilities of the recipients of nursing?
3. What are the governing ethical principles in the delivery of nursing care and the conduct of research in nursing?
4. What are your beliefs about the educational requirements for the practice of the profession?
5. What are your beliefs about the teaching-learning process?
6. What are your beliefs about the essential roles for the implementation of the nursing process?

The greatest opportunity for the beginning development of answers to all the above questions is provided in the educational experience of the nurse. Built on the entire life experience of the nurse as well as the professional education experience, the nurse develops a professional self--concept in which a dynamic philosophy of nursing can be operationalized.

QUESTIONS OF PHILOSOPHY THAT ARE ESSENTIAL TO THE PRACTICE OF THE NURSING PROFESSION

Philosophy is concerned with several essential questions in its quest for understanding the correct procedure for reasoning, being certain of truth, understanding what is reality and what is ultimate truth about humans, deities, and the world, and considering what is the right way of conducting life. The five essential questions that can be directly related to nursing are organized around logic, ontology, cosmology, philosophical psychology, and ethics or moral philosophy (Glenn, 1947).

What is Logical? (Logic)

Logic helps one understand the procedure of reasoning. The function or the action of reasoning is the critical element of the mind, considered to be the source of the human power for knowing. The mind exhibits this power of reasoning through its ability to attend, to abstract, to judge, and to infer. "Reasoning is the process of thinking things out" (Glenn, 1947, p. 164).

Ideas

To understand reasoning, one must accept that an idea is the "representation of the essence of a thing in the mind" (Glenn, 1947, p. 168). People have a great tendency to express their ideas. Generally, that expression is through language. Since ideas may be unclear or obscure in the mind of the conveyor or in the expression to another person, there are two means of clarifying ideas: definition and logical division, both elements of logic. Nursing as a scientific discipline and as an interpersonal process with clients emphasizes the importance of *clear definitions* and *accurate categorizations of infinite numbers of ideas.*

Judgements and Propositions

In logical terms, *judgement* is the intellectual process of pronouncing agreement or disagreement of two or more ideas by comparison and analysis. If the judgement made is in agreement with reality, that judgement is called logical truth. When judgement does not square with reality, it is called a logical falsity (Glenn, 1947, p. 175). Judgements are expressed outwardly as propositions. A proposition is "a formula of terms which expresses the agreement or disagreement of a predicate idea with a subject idea" (Glenn, 1947, p. 176). Nurses constantly express judgements through propositions in statements such as: "His response to the painful stimuli indicates that he is still unconscious." If the nurse is correct on both ideas (response to painful stimuli and level of consciousness), the judgement made will be a logical truth. If the nurse is wrong on either idea, a logical falsity is more likely to occur.

The Process of Reason

Reasoning is the final and most complex step in the operation of logic. It is a mediative way of reaching a judgement that cannot be made immediately or the process in which the relationship between two ideas is inferred from their respective relation to a common third idea. Reasoning requires three judgements. The two judgements relating two ideas to a common third are called antecedents. The judgement that is latent in the antecedent is the consequence or the conclusion. An example follows:

Two Premises:
Antecedent. . . . "A sign of anxiety is hyperirritability."
Observation. . . . "Mary is hyperirritable."
Conclusion:
Consequence. . . . "Mary is anxious."

The rules of reasoning state that if the antecedent is true (congruent with reality), the conclusion must be true. These rules also state that if the antecedent is false, the conclusion may be true or false. For conclusions to be valid, they must proceed from premises known to be certain. "Reasoning is deductive when its course is from the more general to the less general; it is inductive when its course is from the less general to the more general" (Glenn, 1947, p. 183). The expression of reasoning is called the argument. To argue from the fact that all preoperative patients have increased anxiety, to the fact that this preoperative patient has increased anxiety is deduction. To argue from the fact that this preoperative patient has increased anxiety to the conclusion that all preoperative patients have increased anxiety is induction. If conclusions proceed from invalid premises, a state of logical fallacy exists (Glenn, 1947).

Thus, what is logical in nursing must meet the following criteria:

1. The ideas must be clear in definition and correct in categorizations.
2. Judgements and propositions must have agreement between subjects and predicates.
3. In reasoning, conclusions must be drawn from valid premises only.

What is Being? (Ontology)

The heart of philosophy is the question of reality in its most profound sense—being. The *essence* of something is its fundamental make-up and its basic character. The *nature* of something defines what it does or can do. The Greek word *ontology* means "the science of being," thus ontology is that part of metaphysics that deals with "being" as such. The term *being* means thing or reality. "It means anything that exists or can be thought of as existing" (Glenn, 1947, p. 232). Humans often understand the term "being" best by contrasting it with its opposite—nonbeing or nothingness. In that sense, "being" is defined as "that which is."

The Categories of Being

Classically, philosophy has identified four types of being, *real being, logical being, actual being,* and *potential being,* which are defined below:

1. Real being—anything that exists in reality independently of one's mind (*e.g.,* humans).
2. Logical being—anything that depends for its existence on one's mind (*e.g.,* death).
3. Actual being—a real being that exists. (*e.g.,* the reasoning student).
4. Potential being—a real being that can exist but does not. Again, an example can be the reasoning student. (Glenn, 1947, pp. 234–235)

Concepts of Being and Becoming

The idea of change has its basis in the relationship between actual being and potential being. Change, sometimes referred to as becoming in philosophical terms, is the transition from potentiality to actuality. Early philosophers identified four types of change (Glenn, 1947, p. 235):

1. Change of substance—such as living body to dead body.
2. Change of quantity—such as the height of the child—growth.
3. Change of quality—such as from satiated to hungry.
4. Change of place—such as a move from east to west.

Nurses are concerned particularly with human *beings*—all four kinds (real, logical, actual, or potential)—especially with the actual or potential being. All nursing conceptual models agree that a primary purpose of nursing is to help the human move to higher levels of health—to potentiate human health. Nursing is so involved with the real existence of humans that it is not surprising that many professional education programs intentionally prepare nurses to act as agents of change.

All four types of change are important to the nursing process in every nurse-client-environment relationship. In focusing on the human's responses to threats to health, one clearly identifies the "being" for whom the nurse is accountable as the whole person/environment, not the threat itself (such as a noxious agent, a disease). This is not to say that the nurse is never concerned with specific aspects of the whole human. Indeed, the nurse does focus on parts, but in the context of trying to change the client environment.

Cause and Effect

Becoming is a process of cause and effect. "A cause is anything that contributes in any manner to the producing or the maintaining of a reality" (Glenn, 1947, p. 253). Beings or states of being that "become" by reason of change are "effects." This is an important concept for nursing to consider because nurses generally have a goal of contributing to the client's (being's) maintenance or changing of some reality. However, one must be careful not to equate "change agent" with "causative agent." If one believes that change occurs through the nurse-client relationship in which responsibility is shared, then the nurse and the client are both "causative" beings and "effect" beings (changed beings). Earlier frameworks for nursing generally presented the nurse as the causative agent and the patient status as the effect. In most frameworks today, both the nurse and the client are believed to be "becoming" or actualizing their potential.

Because humans live in the context of an environment, the nurse in a professional and personal environment and the client in his environment, the nurse must understand the nature of the world. That knowledge needs to include principles about the earthly environment, and perhaps, in the not so distant future, the environment of other planets and intergalactic space.

What is the Nature of the World? (Cosmology)

In approaching the cosmologic question, the philosopher is concerned with "the nature of bodily substance, its ultimate constitution, its first origin, its development and goal" (Glenn, 1947, p. 258). Cosmology studies bodies as material real beings with or without life. A body then is a material substance that extends into space by multiple dimensions (*e.g.,* length and width). Although it is primarily concerned with living bodies, nursing must be concerned with all material beings. Regardless of one's chosen conceptual model, each nurse theorist pays much attention to the interaction of all bodies in a space-time perspective.

Characteristics of Bodies

The world itself and every material body within the world possess the characteristics of composition, changeability, and contingency. *Composition* means that all bodies are composed of matter or substantial form. Larger bodies are composed of smaller bodies or parts. Anything that is composed of substance is subject to change and that change goes on constantly. *Change* can be thought of as an emergent process, that is, when one substance ceases to be, another emerges. A new substance is generated. The classic example of this is the process of *food* being eaten and becoming living flesh. Other changes that occur with bodies are changes in quantity and changes in quality. To increase or diminish is to change in quantity.

To change in quality is to demonstrate alteration in form. The characteristic of *contingency* means that all beings are dependent to some extent on causes to produce their being and on factors to maintain their being. All nursing theorists support the characteristic of contingency by acknowledging humans' dependent or interdependent relationship with the environment. All conceptual frameworks in nursing consider the composition, the changeability, and the contingency of nurses and clients and their environment (Glenn, 1947, pp. 258–261).

Dynamics of Bodies

In describing material beings in the world, whether they are living or nonliving beings, one considers the following dynamic qualities: quantity and activity. "*Quantity* is that property of bodily substance which extends it" (Glenn, 1947, p. 261). This extension refers first to the bodily substance itself and secondly to the place that the bodily substance normally occupies, or, to simplify the concept of extension, humans have size, motion, and place. All of these characteristics can be quantified. *Activity* means that the body is doing something, is operating, or is responding. Every nursing theorist accepts the premise that humans are continuously active and interactive with the environment.

Philosophy, specifically cosmology, has played an important role in the development of nursing theory. Environment is an essential element of every conceptual model. Cosmology has helped nurses look at the nature of that environment and the relationships between all material bodies.

Although all nurse theorists describe their perceptions of humans, Rogers has described the characteristics of the life process. Thus, Rogers' assumptions in the following paragraphs may be readily integrated in all nursing models.

What is Life? Living? (Philosophical Psychology)

In philosophical terms, life can be thought of as both a capacity for and exercise of activity (Glenn, 1947, p. 295). Rogers, believes that "man and environment are continuously exchanging matter and energy with one another" and that this is the essence of the life process, which is evolving "irreversibly and unidirectionally along the space time continuum" (Rogers, 1970, pp. 54 and 59). Philosophers approach "life" in three ways: as a biologic phenomenon, as a sentient phenomenon, and as an intellectual phenomenon.

Biologic Life

A living body is made up of cells, grows by the multiplication of cells, is characterized by a nutrition process, and has the tendency to reproduce (Glenn, 1947, p. 298). Rogers supports the characteristics of growth throughout the life process and the capacity of life to transcend itself, that is, for new forms to emerge (Rogers, 1970, p. 56).

Sentient Life

Humans have the capacity for sensation and consciousness, and experience feelings. These capacities make humans sentient beings. Rogers (1970) attributes to humans alone the capacity to sense or to be aware of one's own mortality. She suggests that feelings are an integrating force equally as significant to life as rational thought. She says: "Man's capacity for experiencing himself and his world identifies his humanness" (Rogers, 1970, p. 72). To support the idea that humans are sentient beings, Rogers assumes: "Man is characterized by the capacity for abstraction and imagery, language and thought, sensation and emotion" (Rogers, 1970, p. 73). To the extent that individuals participate in the nursing process, they need to consciously focus on the influence of their own perceived feelings and knowledge. Rogers suggests that the capacities for thought and feelings account for humans' abilities to understand and to perceive relationships (Rogers, 1970, p. 71). Thus, sentience provides the nurse with essential information and the sense of satisfaction/dissatisfaction. The power of sentience in shaping the way one experiences himself is marked. Since the nursing process is an interpersonal one, humans' feelings and thoughts are critical determinants of the effectiveness of the nurse/client relationships. Both feelings and thoughts determine the establishment, maintenance, and termination of the relationships between nurses and clients. Thus, sentience is the characteristic of humans that supports the absolute necessity for the nurse-person to deliver nursing care rather than the nurse-machine.

Intellectual Life

The *intellect* is the "knowing power" of life (Glenn, 1947, p. 320). Rogers (1970, p. 71) states: "A growing capacity to perceive relationships between events and to hypothesize new relationships marks man's evolution through time. Concept formation—the ordering of thought—is basic to organized action." Intelligence is the power or act of understanding (Webster, 1949, p. 437). Intelligence gives humans the ability to meet any situation, especially novel situations, successfully by adjusting their behavior. Intellect permits humans to understand interrelationships of facts in such a way as to guide actions toward a desirable goal.

The philosophical question, "What is life?" can be answered by the deduction that life is a state of being for the human that is characterized by a biologic status, a sentient status, and intellectual status, none of which can be separated. The person responds as a unified human. Thus, in assuming responsibility for the nursing process, the professional nurse must be able to approach the client as a unity who thinks, knows, and feels (Curtin, 1979, p. 3). The "being" may be composed of a body, sentience, and intellect, but the "being" cannot be fragmented by viewing any single part. This assumption about "being" serves as the basic element in professional nursing. With the emergence of nursing as a scientific discipline, professional nurses need to examine the interrelationships that exist among the biologic body, sentience, and intelligence in the human. Better understanding of those interrelationships would indeed help professional nurses construct their own answers to the questions: "What is life and how can nurses respond to the life process in a helpful manner?"

What is Right? (Ethics—Moral Philosophy)

The ethical question is the question of *right* and *wrong* and of *duty.* It is the question of morality in humans as they make decisions and carry out their responsibilities. Curtin believes that nursing is a moral art. She states: "The end purpose of nursing is the welfare of other human beings. This end is not a scientific end, but rather a moral end. That is, it involves the seeking of good and it involves our relationship with other human beings" (Curtin, 1979, p. 2). That mutually agreed-on "good" in the nurse-client relationship is health.

Principles of Knowledge, Freedom, and Choice

Action is the keystone of the nursing process. The sharing of the action between the nurse and the client in the nursing process indeed makes nursing a moral art— a matter of ethics. Some philosophers have believed that there are three essentials of every human act: knowledge, freedom, and choice (Glenn, 1947, p. 368). Generally accepted principles are:

1. To the extent that one is knowledgeable, one is responsible for his acts. Curtin states, "A person could be wrong . . . but must act with integrity . . . according to the knowledge he possesses in keeping with his obligations . . . in the search for a satisfactory outcome" (Curtin and Flaherty, 1982, p. 59). In her model for critical ethical analysis, Curtin views knowledge as an important step. Knowledge is critical in the analysis of the background information, the selection of relevant information, and analysis of the abilities of the decision-makers (Curtin and Flaherty, 1982, pp. 60–62).

2. To the extent that one is free, one possesses rights and privileges as well as responsibilities. To some extent, freedom also means that one is exempt from the responsibility for actions over which he has no control. Curtin acknowledges freedom as an essential component of ethical analysis by identifying a stage in which the rights, duties, authority, and capabilities of the decision-makers are established (Curtin and Flaherty, 1982, p. 61). In the nursing process, freedom must be conceptualized by the professional nurse in order to understand and implement the client's rights, the nurse's rights, the responsibilities and abilities of the client, the responsibilities and duties of the nurse, the accountability of each to himself, to the other, and to the health care delivery team, and the establishment of authority for various actions planned, implemented, and evaluated in the relationship.

3. There are times when the client needs and should have full choice in decision-making. There are times when the nurse should have more choices in the decision-making. Most of the time, however, the nurse and the client are able to and should share mutual responsibility for decision-making. Since the nurse possesses expert knowledge, the nurse needs to play a major role in decision-making. However, since the client has control of the self and seeks help from the professional, the client has major responsibility in all decision-making.

Social Norms, Rights and Responsibilities

It is an accepted social norm that the human rights of freedom, respect, and integrity are essential for the fullest development of humans. Society has recently begun to champion these human rights for "all persons—young and old, black, white, red and yellow; healthy and sick" (Curtin, 1979, p. 3). Curtin elaborates that these human rights are derived from real and fundamental human needs. She clearly differentiates between desire (what a person wants) and need. Real needs are the basis of human rights. "If human beings have any natural rights at all, they have the right to be recognized and respected as human beings" (Curtin and

Flaherty, 1982, p. 7). Rights are related to the concept of freedom that Curtin says is not really absolute in all conditions. For example, one person's expression of freedom is not justified if it endangers the fundamental rights of others. "If there is such a thing as human freedom, it must include an option, a choice, to exercise rights or to refrain from exercising them" (Curtin and Flaherty, 1982, p. 9). Humans have the right to choose a certain course of action if they are willing to accept the consequences. Human rights and values are sometimes thought to be the outcomes of collective opinion—or societally determined. For example, a segment of society today believes that health care is a right for all.

Human rights are also sometimes the outcome of laws. Human rights then become legal rights because they are derived from the state and the human is protected by the law. Curtin believes that it is not likely that nurses will blatantly transgress the human rights of clients in terms of dramatic/legal areas. She says, however: "It is in our ordinary, day-to-day contacts with patients or clients that we are most likely to fail to respect them as human beings. We are too busy or too caught up in 'important' technicalities to take time to discover and respect the humanity of each individual" (Curtin and Flaherty, 1982, p. 15).

Various nurses have suggested the ethical responsibilities inherent in the special duties of the professional nurse in meeting health needs of humans. Curtin believes that the professional responsibility of nurses is the application of human advocacy. They must ". . . as human advocates—assist patients to find meaning or purpose in their living or in their dying. . . . Whatever patients define as their goal, it is their meaning and not ours, their values and not ours, and their living or dying and not ours" (Curtin, 1979, p. 7). Carper believes that the primary responsibility of the professional nurse is to actualize the process of caring in the therapeutic relationship (Carper, 1979). She suggests that caring raises four ethical issues:

1. The nature of the health care provider-patient relationship
2. Informed consent
3. Determination of the quality of life
4. Determination of ethical participation in decision-making (Carper, 1979, pp. 15–16)

In dealing with each of these ethical issues, the primary responsibility of the professional nurse in caring for the client is to always respect the human as a unified being. The Bandmans (1979) believe that a significant responsibility for professional nurses is protecting the patient's right to live or die. They say this ". . . needs to be done formally, rationally and openly at the level at which the patient's wishes, the family's wishes, medical considerations of feasibility and prognosis, and universal principles of justice such as fairness are considered" (Bandman and Bandman, 1979, p. 34). Pardue suggests that the primary responsibility for the professional nurse is to assume the major impetus for change. Assuming such control, the nurse "would purposefully plan and work toward specific and identifiable professional goals, as well as work with a larger group of nurses toward realizing goals for the nursing profession" (Pardue, 1980, p. 19). DeMaio (1982, p. 15) says that since self-determination is the right of a profession, professionals today must "develop strategies which will protect nursing's right to self-determination and let nursing practice emerge unimpeded." Despite the differences in definitions of responsibility in nursing, all nursing leaders would probably agree to the structure of the professional nurse's responsibility to self, to clients, and to the profession, always for the purpose of improving the health of people.

Morality

"Morality is the relation of human acts to the norm or rule of what they ought to be" (Glenn, 1947, p. 376). Since nursing decisions always involve choices to be made by the nurse and the client, morality is an important characteristic. To say that the nurse acts morally implies that the nurse acts "according to the rules of right conduct" (Sigman, 1979, p. 41). The decisions to be made are matters of conscience. "Working through a moral problem causes normative questions to arise that reaffirm a norm by which both the 'rightness' and 'wrongness' of an act and the values attached to objects of the act can be judged" (Sigman, 1979, p. 42). Glenn defines the determinant of morality as "the act performed and the circumstances of the act performed" (Glenn, 1947, p. 378). Some acts have intrinsic morality, that is they are intrinsically good or evil. An example is killing, always evil, thus never permissible. If the act itself does not do so, the circumstances of the act define its morality. Examples of circumstances are the person performing the act, the intensity of the act, its place, its time, its manner, and its intention. The profession of nursing establishes standards of acceptable practice, education, and research. In reality, those standards serve to determine the morality of nursing acts themselves and the circumstances involved in the conduct of nursing.

A PHILOSOPHY OF NURSING—THE BELIEF SYSTEM FOR THIS BOOK

Following is a brief statement of a philosophy of nursing. This statement of beliefs about the essential elements of nursing (humans, environment, health, nurse and nursing) provide the basis for the further organization and development of this book.

Humans

This book is based on the premise that nursing's central concern is humans interacting with their environment, holistically striving for balance and a sense of well-being. Humans are integrated organisms reflecting abilities to exist as biologic, thinking, and feeling beings.

Society—Environment

Human society is composed of individual beings, families, and community systems. All elements of humans and the society within which humans live constitute the environment. As systems increase in size and function, increasingly complex interactions occur. Through continuous interaction and energy exchange within the internal environment and between the internal and external environments, the individual, family, and/or community systems develop patterns of behavior to maintain balance.

Health

Successful maintenance or restoration of balance in the interactions between humans and the environment constitute well-being, and are components of health. Lesser states of well-being (which some might call illness) result when balance remains disturbed in any system. In well-being, the human maintains or restores balance, thus freeing energy for systems interactions. When humans are in a lesser state of well-being, energy for interaction with other systems is restricted. There are multiple determinants of the human's state of well-being. Well-being is a subjective perception of balance, harmony, and vitality.

Nurse

The nurse is a professional practitioner who is accountable for nursing care, which promotes, maintains, and/or restores health of individuals, families, and communities in a variety of settings. The nurse is a collaborator in leadership roles within a changing health care delivery system. The nurse is socialized into a professional image by growing self-awareness and development of respect for her own abilities as a professional nurse, appreciation of the need for continued education, and integration of both cognitive and interpersonal elements of a professional self in professional nursing roles.

Nursing

Nursing is a process that includes all judgements and actions that are aimed toward maintenance, promotion, and/or restoration of balance in human systems. The nursing process is implemented through a collaborative nurse-client relationship that involves interpersonal communication between the practitioner and the client, others significant to the client, and/or others in the health care delivery system. Among others, the significant emerging roles for the professional nurse are change agent, advocate, and contributor to the profession. These roles are based on the philosophical assumption that the professional nurse's goal is to facilitate health, that change must occur to promote well-being, and that leadership is a process whereby the nurse and the client mutually effect change. Thus, responsibility in the nursing process is shared between the nurse and the client.

The following chapters describe the conceptual bases that operationalize this philosophy.

REFERENCES

Bandman EL, Bandman B: The nurse's role in protecting the patient's right to live or die. Adv Nur Sci 1:21–35, 1979

Carper BA: The ethics of caring. Adv Nur Sci 1:11–19, 1979

Curtin LL: The nurse as advocate: A philosophical foundation for nursing. Adv Nur Sci 1:1–10, 1979

Curtin LL, Flaherty MJ: Nursing Ethics—Theories and Pragmatics. Bowie, Maryland, Robert J Brady, 1982

DeMaio D: Self-determination—The right of a profession. JNYSNA 13:8–17, 1982

Glenn PJ: An Introduction to Philosophy. St Louis, B Herder, 1947

Kahn H, Wiener AJ: The Year 2000—A Framework for Speculation on the Next Thirty-Three Years. (The Hudson Institute). New York, MacMillan, 1967

Mappas TA, Zembaty JS: Biomedical Ethics. New York, MacMillan, 1981

Pardue SF: Translating professional potential into action. Image XII:17–19, 1980

Rogers ME: An Introduction to the Theoretical Basis of Nursing. Philadelphia, FA Davis, 1970

Rustow DA: Introduction to the issue "Philosophers and kings: studies in leadership." Daedalus 97:683–694, 1968

Schlotfeldt R: A Brave, New Nursing World—Exercising Options for the Future. Washington, DC, Am Assoc Coll Nur, 1982

Sigman P: Ethical choice in nursing. Adv Nur Sci 1:37–52, 1979

Silva MC: Philosophy, science, theory: Interrelationships and implications for nursing research. Image 9:59–63, 1977

Thompson JB, Thompson HO: Ethics in Nursing. New York, MacMillan, 1981

Webster N: Webster's New Collegiate Dictionary, ed 2. Springfield, G&C Merriam, 1949

Chapter 3

Socialization for Professional Practice

THOUGHT QUESTIONS

1. How does initial socialization into nursing differ from resocialization in a work or educational setting?
2. What are the characteristics of professional practice?
3. How does the Code for Nurses affect a nurse's practice?
4. What determines the legal parameters of professional nursing practice?

PROFESSIONAL SOCIALIZATION

Socialization to professional nursing involves a process of learning content and skills and internalizing a self-identity appropriate to specific roles. Most students enter nursing with a service orientation in which they view themselves as doing things that will help sick people recover. In contrast, "the professional educational imagery of the nurse is generally of one who (1) defines clients in terms of health and maintaining health, (2) views the relationship between the nurse and clients therapeutically and analytically, (3) approaches technical mastery of tools and procedures from the viewpoint of knowledge principles that guide their use, (4) uses critical inquiry processes to creatively manipulate knowledge in relation to clients' concerns, and (5) accepts responsibility/accountability for patient care decisions" (Hinshaw, 1976, p. 5). Clearly, the socialization process involves changes in knowledge, attitudes, values, and skills. These changes are associated with conflict and strong emotional reactions.

Initial Socialization into Nursing

Much of the literature on socialization has focused on childhood development of the values and standards of the social group. Socialization has been viewed as an early and terminal process, with the family exerting primary influence through role modeling and reinforcement of desired behavior. However, increasing attention is now being paid to adult socialization as a continuing and reoccurring process with important implications for the development of attitudes toward a professional career.

Brim (1966) identified four major differences between socialization of the child and the adult:

Adult Socialization	*Childhood Socialization*
1. Purpose is to learn new overt role behaviors.	1. Purpose is to learn values and motives of society.
2. Resynthesis of previously learned material.	2. Acquisition of new material.
3. Concerned with realism.	3. Concerned with idealism.
4. Learning how to mediate conflicts between and among different role expectations.	4. Learning basic role expectations.

Knowles popularized the term *andragogy* as the "art and science of helping adults learn in contrast to pedagogy as the art and science of teaching children" (Knowles, 1980, p. 43). See Table 3-1 for a comparison of Knowles' assumptions about pedagogy and andragogy. Knowles assumes that adult learners have a *self-concept* that is moving toward that of a self-directed human; have accumulated *experience* that is a rich resource for learning; have a *readiness to learn* that is oriented toward the developmental tasks of their social roles; and have an *orientation to learning* that is shifted toward immediacy of application in performance (Knowles, 1980, pp. 44–45).

A number of implications for adult education (Knowles, 1980, pp. 45–58; Cooper and Hornback, 1973, pp. 63–79; Merritt, 1983, pp. 367–372) are indicated below:

1. The learning climate should be based on an atmosphere of respect and mutuality between the teacher and learner. The physical environment should be informal and comfortable.
2. The learner should be involved in diagnosis of learning needs, planning of the learning process, and self-evaluation of the effectiveness of learning (rediagnosis of needs). The teacher should be a resource and guide.
3. Feedback and reasonable time limits for achievement should help the learner to overcome fear of failure and the possible perception of not being very smart carried over from childhood learning experiences.
4. Support from peers and teachers can help to overcome possible guilt at leaving the family while studying or lack of confidence in learning capacity.
5. Emphasis should be placed on practical application of information. Content should be relevant to the learner's needs.
6. Participation in learning should be encouraged. Techniques such as discussion, simulation exercises, field experiences, and problem-solving situations should be used.
7. Learners should be grouped on the basis of needs rather than content areas. The timing and sequence of material should be congruent with the developmental tasks of the learners.

TABLE 3–1.   A Comparison of the Assumptions of Pedagogy and Andragogy

Regarding:	Pedagogy	Andragogy
Concept of the learner	The role of the learner is a dependent one. The teacher determines when, how, and what is to be learned, and if it has been learned.	Movement from dependency toward increasing self-directedness occurs at different rates for different people. Teachers encourage and nurture this movement.
Role of learners' experience	Experience is of little worth. Primary educational techniques transmit knowledge.	As people develop, they accumulate a rich reservoir of experience that is meaningful to them. Experiental techniques are more effective than passive methods.
Readiness to learn	People of the same age are ready to learn the same things. Learning should be organized into a standardized curriculum.	People become ready to learn when they have a need. Learning should be sequenced according to the learner's readiness to learn.
Orientation to learning	People are subject-centered. Education is a process of gaining knowledge that will be used later. The curriculum should be organized by courses that follow a logical development of the subject.	People are performance-centered. Education is a process of developing increased competence. Learning should be organized around competency development categories.

(From The Modern Practice of Adult Education, copyright 1980 by Malcolm Knowles. New York: Cambridge, The Adult Education Company. Reprinted with the permission of the publisher.)

8. "Unfreezing" may be needed before the individual is ready to learn. Learning from experience should be encouraged.
9. Learners represent different learning styles, orientation, and readiness to learn. Learning experiences should be individualized as much as possible.
10. Teachers should be sensitive to the heavy demands placed on learners by tasks of daily life and personal expectations. At times, resources (physical, intellectual, social, and economic) may not be sufficient to meet these demands and also address the demands imposed by the learning situation.

Simpson suggested that socialization of an adult into an occupational role involves a sequential process. She hypothesized three distinct phases: "During the first phase, the person shifts his attention from the broad, societally derived goals which led him to choose the profession to the goal of proficiency in specific work tasks. During the second, certain significant others in the work milieu become his main reference group. Third, he internalizes the values of the occupational group and adopts the behaviors it prescribes" (Simpson, 1967, p. 47).

Davis (1966, as quoted by Hinshaw) suggested a six-stage model for the process of educational socialization. In stage one, initial innocence, individuals enter an educational program. Students have an image of what they expect to become and of how they "should" behave. However, educational experiences (theory and clinical) are often directed toward behaviors that are different from the students' expectation. For example, in some schools, early learning experiences focus on communication with relatively healthy clients. Students, who expect to give bed baths to sick patients, may express disappointment and frustration and question the value of the educational experience.

In stage two, incongruencies between initial images and apparent expectations of the educational system are identified, articulated, and shared among students. At this point students may question whether or not they wish to continue in the program. Students who do continue enter stages three and four, where they identify what behaviors they are expected to exhibit by "psyching out" the faculty, and then, through role simulation, begin to practice the behaviors. Over time, these behaviors become a part of the individual. However, there may be a feeling of "playing a game" and not being "true to oneself" that can result in feelings of guilt and confusion.

In stage five, students vacillate between commitment and performance of behaviors reflecting both the new professional image and the old lay image of nursing. It is hoped that increasing identification with professional role models such as the faculty, and increasing ability to use professional language will lead to reinforcement of the professional image. The student then moves toward stage six, and stable internalization of the professionally/educationally approved model. As Hinshaw (1976, pp. 6–7) indicates however, preparation of the student for the work setting is only the initial process in socialization.

Resocialization in the Work Setting

When the new professional enters the work setting, another socialization process occurs. The nurse is faced with the need to operationalize professional values in primarily bureaucratic settings. Kramer (1974) describes a postgraduate resocialization model for the resolution of value and role conflict between the generalized knowledges and skills acquired in the educational program and the specific behaviors required for the work setting.

Stage one is skill and routine mastery. New graduates arrive in the work setting with "principles" and are confronted with the need to function in a specific manner. Initially the new graduate feels inadequate and frustrated, and responds by "throwing" herself into the mastery of specific skills and techniques. Certainly the development of technical expertise is desirable. However, a potential problem at this stage is that the nurse may fixate on technical skills and be unable to refocus on the other important aspects of nursing care.

Stage two is social integration. The nurse's major concern at this stage is getting along with co-workers and being accepted into the group. This probably requires having mastered the skills and being perceived as competent and efficient. The potential problem at this stage is that the nurse may fear that if she begins to apply the knowledge and orientation gained in the educational setting that she will alienate her newly acquired colleagues.

Stage three is expressed as moral outrage. At this stage the incongruencies between the professional/educational imagery of how nurses "ought to" behave and the reality of behavior in the work setting are realized. The new graduate feels frustrated, angry, and inadequately prepared. At stage four, conflict resolution, individuals either capitulate their behaviors or their values or integrate the professional and bureaucratic systems. Those who choose behavioral capitulation change their behavior but keep their values. They usually leave nursing altogether, or choose a work situation outside the organized service settings. A second type of conflict resolution is value capitulation in which the values of the bureaucratic system are accepted and the values gained in the educational program are given up. A third type of resolution is to give up both values and behaviors and simply conform enough to maintain a working position. It is the fourth type of resolution, which Kramer labeled biculturalism, that is suggested to be the healthiest and most successful resolution of conflict (Kramer, 1974, p. 162). The nurse realizes that she is not just a target of influence and pressure from others, but that she has the ability to influence others as well. "In essence, these new graduates are able to identify and utilize the values and behaviors of both the professional and bureaucratic work systems in a politically astute manner (Hinshaw, 1976, p. 8).

The issue of whether or not new graduates from any basic educational program are sufficiently prepared for the work setting has been debated for some time. Educators take the position that students are prepared for beginning practice. Employers charge that new graduates are not competent until after an expensive orientation period that may last as long as a year. Everyone agrees that the "old diploma program" was unmatched in preparing a nurse for realistic work responsibilities in the hospital setting, but there is a growing consensus that baccalaureate degree graduates function at a "more complex level" than do graduates of diploma or associate degree programs after completing a period of orientation to the setting.

What are the criteria by which new graduates are judged to be inadequate for the work setting? Are psychomotor skills valued above cognitive and affective skills? Do students have sufficient educational practice time for competence in psychomotor skills? Does a perception of psychomotor inadequacy on the part of the new graduate interfere with the professional socialization from the educational program? Nursing educators and service administrators must design collaborative strategies to address these issues, or the impasse will continue to have divisive effects on the profession.

Resocialization through Education

An increasing number of students are choosing an "educational mobility" route to nursing education (see Chapter 17, The Contributor to the Profession Role"). This may involve moving from practical nursing into an associate degree program for registered nursing, or it may involve baccalaureate education following initial nursing education at the associate degree or diploma level. At each level resocialization is needed to help the student to synthesize the changed theory base and new role expectations. But the resocialization may not be fully effective, and the student may finish the program with more knowledge, but without changes in behavior reflective of an internalized professional self-image.

Kelman (1961) has identified three processes of social influence: compliance, identification, and internalization. In the process of compliance the individual has not accepted the values or expectations of the influencing person or group, but behaves in an expected way in order to get positive responses. In the process of identification there is selective adoption of certain behaviors that are perceived as acceptable because they are associated with a role relationship that forms a part of the person's self-image. However, this does not necessarily include an acceptance of values. It is only in the process of internalization that the individual accepts the norms and standards of the new role because she believes in them and they have become a part of the individual's own value system. An area that needs further study is the effect of the level of opinion change on the course and extent of later resocialization.

Shane (1980) describes the positive and negative emotional states experienced by registered nurses who return to school for baccalaureate education. She labels these states the "returning to school syndrome." The first phase, the honeymoon, is very positive. The nurse is attuned to the similiarities between her previous education and her present experience, and these similiarities tend to reinforce her original role identity as a nurse. However, typically during the semester of the first nursing theory or practice course, this phase ends.

The next stage, conflict, is characterized by turbulent negative emotions. The nurse feels increasingly inadequate to meet the new professional demands because she can no longer trust her experience and knowledge to provide her with appropriate responses. She is acutely aware that the old rules are no longer valid, but she has not yet understood or accepted the new ones. This stage is often associated with depression and bursts of anger, feelings of helplessness, and academic difficulties.

The beginning of reintegration is characterized by a strong rejection of "the new culture," the baccalaureate program. The most common behavior expressed during this stage is hostility, which in its extreme form may result in the student "dropping out" of the program to return to the familiar "culture." Shane indicates that, "the length of time any individual spends in the hostility phase and the mode of resolution probably depends on the overall resiliency of the individual, the intensity of the emotions and experiences she is feeling, and the interpretation and guidance provided by those significant others (faculty, peers, family) surrounding her" (Shane, 1980, p. 123).

Achievement of the ability to integrate the original work culture with the new culture of school is the positive resolution of the returning-to-school syndrome. The student recognizes her own strength and growth, and recognizes that she will function in a different way when she graduates. Her sense of "what nursing is" is forever altered, but contains elements of both worlds. She has not denied her original values and orientation, but she is now directed toward getting as much as possible from her academic experience.

Unfortunately, there are two maladaptive dead ends in which some individuals become trapped as a resolution to the conflict stage. One is "false acceptance" in which the student pretends to the faculty and herself that she believes in the value, worth, or validity of the baccalaureate program in order to complete the program. In the other, "chronic hostility," the student does not drop out of school, but persists in vigorous fighting to defend her original nursing ego-identity. This student has resisted the opportunity for real growth and positive change.

Some research data are available that document the effectiveness of resocialization in baccalaureate programs for registered nurses. Brian (1980, p. 51), in a study of graduates of six programs found that "the programs seem to have accomplished their goal of improving the professional orientation of their graduates." The programs were associated with a significant ($p = .001$) difference in the graduates attending meetings or workshops, acting as a resource person, acting as a leader or coordinator, reading nursing journals, doing nursing research, being interested in nursing organizations, writing nursing articles, and belonging to nursing organizations.

Leddy (1982) found that a baccalaureate degree program for registered nurses was associated with significant ($p=.01$) change in five personality variables: decreased need for abasement, increased need for change, dominance, sentience, and harm avoidance. The personality changes persisted when subjects were retested 2 to 4 years after completion of the program.

Data are needed about the factors that facilitate the socialization process. Wysocki (1982) found that reinforcement was more important than role models or perceived professional commitment as a causal factor. If so, is reinforcement of technical skills and knowledge a desirable base for professional socialization (Estok, 1977)? The educational mobility issue is discussed in Chapter 17, "The Contributor to the Profession Role."

Registered nurses who return to school for a baccalaureate degree are confronted with the need to learn and internalize new information, new ways of thinking, and new roles. In addition, many have full-time jobs as well as family responsibilities, and some have been away from school for some time. Also, many nurses have to deal with their perception of nursing as a "good job for a woman." "Nursing has provided an occupation for large numbers of women and a career for a few" (Yeaworth, 1978, p. 73). There is a belief that nursing is good preparation for a family, and that a nurse can always reenter the work force. Many nurses equate the importance of marriage and family responsibilities with professional responsibilities. Women in the United States may be educated for occupations or even for careers, but they are still effectively socialized to be wives and mothers" (Yeaworth, 1978, p. 71). Thus, they are affected by the prevalent views of "appropriate" female behavior.

So-called feminine traits include being caring, tender, compassionate, having the presumed intuitive ability to relate to people, to be supportive of others' needs and wants, and thus be especially able to nurture others, being submissive, passive, subjective, and emotional. These are in contrast to so-called masculine traits of being decisive, able to take the initiative, objective, persistent, aggressive, rational, brave and dominant (Heide, 1973). The roles of males and females in health care have also been institutionalized. The cure role (male) of diagnosis and prescription is active, manipulative, and intellectual. The care role (female) of nurturance and compassion is passive (Kjervik and Martinson, 1979, p. 39). "Women who conform place much emphasis on the behaviors of collaboration, team work, and mutual agreement rather than on dominance, their enormous potential power, or change" (Kjervik and Martinson, 1979, p. 40).

There is evidence that the expectations of others contribute to a sharing of attitudes and beliefs, and lead to an occupational identity that is collective as well as individual (Moore, 1969). If socialization in baccalaureate nursing is to be successful, the process must include a reconceptualization of what it means to be a professional. The next section explores this issue.

CRITERIA FOR A PROFESSION

Although nursing has been called a profession for many years, an assessment in relation to criteria for a profession indicates that nursing should more accurately be considered an "emerging profession." A number of criteria to evaluate a profession have been proposed. These criteria for a profession can be categorized into intellectual characteristics, practical components, service to society components, and autonomy.

Intellectual Characteristics

The category of intellectual characteristics really has three different components: a body of knowledge on which professional practice is based, specialized education to transmit the body of knowledge, and use of knowledge in critical and creative thinking.

Body of Knowledge

Professional practice is based on a body of knowledge. This base contributes to judgement and a rationale for modifying actions according to the situation. However, nursing education has often emphasized "tried and true" methods for responding in particular kinds of situations. This approach to education may explain why many nurses seem unwilling or unable to apply knowledge in clinical problem-solving. They seek the "right answer," and do things the way they have always been done. Thus, patients are still discharged without teaching because "the doctor didn't write an order," and pain medication is withheld because "it isn't 4 hours yet."

There are some who question whether nursing has a body of knowledge that is unique to nursing, or whether nursing science is an application of knowledge borrowed from behavioral and physical sciences and medicine. In the past, nursing derived its knowledge base intuitively and experientially and by borrowing from other disciplines. But, in recent years there have been a number of nursing theorists who have developed frameworks that are uniquely relevant for nursing. Some of these models are discussed in Chapter 8, "Models of Nursing."

Specialized Education

Nursing transmits knowledge through specialized education. However, there are five levels of basic education for registered nursing, all of which prepare for one licensing examination, the National Council Licensure Examination for Registered Nursing (NCLEX). Three of the five (diploma, associate degree, and baccalaureate degree) accept high school graduates, while the other two (masters degree and doctoral degree) accept college graduates with a liberal arts major. The competencies expected of new diploma or associate degree graduates are comparable. Some of the competencies expected of new baccalaureate graduates appear similar to competencies expected of graduates of diploma or associate degree programs. However, many of the competencies expected of new baccalaureate graduates are clearly different.

Diploma schools of nursing are controlled by the hospital board of trustees. They range from 2 to 3 years in length, with all or most practical experience provided in the training hospital. Since most diploma schools cannot grant college credit for nursing courses, many are affiliated with a college for liberal arts and/or science credits. Others integrate physical and behavioral science content into their nursing courses. In a few states hospital-based associate degree or baccalaureate degree programs have been developed. In these cases the state charters a hospital to provide the academic degree. The emphasis of education in diploma schools is on the skills needed for hospital care of the acutely ill patient.

Minimal competencies (NLN, 1982, p. 18) expected of new graduates of diploma programs include:

1. Establishes a nursing data base for individuals with well-defined health needs having predictable and unpredictable outcomes.
2. Develops individual nursing care plans through use of the nursing data base incorporating principles of organization and management.
3. Performs independent nursing measures including preventive, habilitative, and rehabilitative measures according to the needs demonstrated by individuals and families.
4. Initiates efforts to improve nursing practice by evaluating the effectiveness of nursing care and taking the appropriate action(s).

Most *associate degree* programs are located within a community college, although some are based within a senior college or university. They are usually 2 academic years in length, and the student earns around 60 college credits, approximately half in nursing and half in liberal arts and science. The student has practical experiences in a number of institutions (acute and long term) with emphasis on the care of individuals with predictable health restoration needs.

Minimal competencies (NLN, 1982, p. 18) expected of associate degree program graduates include:

1. Establishes a nursing data base for individuals with common well-defined health needs having predictable outcomes.
2. Develops individual nursing care plans through use of the nursing data base in consultation with other nursing personnel.
3. Performs nursing care by implementing nursing care plans according to a priority of needs and established nursing protocols.
4. Participates in the evaluation and redirection of the total nursing care plan, using established criteria.

Baccalaureate degree programs are 4 or 5 academic years in length (120–140 credits). Approximately one half to two thirds of the curriculum is liberal arts and science and supporting courses, with the remainder alloted to nursing. The graduate is prepared to care for individuals, families, and groups in a variety of institutional and community settings, to prevent illness and maintain health as well as restore health.

Minimal competencies (NLN, 1982, p. 18) expected of graduates of baccalaureate degree programs include:

1. Synthesizes nursing data base to determine health needs and potential health status for individuals and social groups.
2. Develops individual nursing care plans through use of the data base in structured and unstructured settings for both well and ill individuals and social groups in collaboration with members of the health team.
3. Implements nursing care in accord with the current health status and future health potential of individuals or social groups based on nursing theory and research.
4. Evaluates effectiveness of nursing care plans and nursing intervention and revises or considers alternative approaches if indicated.

Power, authority, and professional status are usually associated with a postgraduate educational base, yet in 1980, less than 30% of actively practicing nurses had baccalaureate or higher education.*

How can nursing be considered truly professional while a high school diploma gains entry into three different kinds of educational programs, with the majority of graduates possessing an associate degree or less? Yet, a comparison of expectations of graduates shows many similiarities. Much controversy has focused on presumed quality of the various kinds of education patterns rather than on their differences of purpose. Nurses must refute the persistent assumption that "a nurse is a nurse . . ." and move toward an unambiguous acceptance of the nature of professional practice as differentiated from supporting practice in nursing roles. Education for entry into nursing practice is discussed in greater depth in Chapter 17, "The Contributor to the Profession Role."

Critical and Creative Thinking

A logical and critical thinking process is the essence of professional practice. The "nursing process" is really the problem-solving approach, a system to collect and organize information, decide what is needed, select and implement one approach from among many possible approaches, and evaluate the results of the process. Most nurses solve problems each working day. The main weaknesses, however, seem to be "jumping in" to act on the basis of inadequate information, and insufficient brain storming for alternative approaches.

For example, PROBLEM: what would you (the nurse) do with a hospital patient who keeps his television on after "lights out?" POSSIBLE ACTION ONE: Tell him that he must adhere to hospital policy and turn off the television. POSSIBLE ACTION TWO: Allow him to watch as long as no one else is inconvenienced.

DISCUSSION: Both actions have been taken before enough information has been collected to know *why* the patient keeps on the television. If it turns out that he is anxious, nursing intervention should be directed toward relieving his anxiety, or at least helping him to relax and sleep despite it, instead of on the symptom (the television). If he is not tired because his sleep-wake pattern is different than hospital policy, the television might be allowed, with an effort to let the patient sleep later in the morning. The point is that the appropriate action depends on the reason for the problem (see Chapter 5, "Scientific Thought and Theory Development," for a more detailed discussion).

Practical Components

There is no question that nursing involves "specialized skills essential to the performance of a unique, professional role" (ANA Standards for Nursing Education, 1975, p. 3), although the skills that comprise nursing practice have changed over the years. Some of the skills required for present day professional responsibilities include coordination of care given by a variety of allied health workers; critical thinking and judgement in ambulatory as well as acute care settings; communication and collaboration with clients, their families, and members of the health care delivery team; advocacy and leadership to bring about needed changes in the

---

*In 1980, of practicing nurses, 51% were diploma prepared, 29% baccalaureate or higher degree prepared, and 20% associate degree prepared. The projection for 1990 is that 36% of practicing nurses will have a diploma, 28% an associate degree, and 36% a baccalaureate or higher degree (Institute of Medicine Study, p. 77).

health care delivery system; expanded assessment skills to establish baseline data for the nursing process; and competence in diagnostic and therapeutic nursing techniques.

Service to Society

Since the days of Florence Nightingale, nursing has been associated with service to others. Many students still enter nursing "to help people," an image of the nurse that is shared by the public. This altruistic image is an untapped resource that nursing could translate into legislative power to increase legal autonomy and provide for third-party reimbursement for nursing services (see Chapter 17, "Contributor to the Profession Role").

Professional service to society requires integrity and responsibility for ethical practice and a lifelong commitment. Nursing has been viewed by many of its practitioners as a job rather than a career. The 1980 American Nurses Association (ANA) statistics indicate that 75% of registered nurses are actively employed in nursing (Johnson and Vaughn, 1982, p. 499). Many nurses "drop out" to raise a family, or work primarily to supplement family income. Under these circumstances, the tendency is to seek job security and avoid "rocking the boat." This attitude is easily exploited by the employing agency. Regardless of a high patient to nurse ratio, rotating shifts, reassignment to "cover" other units (floating), and constant change in patient assignments, some nurses will make do and maintain the status quo. For those nurses the service orientation has shifted from the welfare of patients to the welfare of the employing institution.

Service to people involves ethical responsibility. In other words, the nurse must have the integrity to do what is right, often in situations that cause real moral dilemmas. Codes for nurses have been developed by the International Council of Nurses and the ANA. Intrinsic to these statements is the belief that the recipient of nursing care has basic rights and that the nurses' primary responsibility is to the client. The ANA code is discussed later in this chapter.

Autonomy

Autonomy means that practitioners have control over their own functions in the work setting. Autonomy involves independence, a willingness to take risks, and responsibility and accountability for one's own actions, as well as self-determination and self-regulation.

Most nurses work in institutional settings where authority is vested in administrative positions in a hierarchical organization. This is in contrast to medicine, which has maintained political power and professional credibility through technical competence and specialized knowledge. Nurses seek status through increased rank in the hierarchy rather than through expert practice.

Nursing lacks a collective professional identity. United action by over one million practitioners is enormous potential power. However, nursing has been fragmented by internal dissention and rivalry. Instead of presenting a united front, each subgroup maintains its own turf. The result is political impotence and professional powerlessness.

This section has focused on the composite character of the profession. The next section examines characteristics of the individual as a member of the nursing profession, what Styles (1982, p. 8) calls "professionhood."

CHARACTERISTICS OF PROFESSIONAL PRACTICE _____

For some nurses work is a job that provides financial return and some degree of satisfaction. Professional practice, on the other hand, requires a "deep and abiding awareness of purpose and direction in place of a specific set of objectives or standards" (Styles, 1982, p. 57). For a professional, work is a component of a career plan and an integral part of the person's being.

Styles has explored the idea that involvement, commitment, and motivation are separate components of the individual's sense of vocation. *Involvement* is viewed as a quantitative measure. For example, how much time or energy does the individual devote to nursing? *Motivation* is the driving force, the "what's in it for me." Motives might be for prestige, financial gain, or to "keep busy," or they might include the opportunity for self-expression and the achievement of excellence. *Commitment* is seen as the "intimacy of the perceptions about nursing to the very core of the self" (Styles, 1982, p. 107). It is unlikely that a professional self-identity could be achieved without sizable involvement and a sense that nursing is a major component of the person's life.

Styles suggests that it is time to "reinstate the service ideal in its proper primary relationship to our science and practice, on the one hand, and to our legitimate claims to self determination and reward, on the other" (Styles, 1982, p. 60). Components of the service ideal include a sense of purpose, a sense of capability, and a concern for others demonstrated as *caring.* According to Griffin (1980, p. 265), caring is the "moral emotion of respecting the dignity and autonomy of another human being." It is expressive, and consists of nurturing, helping, comforting, and guiding (Bates, 1970, p. 129). This concern for others is basic to a service ideal. It is not sufficient in itself to form a professional purpose, yet it is questionable if a person could be a professional nurse without possessing a genuine warmth and caring about others.

The concept of a professional includes legal and moral *accountability* for the individual's own actions. Accountability means that the person is answerable for his own behavior. This concept is closely aligned with *responsibility,* which is the expectation that something that has been assigned will (or will not) be done (Fiesta, 1983, p. 24). This sense of self-imposed responsibility is critical to the exercise of professional autonomy. *Autonomy* means that the individual has the freedom and the authority to act independently. For example, an autonomous nurse would make a judgement about a client's possible health problem, and would work with the client to resolve the problem through use of the nursing process. Autonomy means "identity (form, not shadow), independence (ability to stand alone), and authority (theory and rationale for practice acknowledged by others" (Fiesta, 1983, p. 1).

"Autonomy operationally is power" (Fiesta, 1983, p. 1). Power is defined as "one person's degree of influence over others, to the extent that obedience or conformity are assumed to follow" (Shiflett and Mc Farland, 1978, p. 19). Collectively however, nurses have been characterized by feelings of inadequacy, powerlessness, frustration, and pessimism. Competition for status has interfered with a spirit of *collegiality* and shared respect. As a result, nursing is largely a labor force, rather than a significant influence on the health care delivery system.

Collaboration with members of the health professions, especially physicians, has been promoted as an appropriate approach to teamwork. True collaboration involves the potential for equal input, equal leadership, and equal value between the parties (Fiesta, 1983, p. 23). However, the typical medical curriculum has provided the physician with little experience or knowledge of the potential contributions of colleagues in other disciplines. Most nurses have much less education than do physicians, and thus are usually not viewed as their equal colleagues. Under such circumstances, "coordination, cooperation or collaboration, however desirable, do not provide lasting solutions in power struggles" (Shiflett and Mc Farland, 1978, p. 22). By emphasizing "cooperation" and "collaboration," nurses have used their potential power to "maintain the very system which has oppressed . . . rather than change the system" (Ashley, 1973, p. 638).

Nurses are not ready *risk takers.* Seeking to cooperate with other health professionals may represent less risk than autonomous practice, but professionals need the ability to manage ambiguity and diversity in order to make sound judgements and decisions in practice. They also need knowledge and skills to use the political process for power. The lack of willingness to take risks (based on sound knowledge) and use political power are the greatest barriers to autonomous and assertive nursing practice.

MORAL DIMENSIONS OF PROFESSIONAL PRACTICE

Ethical Systems

Ethics is the philosophical study of morality. Where morals are "oughts and shoulds of society, ethics are the principles behind the shoulds, the whys of moral code or statement" (Thompson and Thompson, 1981, p. 1). Ethics are standards for determining right or wrong, and for making judgements about what should be done to or for other humans. Since there is no arbitrary standard of right and wrong, the study of ethics helps each individual nurse to identify her own moral positions and biases (Thompson and Thompson, 1981, p. 3), in preparation for decision-making in ethical dilemmas.

Since there often is no clear-cut single answer for a given moral dilemma, and since people may disagree on the "best" decision, many moral decisions require an agonizing personal choice between imperfect alternatives. "The basic categories of moral life are conflict, choice and conscience. Conflict and choice constitute the two interdependent factors of the moral process in its developed stage. Neither factor can function properly without the other, the moral process itself being precisely the product of the two" (Romanell, 1977, p. 852).

Standards for Ethics

It is important to remember that the "basic moral concern (of nursing) is with the welfare of other humans" (Curtin, 1978, pp. 4–5). There is a "need for practitioners to view care as the primary objective of service and the consumer of care as the ultimate source of legitimate authority" (Fenner, 1980, p. 47). This principle may be helpful in considering controversial moral decisions that arise in relation to institutional policies and physician orders about medical care. It is the basis for the Code for Nurses, first developed by the ANA in 1950, and periodically revised since. This code "serves to inform both the nurse and society of the profession's expectations and requirements in ethical matters" (ANA, 1976, p. 1).

Code for Nurses

The ANA Code for Nurses (1976) is as follows:

1. The nurse provides services with respect for human dignity and the uniqueness of the client unrestricted by considerations of social or economic status, personal attributes, or the nature of the health problems.
2. The nurse safeguards the client's right to privacy by judiciously protecting information of a confidential nature.
3. The nurse acts to safeguard the client and the public when health care and safety are affected by the incompetent, unethical, or illegal practice of any person.
4. The nurse assumes responsibility and accountability for individual nursing judgements and actions.
5. The nurse maintains competence in nursing.
6. The nurse exercises informed judgement and uses individual competence and qualifications as criteria in seeking consultation, accepting responsibilities, and delegating nursing activities to others.
7. The nurse participates in activities that contribute to the ongoing development of the profession's body of knowledge.
8. The nurse participates in the profession's efforts to implement and improve standards of nursing.
9. The nurse participates in the profession's efforts to establish and maintain conditions of employment conducive to high quality nursing care.
10. The nurse participates in the profession's effort to protect the public from misinformation and misrepresentation and to maintain the integrity of nursing.
11. The nurse collaborates with members of the health professions and other citizens in promoting community and national efforts to meet the health needs of the public (ANA, 1976, pp. 1–20).

The Interpretive Statements distributed with the Code emphasize eight major ethical themes:
The *client's right* to:

1. Be fully involved in the planning and implementation of his own health care.
2. Nursing care based on need, irrespective of social and economic status, personal attributes, or the nature of the health problem.
3. Privacy and confidentiality of information.
4. Protection from unsafe or unethical health care practice.

The *nurses' responsibility* to:

5. Assume accountability and responsibility for giving safe and competent care, delegating activities to others, and maintaining the integrity of nursing.
6. Participate in research while protecting the rights of human subjects.

7. Establish and maintain employment conditions that are conducive to high quality nursing care.
8. Promote collaborative planning for availability and accessibility to quality health services for all citizens.

Reexamination of Ethical Standards

The Code and the Interpretive Statements "together provide a framework for the nurse to make ethical decisions and discharge responsibilities to the public, to other members of the health team, and to the profession" (ANA, 1976, p. 1). An ethical code defines a professional standard, but it does not provide specific guidelines for how the nurse should act in a given situation nor is it legally binding. Individual decisions, if moral, are based on ethical principles and can only be enforced by the individual's conscience.

Ethical Principles

Autonomy of the individual is one of the basic ethical principles. An autonomous person is capable of making rational and unconstrained decisions and acting on those decisions. Belief in autonomy means that the nurse respects the client and the choices that he may make as a rational person.

An individual is considered to be rational when he is capable of choosing the best means to some chosen end (Mappes and Zembaty, 1981, p. 8). A person's rationality may be diminished by a number of factors, including fear, laziness, lack of intelligence, pain, drugs that affect reasoning ability, and disease. However, regardless of rationality, some people believe that there are a few situations that justify constraints on autonomy. Some of the most widely accepted situations include preventing harm to others (private harm principle), preventing offense to others (offense principle), and preventing impairment of institutional practices that are in the public interest (public harm principle). Some situations in which the moral legitimacy is a matter of dispute include preventing self-harm (principles of paternalism), benefit for the person who is being constrained (principle of extreme paternalism), and to benefit others (social welfare principle) (Mappas and Zembaty, 1981, p. 11). Interference with an individual's autonomy, whatever the reason, is called *paternalism.*

A person can be constrained from acting autonomously through lack of knowledge just as well as by coercive force. Thus, the nurse is obligated to share all relevant information and alternatives for action with the client so that informed choices can be made. The nurse is also obligated to respect the decisions made by the client even if the nurse does not happen to agree with the decision. This may mean that the nurse may be forced to choose between doing what she believes is in the patient's best interest and respecting the patient's decision to do otherwise.

Another ethical principle is that of *beneficence.* This principle is related to the nurses' duty to help clients further their legitimate interests within the boundaries of safety. This principle is closely related to the principle of *justice,* which specifies that all patients be provided with high-quality nursing care irrespective of social conditions, economic status, personal attributes, or the nature of health problems (Fry, 1982, p. 365).

The preceding principles are based on the assumption that all persons have certain ethical rights. Smith has described three types of ethical rights:

1. A conventional ethical right is a claim derived from customs, traditions, and expectations. An example is the right of the client to confidentiality of information.
2. An ideal ethical right is a claim of what ought to be, but it may not actually exist. An example is the right of all citizens to equal access to excellent health care.
3. A conscientious ethical right is a claim based on principles of conscience. Such claims may not be recognized as valid by others. An example is terminating life supports on a person who is "brain dead" (Smith and Davis, 1980, p. 1465).

Individual rights are associated with a number of concerns. For example, what kinds of entities have rights and what kinds do not (*e.g.,* does the fetus have rights)? When there is a conflict of rights, how should the conflict be resolved? Obligations to clients may seem to conflict with obligations to the physician or to the institution. This is not really a moral dilemma, although the decision may be an agonizing one. There is an important distinction between doing what is morally right and what is least difficult practically. As a professional, the primary ethical obligation of the nurse is to her client. However, she may have legal obligations to both the client and the institution. These legal obligations are discussed in the next section.

LEGAL DIMENSIONS OF PROFESSIONAL PRACTICE

Licensure

The United States government defines licensure as "the process by which an agency of government grants permission to persons to engage in a given profession or occupation by certifying that those licensed have attained the minimal degree of competency necessary to ensure that the public health, safety, and welfare will be reasonably well protected" (USDHEW, 1971, p. 7). Thus, a license is a legal document that certifies that minimal standards for qualified practitioners have been met.

Requirements for licensure as a registered nurse are included in each states' nurse practice act. Each act "contains a definition of professional nursing; outlines requirements for licensure and provides for endorsement for persons licensed in other states; specifies exemptions from licensure; lists grounds for revocation of licensure; provides for a board of examiners and outlines its responsibilities; and sets penalties for practicing without a license" (Kelly, 1974, p. 1314).

The state board of examiners may also be called the "state board" or the "nursing board." This board sets up requirements for and grants state approval to nursing schools, conducts examinations, issues and renews licenses and certificates of registration, and prosecutes violators and revokes licenses and certificates (Creighton, 1981, p. 20). All states use the National Council Licensure Examination (NCLEX) for licensure purposes. To be eligible a student must be a graduate of a state approved school of nursing. The examination is given on the same day, at the same time, in numerous sites throughout the country. Thus, "passing" the examination not only permits licensure and registration in the state in which the examination is written, but also permits later registration (listing on the official roster) in other states if desired. While licensure is permanent (unless the license is revoked for illegal or immoral behavior), registration must be renewed periodically (usually every 1 to 2 years) by payment of a fee to each state in which current registration is desired. All that is needed is to fill out forms and pay the required fee to become licensed "by endorsement."

The 50 states have mandatory licensure. This means that anyone who practices nursing according to the definition of practice in the law must be licensed, except for students in their course of study, employees of the federal government, and when performing in an emergency situation.

In 1983, 11 states required continuing education as a precondition for registered nurse license renewal. In another five states, continuing education was mandatory for nurse practitioners only. The number of contact hours required for reregistration of registered nurses ranged from a low of 5 every year to a high of 30 every 2 years (CE, 1982, p. 1668). Mandatory continuing education has proved expensive to monitor, and the momentum toward its enactment has slowed considerably.

Most states have revised their nurse practice act several times since the first acts were written in the early 20th century. In 1982, the National Council of State Boards wrote a model nursing practice act that will probably be the basis for the next set of revisions. For example, in 1983, Wyoming revised its nurse practice act using the model act as a guide. The Wyoming Nursing Practice Act defines the practice of nursing as "assisting individuals or groups to maintain or attain optimal health throughout the life process by assessing their health status, establishing a nursing diagnosis, planning and implementing nursing care to accomplish defined goals, and evaluating responses to care and treatment."

Legal Responsibility

Licensure as a registered nurse carries with it the responsibility for safe and competent practice. If injury, unnecessary suffering, or death should occur as a result of care given by a nurse, she may be held legally responsible. *Negligence* is defined as "the omission to do something that a reasonable person, guided by those ordinary considerations that ordinarily regulate human affairs, would do, or as doing something that a reasonable and prudent person would not do" (Creighton, 1981, p. 154). *Malpractice,* on the other hand, has been defined as "any professional misconduct, unreasonable lack of skill or fidelity in professional or judiciary duties, evil practice, or illegal or immoral conduct" (Creighton, 1981, p. 154).

Some of the most common acts of negligence by nurses involve burns; falls; wrong dosage, concentration, or kind of medication; mistaken identity; administration of blood; failure to communicate effectively with the client, the client's family or health team members; failure to observe and take appropriate action; defects in equipment; and failure in reasonable judgement.

The nurse is legally responsible for her own actions. However, since in most cases the nurse is also an employee of an institution, the question may arise as to whether the institution and the patient's physician are also legally responsible. This is due to the legal "respondeat superior" (master-servant) rule that states that the master is responsible for the acts of his servants. Whomever is the nurses' employer is also held responsible for the acts of the nurse.

A person becomes an employee "when he performs services for another who has the 'right to control' what is done and how it is to be done. An employee is one who works for wages or salary in the service of an employer" (Creighton,

1981, p. 75). The registered nurse who is also a student is usually considered an employee. She must "act as a reasonable prudent person under the circumstances. The amount of experience and education, her record, and her grades are some of the matters considered. Responsibility increases as a nurse progresses in professional knowledge and experience" (Creighton, 1981, pp. 74–75).

Ethical and legal considerations may at times overlap. The Tuma case, which was reported in the literature in the early 1980s, is an example. Ms. Tuma was a registered nurse employed as an instructor in an associate degree nursing program. A student was assigned to care for a woman who had been told the day before by her physician that she was dying of leukemia and that the only hope for prolonging life was chemotherapy. The patient had consented, and Ms. Tuma and the student were to begin the treatment.

The patient was very upset, as she had lived with her disease for 12 years with the help of prayer and natural foods. While the treatment was being started, Ms. Tuma discussed alternative treatments with the patient who asked her to return that evening to continue the discussion with her children. Ms. Tuma did return, but did not discuss her intervention with the physician and asked the student to "forget" that she had heard the discussion. The patient's children told the physician, who complained that the nurse had interfered with the patient-physician relationship. As a result of the complaint, Ms. Tuma was suspended from her job and had her license to practice suspended for 6 months. Ms. Tuma appealed her case up to the state supreme court, which upheld her appeal on the grounds that the state's practice act did not define unprofessional conduct.

Concern was raised by this case because it seemed to indicate that the nurse did not have a legal right to give information about medical treatment to a patient even though the patient had requested that information; but that was not the issue in this case. Ms. Tuma not only gave the requested information, but she deliberately withheld information from the physician. She was aware that the consent that the physician had received was not informed consent, but she did not alert the physician to the patient's concerns nor did she refuse to start the treatment. The nurse must know and function within the legal parameters of practice in her state. If she has moral or legal concerns about medical treatment she must share her concerns and their rationale with the physician and, if necessary, with nursing, medical, and/or hospital authorities. She may refuse to carry out the treatment. But she must not attempt to circumvent the physician by interfering with treatment without his knowledge. The goal should be collaboration, not competition.

SUMMARY

The process of "becoming" a professional nurse involves change and growth at various stages throughout an individual's career. Through educational and occupational experiences, the nurse is socialized and resocialized to the attitudes, beliefs, knowledges, and skills which, when integrated with moral and legal standards, characterize competent and committed professional service.

REFERENCES

American Nurses Association Commission on Nursing Education: Standards for Nursing Education. Kansas City, American Nurses' Association, 1975

American Nurses Association: Code for nurses with interpretive statements. American Nurses Association Pub No G-56, 1976

Ashley J: This I believe about power in nursing. Nurs Outlook 21:637–641, October 1973

Bates B: Doctor and nurse: Changing roles and relations. New Engl J Med 283:129–134, July 16, 1970

Brian S: The bottom line: Graduates and careers. In Jako K (ed): Proceedings of Researching Second Step Nursing Education, pp 45–54. Rohnert Park, Sonoma State University, March 1980

Brim OG Jr: Socialization through the life cycle. In Brim OG Jr, Wheeler S (eds): Socialization After Childhood: Two Essays, pp 24–33. New York, John Wiley & Sons, 1966

CE Now Required for Relicensure in Sixteen States. Am J Nurs 82:1668, November 1982

Cooper SS, Hornback MS: Continuing Nursing Education. New York, McGraw-Hill, 1973

Creighton H: Law Every Nurse Should Know. Philadelphia, WB Saunders, 1981

Curtin LL: Nursing ethics: Theories and pragmatics. Nurs Forum 17:4–11, 1978

Estok P: Socialization theory and entry into the practice of nursing. Image 9:8–14, 1977

Fenner KM: Ethics and Law in Nursing: Professional Perspectives. New York, Nostrand, 1980

Fiesta J: The Law and Liability: A Guide for Nurses. New York, John Wiley & Sons, 1983

Fry ST: Ethical principles in nursing education and practice. Nurs Health Care: 363–368, September 1982

Griffin AP: Philosophy and nursing. J Adv Nurs 5:261–272, 1980

Heide WS: Nursing and women's liberation: A parallel. Am J Nurs 73:824–827, May 1973

Hinshaw AS: Socialization and resocialization of nurses for professional nursing practice, pp 1–15. National League for Nursing Pub No 15-1659. November 1976

Institute of Medicine: Nursing and Nursing Education: Public Policies and Private Actions. Washington DC, National Academy Press, 1983

Johnson WL, Vaughn JC: Supply and demand relations and the shortage of nurses. Nurs Health Care: 497–507, November 1982

Kelly LY: Nursing practice acts. Am J Nurs 74:1310–1319, July 1974

Kelman H: Processes of opinion changes. Pub Opin Quar 25:57–78, 1961

Kjervik DK, Martinson IM: Women in Stress: A Nursing Perspective. New York, Appleton-Century-Crofts, 1979

Knowles MS: The Modern Practice of Adult Education: From Pedagogy to Andragogy. Chicago, Association Press, 1980

Kramer M: Reality Shock: Why Nurses Leave Nursing, pp 154–164. St Louis, CV Mosby, 1974

Leddy S: Personality changes associated with baccalaureate education for registered nurses (Abstr). J Nurs Ed 21:45–46, October 1982

Mappas TA, Zembaty JS: Biomedical Ethics. New York, Macmillan, 1981

Merritt S: Learning style preferences of baccalaureate nursing students. Nurs Res 32:367–372, November–December 1983

Moore WE: Occupational socialization. In Goslin DA: Handbook of Socialization Theory and Research, pp 861–883. Chicago, Rand McNally 1969

National League for Nursing: Competencies of Graduates of Nursing Programs, p 18. National League for Nursing Pub No 14–1905, 1982

Romanell, P: Ethics, moral conflicts, and choice. Am J Nurs 77:850–855, May 1977

Shane DL: The returning-to-school syndrome. In Mirin S (ed): Teaching Tomorrow's Nurse, pp 119–126. Wakefield, Nursing Resources, 1980

Shiflett N, McFarland DE: Power and the nursing administrator. J Nurs Adm 8:19–23, March 1978

Simpson IH: Patterns of socialization into professions: The case of student nurses. Socio Inquiry 37:47–54, Winter 1967

Smith S, Davis A: Ethical dilemmas. Am J Nurs:1463–1466, August 1980

Styles MM: On Nursing: Toward a New Endowment. St Louis, CV Mosby, 1982

Thompson JB, Thompson HO: Ethics in Nursing. New York, Macmillan, 1981

USDHEW: Report on Licensure and Related Health Personnel Credentialing, p 7. DHEW Pub No (HSM) 72-11, Washington DC, US Government Printing Office, 1971

Wysocki AB: Role modeling in the socialization process of baccalaureate nursing students (Abstr). J Nurs Ed 21:62–63, October 1982

Yeaworth RC: Feminism and the nursing profession. In Chaska NL (ed): Views Through the Mist, pp 71–77. New York, McGraw-Hill 1978

Chapter 4

Development of Professional Self-Concept

THOUGHT QUESTIONS

1. What are three assumptions used to justify the evolutionary nature of the development of the personal or professional self?

2. What is the significance of reflected appraisals to the development of the professional self-concept?

3. Explain the influence of society's image of the profession on the individual nurse's professional self-concept.

4. What are the goals associated with each stage in the development of the professional self?

5. If the nurse does not view self as an autonomous professional being, what are some of the outcomes in the professional self-concept?

6. What is the relatedness between the personal self-concept, the professional self-concept, and the quality of the nursing process?

Nursing's primary concern is with man (Rogers, 1970, p. 41). Man is used here and throughout the book in a nonsexist way. Man is used to mean humans. Humans experience the process of life along with other living systems. Man, however, shows the greatest complexity in the sequential development of behavior, and possesses one attribute believed to be missing in other living systems: the capacity for conscious awareness of self and the world. This consciousness provides the basis for man's rationality, creativity, and humanness. "People are thinking, feeling beings." (Rogers, 1970, p. 41). This awareness of self is the basis for the self-concept.

As the human develops patterns of behavior, the self-system becomes organized and strives to maintain itself, although it is continually undergoing change, being repatterned, and affecting the environment in a significant way. These interactional experiences with the environment provide the substance from which a view of the self emerges—the self-concept. The nurse, as a person, is continually interacting with the personal environment; as a professional, she is continually interacting with the professional environment. Since the human develops the personal self first, that personally organized set of behaviors forms the basis of the self brought into the profession. Thus, that personal self is highly influential on the emerging professional self.

Several assumptions can be made about the development of human self-systems.

1. The human is an open system, constantly affecting and being affected by other humans and nonhumans in his world (his environment).
2. "Man interacts with his environment in his totality" (Rogers, 1970, p. 44).
3. As open systems, humans demonstrate continuous interaction with their surroundings. Energy and materials are constantly being interchanged. The human system both shares with and takes in energy and materials in the environment (Rogers, 1970, p. 49).
4. "Man-environment transactions are characterized by continuous repatterning of both man and environment" (Rogers, 1970, p. 53).
5. "It is in the mutual changing and being changed that evolution proceeds" (Rogers, 1970, p. 54).
6. The evolutionary process is descriptive of or analogous with the development of the self-system, both personal and professional.

THEORETICAL BASES OF SELF-CONCEPT: INTERACTION

Known as the father of the interpersonal school of thought in psychiatry, Sullivan attributed great power to the interactional process between the developing person and the "mothering one." He theorized that the self-system—"the system involved in the maintenance of felt interpersonal security" (Sullivan, 1953, p. 109) emerges from the interpersonal cooperation in acculturation and the socialization process for the human. "The self system . . . is an organization of educative experience called into being by the necessity to avoid or to minimize incidents of anxiety" (Sullivan, 1953, p. 165). In humans anxiety is viewed as "anticipated unfavorable appraisal of one's current activity by someone whose opinion is significant" (Sullivan, 1953, p. 113). The self-concept can be seen as the personal view of oneself developed as the result of interaction with significant others.

Using Sullivan's view of development, Lancaster and Lancaster state that the self is formulated through conscious and unconscious perceptions of one's experiences, including achievements, failures, conflicts, embarrassments, and accomplishments. The self is constantly reinforced by feedback received from significant persons in one's environment (Lancaster and Lancaster, 1982, pp. 72–77). When the message received is a positive appraisal, the part of the self reinforced is the "good me"; when the message received is a negative appraisal, the part of the self reinforced is the "bad me"; and when the message received is associated with over-whelming anxiety, the part of the self reinforced is the "not me" (Sullivan, 1953, pp. 161–164).

The Significance of Reflected Appraisals

As noted above, the view of the personal self is directly related to the appraisals that occur in the personal relationship with the significant other person(s). As humans develop over the life span, the significant other person(s) changes. In infancy, the parent most directly involved in caretaking is the significant other; that later changes to both parents in early childhood, to other adults next; then to peers of the same sex; then to peers of the opposite sex; and finally to the partners of the mature adult. In all stages of life, the relationship between the person and that person's significant other is central to acculturation and socialization since learning is dependent on the view of self and the existing level of anxiety. An inverse relationship exists between awareness of self and the level of anxiety experienced in the person-significant other relationship. Perceived anxiety in either high dosage or continuous patterns leads to a perception of the self as "bad." Persons with bad views of self have internalized that view of self through patterns of relatedness established with their significant others in circumstances of high anxiety. Positive appraisals result in the perception of self as "good." Persons with good views of self have learned that view of self through patterns of relatedness established with their significant others in circumstances of low anxiety. Sheehy states that people pleased with life (with a good view of self) use the following qualities to describe self: honest, loving, and responsible. She calls these successful navigators of life, pathfinders. They possess high levels of well-being (Sheehy, 1982).

The development of the professional self follows the same path that the development of the personal self takes. In every profession, the professional has significant others. Nurses have had varying significant others during their various stages of growth and development. Those significant others have differed in sex, socioeconomic conditions, education, and cultural background. Those others that are significant in terms of professional self-development are somewhat determined by the nurse's adjustments to changing situations. The professional nurse moves in and out of new situations. Adjusting to the perceived expectations of the significant other in each situation, the nurse tries to be the kind of person the situation demands. Highly related to how successful the nurse is in moving in and out of changing situations is the nurse's personal self-view as well as her sensitivity to the professional significant other. The personal self-concept cannot be separated from the professional self-concept, although the significant others for the professional person are different from the personal significant others.

Sheehy identified two types of significant others who perhaps play very influential roles in the development of the professional self: the mentor and the polestar. The mentor "is a trusted friend and counselor, usually from 10-20 years older, who endorses the apprentice's dream and helps in a critical way to guide him or her toward realizing it" (Sheehy, 1982, p. 231). The polestar is a figure who exerts a forward pull, offers guiding principles, and is a conspicuous guide having a major impact on the road a child takes (Sheehy, 1982, p. 230). Given this framework, the polestars for the professional nurse would be those people who introduced the nurse to the discipline in infancy, childhood, and adolescence as a professional. The mentors would be those selected significant others who were professionally older and wiser and trustworthy in the nurse's adulthood in nursing.

Societal Values of "Nursing" and "Nurses"

The nurse's view of self as a professional is greatly influenced by the image of nursing and nurses as portrayed by the public, the profession-at-large, and the nurse's own polestars and mentors. Nurses, like members of every professional discipline, have established role identifications. "A role consists of performed behaviors or behaviors peceived as acceptable, relative to a given situation" (Brooks and Kleine-Kracht, 1983, p. 51). What particular role a nurse plays is arrived at by mutual validation between the nurse and consumers of nursing care. It has been noted that the public tends to view nurses in terms of personal qualities, not role skills (Brooks and Kleine-Kracht, 1983, and Kalisch and Kalisch, 1983). The recent view of nurses as sex objects attests to the public's attitude about nurses and nursing. It validates that people are more reactive to the personal qualities of the nurse than the professional qualities. The public seems to be concerned primarily about the quality and cost of health care received rather than the credentials of any health group.

Social conditions and developments have markedly influenced the image of nursing that is held by society. For example, since the Victorian era, the Women's Movement has demonstrated ebbs and flows dependent on the major events of the times. Some believe that the kinds of leaders that have emerged in nursing and the consequent image of the group have been primarily affected because they have been treated as an oppressed group. That means that nursing throughout history has been controlled by societal forces that have determined the behavior of nursing's leaders (Roberts, 1983, p. 21). Women constitute the majority in nursing, and women, like blacks, Jews, and others, have been considered to be an oppressed group. They have been controlled by forces other than self and forces that have greater prestige, power, and status. Nursing, controlled by other health disciplines and employing agencies, perhaps has internalized personality characteristics of an oppressed group: self-hatred and low self-esteem (Roberts, 1983, p. 22). Lavinia Dock seemed to validate the idea that nurses have been an oppressed group when she described the nurse of 1890: "The nurse is a soldier. Absolute and unquestioning obedience is the fundamental idea of the military system. . . . Strictness and exactness produce better nurses" (Matejski, 1981, p. 18). Such nurses demonstrate poor professional self-concept behaviors such as showing awe of authority, devotion to routines, and retreating from initiative. They are resistant to change and possess oppressed attitudes. These attitudes on the part of the nurse, along with societal factors and economics, are inevitable elements in shaping the nurse's professional self concept (Matejski, 1981).

Nurses need to deal with the conflicts arising out of social oppression before they will be able to exhibit a professional image of pride and expertise. Nursing leaders have recognized that role behavior of the professional nurse is largely related to the image of the nurse held by the consumer, the public. Thus, there are concerted efforts by the profession to influence the media to present a scholarly image of the profession and a competent image of the practitioner. The media's influence on the consumer perhaps offers the best strategy for changing the professional self-image of nurses. The reflected appraisal of the nurse by the consumer indeed plays a vital role in shaping the individual nurse's professional self-concept.

THE PROFESSIONAL SELF

To a large extent the kind of professional a person becomes depends on the person's self-system. The professional self-system is an emergent from the personal self.

Personal Self-System's Impact on the Professional Self

As noted earlier in this chapter, one's self-concept "results from previous interpersonal relationships" (Simms and Lindberg, 1978, p. 9) and affects one's future relationships. "A person's view of self controls the roles he or she will be able to assume" (Simms and Lindberg, 1978, p. 9). One's self-system determines one's personal characteristics and these personal qualities enable one to carry out professional roles in more or less successful ways.

Sheehy cities several qualities of people who are successful in navigating their roles in life. These qualities are direct outcomes of the development of the self-concept:

1. Willingness to take risks is an outcome of a positive self-concept reflecting the person's ability to trust others, to be confident in assuming responsibilities, and to direct initiative toward changing the self and the environment.

2. The sense of right timing is an outcome of a positive self-concept, reflecting the person's ability to anticipate one's own and others' needs as well as the ability to prepare for the future.

3. The capacity for loving is an outcome of a positive self-concept, reflecting the person's ability to experience happy or sad emotions by sharing experiences with others and by participating in others' lives.

4. Establishment of friendship, kinship, and support systems is the outcome of a positive self-concept reflecting one's ability to establish networks of supportive contacts among friends, family, and other support systems. (Sheehy, 1982, pp. 95–97, 130–141, 163–178, and 206–227)

Simms and Lindberg validate that the professional self is a direct reflection of the personal self-concept. "Responsibility for our own acts—especially toward others—will flourish in an environment which fosters growth of self and independence" (Simms and Lindberg, 1978, p.7). Understanding self and working to view self positively inevitably leads to more productive professional self-concepts. Negative self-concepts are barriers to effective independent functioning, which is vital to the successful performance of professional roles.

Achievement of Developmental Tasks

The development of the professional self is sequential. It follows the same sequence that the developmental process follows in the evolution of the personal self-concept. Like the personal self-development, the professional self-development is based on the achievement of specific tasks in sequential stages. This section describes the stages of professional self-development using the framework of the developmental tasks associated with the development of the personal self.

Identification of Professional Goals Associated with the Tasks of the Developmental Eras

The development of the professional self is the process of personal self-transformation arising from the interactions associated with education, practice, or research in the profession of nursing. The nurse who is ready to enter practice enters the profession with an idealized image of the self, clients, co-workers, other workers in the delivery systems, and all others significant to the profession. Nursing is not unlike other professions in developing the professional self from an idealized image of self and others. That process has been described by Pajak and Blase (1982, pp. 65–72) in regard to teachers. Being a teacher is defined almost entirely within the framework of the teacher-student relationship. Being a nurse can also be defined within the framework of the nurse-client relationship. Teachers have reported that in the first years of their professional practice they expend a great deal of time and energy developing their knowledge, skills, and attitudes to meet the role expectations. Young teachers are said to be preoccupied with their own development in three areas: instructional knowledge, managerial skills, and the establishment of appropriate relationships with students. It has been suggested that it takes approximately 3 years to master these skills. Nurses probably are preoccupied with the same developmental problems. However, the demands of the health care delivery system that serves as the nurse's employer generally does not allow or provide for 3 years of orientation. What emerges for the professional teacher or nurse is that the new professional is placed in the position of needing to change her own glorified image of everyone and everything. What occurs in this change is a series of stages in the developmental process for the professional self (Pajak and Blase, 1982). The maturation of the professional self ensures that the professional does not mistake ideals and illusions for reality (Pajak and Blase, 1982, pp. 71–72).

Table 4-1 outlines the stages of professional development. Each stage, with its associated tasks and goals, is modified from Erikson's stages of the life cycle (Erikson, 1982, pp. 55–82).

The degree of achievement of each of the goals in each of the stages of professional development influences what the person as a professional is like. A positive concept of the self as a professional person is essential to the nurse in effectively meeting the health needs of the population that nursing serves. Following is a discussion of the outcomes for the professional self-system when developmental tasks of each stage are more or less satisfactorily negotiated through the achievement of specific developmental goals.

Outcomes for the Professional Self-System Related to Negotiation of the Developmental Tasks

All developmental theories are based on the assumption that the growth and development of the human is sequential and that successful negotiation of earlier developmental tasks are critical to the negotiation of later developmental tasks. This means that the development of the professional self is greatly influenced by the quality of goal achievement in each of the developmental eras. In the following discussion the task of each era is stated and followed by a discussion of the outcomes of satisfactory and incomplete or unsatisfactory achievement of goals of the era.

The Beginning Professional Nurse During the Orientation Period
Task: Trust   Emerging Strength: Hope

Goals: To trust one's own mentors and polestars to effectively develop abilities to fulfill professional role requirements, to count on others to assist in the pursuit of professional objectives, to experience gratification in a new role, and to count on recognition from employers and clients for effectively delivering a needed service.

These goals require that every professional nurse have readily accessible a number of guides and teachers on whom the nurse can count—relationships characterized by positive appraisals and relationships in which the nurse's professional needs can be satisfied without undue anxiety.

Outcomes of Satisfactory Achievement: The professional nurse who has been able to count on those who have assisted her in developing nursing skills and knowledge will most likely be able to trust her own professional and interdisciplinary peers in

TABLE 4–1.   Stages of Professional Development

Stage	Task	Goals
Infancy— *The Beginning* *Professional—* *Orientation*	Trust	To trust one's own mentors and polestars to effectively guide oneself to develop abilities to fulfill professional role requirements
		To count on others to assist in the pursuit of professional objectives
		To experience gratification in a new role
		To count on recognition from employers and clients for effectively delivering a needed service
Childhood The Beginning Professional Nurse— Postorientation	Autonomy	To depend on more mature professionals for guidance some of the time
		To view self as autonomous in practice some of the time, a professional in one's own right, able to stand on own competence in meeting role responsibilities
		To view nursing as an independent body, determining its own policies and regulations, effectively using its power, and in control of its own practice
The Young Professional— Moving into Independence	Initiative	To find rewards in using one's own initiative and imagination to test the realities of nursing roles.
		To independently anticipate professional role responsibilities while being held accountable for own actions.
The Growing Professional— Developing Expertise	Industry	To experience competence in independently performing the tasks of the profession
		To expand one's own knowledge of nursing
		To integrate a sense of accomplishment in one's own work in the profession
Adolescence— The Professional with Own Identity	Identity	To feel self-certain in role as a professional nurse
		To feel competent in role experimentation
		To clearly articulate own ideological commitment to the profession
Adulthood The Maturing Professional	Intimacy	To develop the capacity to commit oneself to collaborative relationships with clients, professional peers, and other colleagues in the health care delivery system as an interdependent professional

(*Table continues on p. 60*)

TABLE 4–1.   Stages of Professional Development (*Continued*)

Stage	Task	Goals
The Productive Professional	Generativity	To be productive for self and others in a professional nursing role, contributing to society through own efforts in nursing education, practice, and research
The Older Professional	Integrity	To find pleasure in the accomplishments of one's own self and others in professional pursuits
		To appreciate the full life cycle of the professional self

Modified from Erickson E: The Life Cycle Completed, pp 55–82. New York, WW Norton, 1982).

their common efforts to assist clients. Such a nurse will feel good about her own abilities, experience satisfaction in relationships with clients, nursing peers, and interdisciplinary team members, and will tend to appreciate the efforts of all concerned in professional experiences. Nurses who have experienced trusting relationships in professional development will be able to focus their professional energies toward meeting client needs rather than having energies tied up in calculating and untrusting relationships. They also are giving in their relationships, willing to serve as mentors and guides for the less experienced or educated nurses. Such a nurse welcomes accountability and responsibility, feeling confident about abilities. This nurse also is optimistic about getting future professional needs met and values lifelong learning as one avenue for professional self-development.

Outcomes of Incomplete or Unsatisfactory Achievement: Nurses who have not been able to count on others to assist them in developing skills and knowledge in the professional discipline continue this pursuit until their sense of need is reduced. Unfortunately, however, the pursuit is usually so tinged with anxiety that the nurse is not likely to be very successful. That nurse has entered the work world where abilities are immediately needed. If the nurse does not feel good about her competence and that feeling is at least partially related to the nurse's perception of her relationships with those teachers and guides she has had, that nurse is unlikely to feel comfortable in future relationships. That nurse will not trust peers or interdisciplinary workers to assist, and the nurse's professional needs remain unmet. Energies will remain tied up in trying to get her needs met, thus reducing what can be given to clients, peers, and others. Indeed, many work environments may reward short-term tasks achievement only, rather than portray any valuing of supportive processes. In this environment, relationships generally need to be calculated rather than open and honest. Relationships with clients are limited to getting the job done rather than including the pleasures and pains of clients and others in the implementation of the nursing process. Such nurses become task-oriented because they have not integrated the feeling that persons can be counted on when you need them. They have integrated the feeling that relationships make them vulnerable to negative appraisals more often than positive appraisals. Unless the professional nurse is successful in finding a significant other professional person who offers a relationship in which the nurse can experience positive appraisals as a person while getting professional needs met, that nurse will probably remain untrusting of others throughout professional practice. That nurse will not be able to be truly gratified in professional role accomplishments. The work environment that does not recognize professional nurses for effectively implementing the nursing process—rather, recognizes quantity of tasks achieved—will continue to contribute to the lack of trust that exists between its workers.

The Beginning Professional Nurse in the Postorientation Period
Task: Autonomy   Emerging Strength: Will

Goals: To view self as autonomous in practice, a professional in one's own right, able to stand on one's own competence in meeting role responsibilities, and to view nursing as an independent body, determining its own policies and regulations, effectively using its power, and in control of its own practice.

Outcomes of Satisfactory Achievement: The nurse who has learned to trust professional leaders, to trust that clients are able to assume responsibility in their own care, and most of all to trust herself as being competent and knowledgable will move into the work world with an excellent potential for feeling autonomous as a professional person. As a beginning practitioner, this nurse bases practice on nursing theory that is perceived to be valid, senses that nursing offers a needed professional service that incorporates a high level of technical competency, judgement, and decision-making, and requires effective interpersonal relationships characterized by an ability to collaborate. To view self as autonomous requires that the "trusting" new professional nurse experience a work environment in which she is encouraged to make judgements, to participate in policy-making for nursing, and to establish and pursue her own professional goals. The autonomous beginning professional nurse will feel comfortable in trying to put into practice what has been learned. Perhaps even more importantly, the autonomous nurse can appreciate the unique role others can play as well as feeling competent in her own role.

Outcomes of Incomplete or Unsatisfactory Achievement: At best, the nurse who does not trust others and does not have a sense of existing in her own right can only view self as a helpmate rather than an autonomous professional person. The handmaiden image is perpetuated if the nurse and nursing are both perceived to lack the right to exist autonomously. Some schools and work environments still portray nursing and nurses as dedicated helpmates to medicine and physicians (Donnelly, 1981). If nursing is believed to be only a part of medical care, rather than a partner in health care, the nurse cannot justify the need to be autonomous. That nurse exists only as an assistant on a medical team, nursing is limited to restorative care of sick people who are under the primary care of physicians, and the nurse spends the majority of time carrying out the orders of others. That nurse cannot feel like a real professional person because a primary criterion for any profession is that it offers a unique and needed service to people and is based on its own body of knowledge. If the beginning nurse comes to the work environment without a strong sense of professional autonomy or even with a fledgling sense of professional autonomy, that professional person needs the help of significant others in the nursing environment. Assistance is needed for young professionals to feel in control of what they are doing (provide for some successes), to provide orientation and resources for developing essential competencies as a professional person, and to enable the beginner to participate on the nursing team as it assumes responsibility for policies and regulations (provide for democratic process in decision-making). The beginning professional who does not have an advocate for a leader may indeed question the belief that nursing is autonomous rather than dependent and will rapidly fall into "caring for" rather than advocating for clients. One who does not feel autonomous does not tend to perceive others as autonomous persons existing in their own right. Without perceiving others as autonomous, the nurse cannot effectively implement nursing in a professional way. At best, that nurse can implement a technical process only.

The Young Professional Who is Moving into Independence
Task: Initiative   Emerging Strength: Purpose

Goals: To find rewards in using one's own initiative and imagination to test the realities of nursing roles and to independently anticipate professional role responsibilities while being held accountable for one's actions.

Clearly the professional needs to have achieved a sense of trust and a sense of autonomy as a professional person before truly experiencing pleasure in behaviors reflecting initiative. In addition, the young professional nurse needs professional leaders who encourage the achievement of mutually agreed on goals by a variety of means in order to assist that nurse to develop initiative. Leaders who insist on singular methods and procedures for achieving goals do not support the professional nurse's development of initiative and creativity.

Outcomes of Satisfactory Achievement: Implementing the nursing process in a variety of settings with a diverse client population requires competency in critical thinking and the ability to make valid decisions. Protocols and procedures cannot serve to organize all professional behavior. Thus, the nurse needs to be able to demonstrate initiative and creativity in effectively participating as the professional in relationships with clients. The professional who has achieved a sense of initiative can readily gather the data needed to assess client needs, can permit the client to participate in the planning for how to best meet that need, can offer creative ideas to the development of alternatives for problem-solving, and can take risks in carrying out the advocacy role for the client. The nurse with initiative will be challenged by the potential and/or need for change. The nurse with initiative can help the health care delivery system respond in a dynamic fashion to meet clients' health needs. The nurse with initiative will be willing to explore and assume new roles as a professional person if those roles are indicated for the improvement of health care. Initiative is a prerequisite for role accomplishment as change agent, client advocate, and contributor to the profession. The nurse with initiative will be able to acknowledge the importance of roles played by other health professionals rather than to feel oppressed or suppressed by others in the system. Finally, if the nurse has felt active in the planning and implementing of the nursing process with clients, that nurse will assume responsibility for the nursing actions. Accountability for nursing actions is readily accepted if the nurse feels responsible for decisions involved in taking the actions.

Outcomes for Incomplete or Unsatisfactory Achievement: The nurse who does not feel a high degree of independent and interdependent abilities and/or opportunities will have difficulty integrating initiative as a real functional part of the professional self. This nurse has developed a sense of shame in being a nurse. Nursing is not perceived as deserving of pride. Nurses are perceived as low-status workers and certainly not equal to the other "professionals" in society (such as lawyers, physicians, engineers). Nurses without initiative need to find their rewards in carrying out the directives of others—being appraised positively for following directions that involve little decision-making on their part. Such nurses have difficulty keeping clients as the central focus of the nursing process. Employers and agency policies assume paramount importance. Conflict arises when client needs cannot be met by procedures and policies or when critical thinking and active participation in decision-making are mandated in order to solve problems. The nurse without initiative in this conflict situation can only feel guilty when client needs cannot be met. Thus, it is clear that professional nurses without initiative are extra-ordinarily limited in the professional services they can offer clients. They may be very skillful in carrying out medical and nursing protocols in the restorative activities that are part of the nursing process, while being very limited in carrying out the less prescribed promotional and preventive activities of the professional process. They will perhaps be able to react well to the client's illness but not the client's response to illness. They may be effective in dealing with parts of the person, but not the person as a whole human. Dealing with the client as a whole integrated human requires the ability to describe, to analyze and compare, and to evaluate and synthesize the complex relationships that exist within and between humans. Since these relationships are continuously changing, the nurse must have the ability to use initiative to test the realities of the situation at any point in time. The nurse who has not achieved that sense of initiative will consequently feel overwhelmed by demands to make independent judgements and will feel more comfortable fulfilling prescribed roles and passing on the accountability for the nursing actions to the persons prescribing the nursing role behaviors. What should be professional behaviors becomes occupational behaviors where the worker assumes primary responsibility for carrying out the directives of an employer. In that perspective, one is rewarded for efficiency with skills and for quantitative outcomes rather than knowledgable judgements and qualitative outcomes. The nurse without initiative feels accountable to the employer primarily and to the client secondarily and perhaps even incidentally.

The Growing Professional Who is Developing Expertise
Task: Industry   Emerging Strength: Competence

Goals: To experience competence in independently performing the tasks of the profession as well as to expand one's own knowledge of nursing and to integrate a sense of accomplishment in one's own work in the profession.

If the professional nurse has developed a feeling of trust in others, a sense of autonomy in practice, and initiative in the nursing process, the nurse is ready to practice in an independent role and to feel accomplished in the profession and to continue a life-long learning process. In addition to the growth of the professional person, the support system for the professional person must value and reward professional accomplishments and must support the continued acquisition of knowledge. Support systems for the professional person, such as staff development people, need to focus on knowledge expansion as a primary role for the growing professional person. The new and young professionals need to use the knowledge with which they come while primarily developing trusting relationships and promoting a sense of competence in their abilities. It is exciting to see staff development programs tailored to the developmental needs of the varying staff members. Such programs are organized around the professional's strengths rather than needs, promoting initiative rather than conformity. In such a setting, professional role achievement assumes priority over bureaucratic structure and function.

Outcomes of Satisfactory Achievement: The professional person who integrates well a sense of industry, that is, feels comfortable and competent to carry out the tasks of the nursing process, is able to identify and carry out the duties inherent in particular roles. The consequent sense of obligation to clients and society creates the desire to know more. Acting on the motivation to know more inevitably translates to an improved quality of care to clients. This professional person experiences pleasure in competence in nursing care and satisfaction in learning. The nurse's own accomplishments with clients and ongoing learning form the basis for the nurse's real feeling of being a true professional who has either the ability or potential for meeting all professional obligations. Continuing education is viewed as a pleasurable professional responsiblity rather than a job or licensing requirement.

Outcomes of Incomplete or Unsatisfactory Achievement: The nurse who for any reason does not feel comfortable and competent in carrying out professional responsibilities cannot develop a pleasurable sense of industry. Rather, that nurse feels inferior, thus incompetent and unable to carry out the nursing activities previously identified as professional expectations. It is not uncommon for the nurse who feels "other-directed" rather than self-directed to experience conflict rather than satisfaction in the work role. For example, the nurse who says "I know I am not doing what I need to do as a professional person because I do not have the time," reflects an inability in negotiating the task of industry. That nurse indeed feels that she has "worked hard" and is industrious, however, that nurse clearly does not feel in control of her professional practice. Someone else is in control and the nurse develops a feeling of inferiority. This nurse may feel competent in fulfilling the assigned tasks but incompetent in fulfilling the "real" professional tasks. Continuing learning in this situation is commonly viewed as a mandate and another assigned task rather than a pleasure. Certainly the nurse who does not feel competent in meeting professional obligations and is not motivated to expand knowledge is limited in what goals can be achieved with clients. At this stage of professional development, the nurse who has not achieved the developmental task of industry inevitably must find some way to receive satisfaction from her work. Unmet professional needs must be negotiated or defended against. Obviously, the profession and the public can only profit from the first alternative.

The Professional with Own Identity
Task: Identity   Emerging Strength: Fidelity

Goals: To feel self-certain in the role as a professional nurse, to feel competent in role experimentation, and to clearly articulate one's own ideological commitment to the profession.

One does not develop a professional identity by completing assigned tasks of a discipline. Rather, one develops a professional identity by accomplishing the responsibilities of a *role* that is perceived to be appropriate to the accomplishment of the goal of the profession. We believe that the profession's goal is to facilitate health of clients, that the nurse plays a leadership role in society for promoting health, and that the significant emerging leadership roles for the nurse are change agent, advocate, and contributor to the profession.

Outcomes of Satisfactory Achievement: The most significant outcome of the successful achievement of a professional identity is that identity makes it possible for the person to carry out role responsibilities. The nurse who feels self-certain in the change agent role clearly is able to implement all the activities involved in a planned change process. Planned rather than accidental change is much more likely to result in improved health habits on the part of the client. The professional nurse who assists clients to take necessary steps to change health behavior often is more effective if the advocate role is also carried out. Finally, the nurse influences other nurses to facilitate change in clients toward better health through responsibly implementing the contributor to the profession role. The person who has a personal sense of a professional identity knows what the role(s) involves, is willing to experiment with role implementation, and is able to begin to articulate a personal belief system about the discipline.

Outcomes of Incomplete or Unsatisfactory Achievement: The obvious outcome of unsuccessful achievement of a professional identity is confusion about role responsibilities and behaviors. A common indictment of nursing today is that the profession is not clear about what it should be doing—in other words, its identity is vague in terms of professional criteria. In terms of occupational tasks derived from employer expectations, the occupational identity of the nurse may be clearer. The most significant outcome of the professional nurse not achieving professional identity is that the health care needs of the public will be incompletely and ineffectively met. Nursing is the only health discipline that clearly states that its primary goal is to facilitate health by *responding to the human's whole response to health and illness.* Since the human responds holistically, some health care discipline must serve that purpose if health care delivery is to be adequate. Otherwise, the public will perceive even more that health care is fragmented and/or unaccessible in this era of high technology. Without a professional identity, the nurse cannot implement nursing processes that respond to the whole person and these human needs will be incompletely or ineffectively met.

The Maturing Professional
Task: Intimacy   Emerging Strength: Love

Goals: To develop the capacity to commit oneself to collaborative relationships with clients, professional peers, and other colleagues in the health care delivery system as an interdependent professional.

After the professional person has clearly developed a professional identity and knows who she is and what she does, that professional is able to function interdependently as well as independently. Being secure in the professional self and professional role responsibilities, the nurse can share some energy within collaborative relationships. Nursing and other health care disciplines thus mutually agree on their common goal: the well-being of the client. They can mutually assess the total health care needs of the client, mutually respect the specific contributions of each discipline, and mutually determine who is best qualified to help with specific aspects of the client's health care needs. Nursing can share particular experiences with health care team colleagues, and contribute to the evaluation of the delivery of health care, keeping the client as the central focus throughout the collaborative process.

Outcomes of Satisfactory Achievement: Intimacy reflects the person's ability to place as much value on someone else's needs as one's own. Thus, the nurse who can invest herself in this way in professional relationships offers the greatest opportunity for affecting change in others. Influence and vulnerability are greatest in intimate relationships. Although the nurse is more vulnerable in such relationships, that nurse is the same person who has learned to trust, to feel confident of self, and willing to take risks in order to enhance her effectiveness. By virtue of their need in the nurse-client relationship, clients are considerably more vulnerable. Thus, it becomes extremely important for the nurse to value the client as a person in his own right deserving of respect and unconditional acceptance. Use of the client's abilities is much more likely to occur in this accepting relationship. If the client has been valued and has actively participated in the nursing process, the achievement of the goals mutually agreed on is likely to occur, and perhaps more important, is more likely to endure. The hoped-for achievement of the highest level of health is enhanced. In the same manner, the nurse who can value professional peers and other health care workers in their own right is clearly more effective in advocacy efforts for clients. Energy can be directed toward collaboration for the benefit of all rather than competition for the benefit of self only.

Outcomes of Incomplete or Unsatisfactory Achievement: Even if the professional nurse has achieved a clear professional identity of self, the nurse who cannot express intimacy limits her own ability to influence clients, peers, and others. Unless one can value others' beliefs, rights, abilities, and responsibilities as much as one values one's own, the professional person cannot maximize the positive outcomes of the nurse-client relationships. Without such respect for others the nurse cannot participate effectively in collaborative relationships, which have been demonstrated to be the most productive of positive changes. Lacking collaborative abilities, the nurse practices in isolation in either competitive or at best cooperative relationships. Thus, professional influence is limited. Although the professional is the expert in knowledge and skill in nursing, the nurse is not the expert in exiencing the client's human responses or determining what the client must or can do. The client is the expert. When nurses or any health care workers feel that their expertise includes all factors related to achieving health, they tend to respond in ways that clients perceive as dehumanizing. The nurse who has not integrated intimacy and thus cannot fully understand the value of other humans will tend to distort professional expertise and behave in ways that dehumanize clients rather than maximize their abilities in collaborative relationships. One can readily understand that nurses who have not felt respected as equals on the health care delivery team will have more difficulty developing their collaborative abilities with clients, peers, and others.

The Productive Professional
Task: Generativity   Emerging Strength: Care

Goal: To be productive for self and others in professional nursing roles, contributing to society through one's own efforts in nursing education, practice, and research.

Once the professional nurse has developed the ability to consistently collaborate with all those with whom she is professionally involved, she moves forward to a developmental stage in which she is most productive. Professional contributions peak and she experiences the most return for investment in professional activities. Nurses who have done well in this stage of professional life influence society's image of nursing most positively. Their activities are viewed as real contributions. They generate contributions to society directly through practice of the profession with clients, education of future professional persons, and the conduct of research that substantiates the significance of nursing in the delivery of health care.

Outcomes of Satisfactory Achievement: If the nurse achieves the task of professional generativity, the public and the professional self are greatly enriched. To feel productive—to feel absolutely essential to the world one knows—is a personal and professional need of every nurse. "Leaving one's legacy" is a human need. As a change agent and an advocate, the mature professional nurse provides the highest quality of professional nursing in her professional experience. That nurse appreciates the value of practice with clients. That nurse also appreciates the value of nursing education, acting as a continuing consumer as well as a contributor in some manner. That nurse appreciates the significance of research in nursing, acting as a consumer of research findings in practice and education and as a participant at some level in the conduct of research. Society's image of the professional nurse depends on the productivity of nurses in this generative stage of professional development.

Outcomes of Incomplete or Unsatisfactory Achievement: Nurses who do not reach the maturity level in the profession characterized by productivity nevertheless "leave their mark" on the professional world. However, their legacy in all likelihood contributes to a societal image of nursing as something less than professional. At best, that image may be a person with technical expertise or competent restorative care abilities. At worst, that image would be of a person who primarily serves as a helpmate to all other health workers, and secondarily serves as an attendant to clients. The image of the nurse as a real professional person depends on the majority of nurses reaching a mature level of professional development. The professionals who do not experience productivity and generativity will experience perhaps long periods of nursing practice in which they feel stagnant, even "burned out," to use a cliche describing persons unsatisfied with opportunities and their own performance in a fast moving, highly technologic environment.

The Older Professional
Task: Integrity   Emerging Strength: Wisdom

Goals: To find pleasure in the accomplishments of one's own self and others in professional pursuits and to appreciate the full life cycle of the professional self.

To paraphrase a concept made real by Dr. Elisabeth Kubler-Ross in her work with people in the terminal stage of life, the older professional has opportunities and obligations to complete unfinished business and to reflect on and cherish her significant contributions and relationships. If this is done successfully, the professional feels well integrated in the profession as long as she lives. This achievement requires an environment that values its older members, that permits tasks adjustments in order for older professionals to continue to actively contribute, and professional peers who call on older members for their wise and sage counsel.

Outcomes of Satisfactory Achievement: The professional who achieves a sense of integrity while growing older in the profession wields an extraordinarily strong influence on shaping the future directions for the profession. For example, the six founders of Sigma Theta Tau (the national honor society in professional nursing), all of whom were probably very successful in achieving the developmental tasks of each professional era, most likely have exerted the most influence on the profession during their older years. In recent years, each of them espoused the integrity of the profession. They never despaired about the potential for nursing to offer a vitally needed service to society. Each of them expressed great pleasure in their own professional achievements and perhaps more importantly in the achievement of those that followed them in the organization they founded. In an environment that truly treasures them, as expressed in the ongoing founders awards program, the surviving founders create the most dramatic moments at the biennial conventions. Their dreams and accomplishments are passed on in the most memorable way, that is, interaction with them and interaction between younger professionals and older professionals who have achieved the highest level developmental task—integrity.

Outcomes of Incomplete or Unsatisfactory Achievement: If the older professional cannot find pleasure in her own accomplishments or is dissatisfied with the professional practice of others, that person cannot achieve a sense of integrity as a professional person. Rather, just as it occurs in personal self-development, the professional self development is characterized by a sense of despair. This person cannot complete unfinished business and recount the accomplishments of self or others in the profession. This nurse cannot appreciate ongoing change and development. The lack of achieving integrity in older professional life is understandable, however, it usually leaves the older nurse alone and unsupported. The sense of despair creates a vicious cycle of alienation. Concurrently, this nurse cannot yield a positive influence on health care and is generally viewed by society in a stereotypic way, characterized by phrases like "You can't teach an old dog new tricks."

Challenging the Personal Self-System in the Development of A Professional Identity

A parallel has been drawn between developmental tasks of the personal self and the professional self. The professional tasks to be achieved for full professional development have been suggested to be identical to the personal tasks identified by social scientists. Thus, it is logical to conclude that those persons with the greatest achievement of personal tasks in the development of the personal self-system have the best potential to achieve more fully the professional tasks. Simms and Lindberg (1978, p. 9) state that the personal self-concept "results from previous interpersonal relationships" and that the resultant self-concept "affects future interactions." They conclude that "a person's view of self controls the roles he or she will be able to assume" (Simms and Lindberg, 1978, p. 9). They view the self-concept as an internal barrier or support for the professional self. During the developmental process that occurs between developing professionals and their significant professional others, it is entirely possible that the established self-system will be challenged. Given the assumption that a person always has the potential to change in a positive way, the developmental professional experience can be used as a corrective growth experience. Just as the individual's personal characteristics influence the professional characteristics one can exhibit, the professional experiences can have an impact on the personal self. Thus, the personal self-system and the professional self-system demonstrate a reciprocal relationship in which both are always open to change in relation to constraints or opportunities experienced by the person.

Donnelly (1981, p. 50) describes how nurses commonly experience conflict between the image of self and the image of the nurse as viewed by others, particularly those nurses who have been taught "that being self-effacing was the best way to avoid conflict with doctors." No conflict exists in this situation if the nurse views self as a helpmate who is less important to clients than the physician. The physician simply gives orders and the nurse follows them. The nurse who incorporates professional values will experience conflict in such a situation. That nurse's self-system will be challenged. Donnelly suggests the following strategies to deal with that challenge:

1. Focus on the client issue at hand rather than personalities. Respond with facts when dealing with doctors.
2. Command respect for yourself by establishing your position in client care as equal to the physician's. Let it be known that client care has top priority

with you even if it means the physician's request for your attention has to be refused. Expect courtesy and equity in interpersonal exchanges with the physician.

3. Know your personal and professional rights.
4. Evaluate requests and directives before responding.
5. Relax and be yourself, functioning at your highest potential. (Donnelly, 1981, pp. 52–53)

Essentially, the nurse who has achieved well the tasks of personal self-development can use that personal strength to achieve the professional tasks. The nurse who has not done as well in achieving personal tasks in the previous developmental eras can use the professional significant others to further develop the professional self.

PROFESSIONAL IDENTITY AND IMAGE

"Nursing has struggled with its identity for at least a century. This crisis, usually described as unresolved tensions between art and science, occupation and profession, practice and theory, is reflected in great debates . . ." states Donley (1982, p. 2). During that struggle, society has perceived nurses as they have practiced in reality and as they are portrayed by the various communication media. Since most people receive far more of their information about nurses from the media rather than actual nurse-client relationships, it is essential to understand the media portrayal of nurses.

Role Behavior

The Kalisches (1983) have extensively documented the image of nursing as portrayed by the media. Fagin and Diers (1983, p. 116) suggest that social perceptions of nursing can be understood by "examining the metaphors that underlie the concept of 'nurse'—metaphors that influence not only language but also thought and action." They describe nursing as a metaphor for mothering, characterized by "nurturing, caring, comforting, the laying on of hands, and other maternal types of behavior, all of which are seen in our society as essentially mundane and hardly worth noticing" (Fagin and Diers, 1983, p. 116). Nursing is also viewed as a metaphor for class struggle. This notion supports the earlier description of nurses as an oppressed group. Nursing is also viewed as a metaphor for equality, with little distance shown between practitioners and clients and others considered to be the working class. Fagin and Diers suggest that nursing may be a metaphor for conscience among physicians, an uncomfortable reminder to them of their fallibility, since nurses generally see everything that goes on in health care. They also believe that nursing is a metaphor for intimacy since nurses deal publicly with the most private aspects of life. Finally, Fagin and Diers believe that a distortion of the fact that nurses deal with most intimate aspects of the person results in another metaphor for nursing, that of sex. These metaphors represent roles that stereotype nursing rather than the roles for which professional nurses are prepared. As such, these metaphors represent partial fact and partial fiction. Professional nurses need not be defensive, rather they need to try to influence the public by taking control of their own professional self-development and responsibility for role behaviors that reflect needed professional services (Fagin and Diers, 1983).

Challenging the Image

Since the current status of the profession relates in some ways to the images of nursing reflected by society as well as the origins of the group, it is important to challenge the distorted images and to differentiate the professional self of nursing. Winstead-Fry (1977) says that generational transmissions suggest that group members can decide to maintain, modify, or overcome the status problems of nursing. She believes that the ability to overcome the status problem demands a clear diffentiation of the professional self. With a clear professional self-concept, the nurse can challenge the myths and assumptions from previous generations. She states that two of nursing's major problems in articulating a clear professional self are nurses' relationships to the hospital (employer-employee) and socialization in the traditional female role. Winstead-Fry (1977) concludes that successful handling of either of these problems will result in successful handling of the other and she suggests some actions that should be effective in challenging the nonprofessional images.

Conveying the Professional Image

Successful challenge of distorted images of nursing can be achieved if professional nurses differentiate their desired professional self by the following behaviors (Winstead-Fry, 1977):

1. Say something directly to persons distorting the professional image.
2. Understand the group's generational linkages to hospitals and the productive and nonproductive outcomes of this linkage.
3. Address the issue of reasonable relationships to hospitals.
4. "Come to grips with what we want to be as a young profession peopled primarily by women" (Winstead-Fry, 1977, p. 1454), which involves dealing with issues of women's liberation that are significant to the profession and differentiating today's professionals from previous generations and from those aspects of nursing's history that interfere with independence and professional autonomy.

All of the above actions directed toward conveying the professional image of nursing need to occur within the peer group of nursing, the larger health care delivery team, and societal groups that influence the image of the profession. The informational sharing that could come out of these actions could act as a strong determinant for nursing to achieve its rightful place in society as a valuable professional discipline offering an essential service to the society it serves.

USE OF SELF IN THERAPEUTIC RELATIONSHIPS: PRACTICE OUTCOMES OF THE PROFESSIONAL SELF-BEHAVIORS

"The real promise for bringing about effective change in nursing lies in our ability to build positive self-images . . . the key to the helping-caring relationship" (Uustal, 1978, p. 2063). Based on knowledge, the nurse purposefully uses the professional self in collaborative relationships with clients to use the client's strengths to maximize health.

The Significance of the Personal Self-System of the Nurse

The process of relating interpersonally with others is based on one's view of self, that is, one's personal self-system. Healthy interpersonal relationships contribute to healthy views of oneself, which in turn helps the professional person relate helpfully to clients. The quality of interpersonal relationships between nurse and client is important to both the nurse's and the client's view of self. These views of self play an integral part in the way persons strive for health and in the degree of health that is attainable. This nurse-client interaction for the purpose of maximizing health is dependent on the knowledge base from which the nurse operates and the effectiveness of communication efforts, determined to a great extent by one's personal self-concept. Nurses constantly have to ask themselves, like Michelangelo did, "How much of what I wanted to say have I managed to convey?" (Stone, 1961, p. 362). Duldt *et al* (1984, p. 271) believe that the significant outcomes of nursing activities with the client are based on the degree of humanizing communications that occur reciprocally between the nurse and the client. Humanizing communication ability is inextricably related to the personal self-system and the degree to which the developmental tasks have been successfully negotiated. In order to understand and respond to the feelings of clients, it is extremely important for the professional nurse to develop awareness of her own self-system and the consequent patterns of relating that may require reinforcement and/or modification in order to effectively meet professional responsibilities with clients. Examples from literature that poignantly illustrate what it is like for clients and how important it is for nurses to understand and respond positively to their feelings are: "When a person knows and can't make the others understand, what does he do?" (McCullers, 1940, p. 59), and "I was put in a hospital because a great gap opened in the ice floe between myself and the other people whom I watched, with their world drifting away. . . .I was alone on the ice. . . .A blizzard came and I grew numb and wanted to lie down and sleep" (Frame, 1961, p. 10).

The Significance of the Professional Self-System

The way one views one's profession and the way one feels about oneself as a professional influences the way one thinks and acts in professional relationships. Nursing has some inherent difficulties in clearly differentiating a professional self that meets all the criteria for a legitimate profession. Barbara Jordan has suggested that all professions that are extensively peopled by women have a common problem: women do not really act out the equality they say they feel. She says:

> The problem remains that we fail to define ourselves in terms of whole human beings, full human beings. We reduce the definition of our lives just a little bit because somewhere in the back of our minds is the thought that we are really not quite equal. So what are women going to do about it? How are we going to change all that? It is going to take long, hard, slow, tedious work. And we begin with our own self concept. We begin to try to internalize how we really feel about ourselves, and proceed to actualize the thinking that we finally evolve from the look inward and the projection outward. (Jordan, 1979, pp. 218–219).

Jordan believes that the true professionalization of women's groups can only occur when women have clearly dealt with their personal self-concepts.

Regardless of the dynamics of the evolution of the profession, it has been assumed that the kind of professional self each nurse becomes makes a substantial difference in what each client can gain from the nursing process. If the majority of nurses achieve mature professional self-concepts (in terms of the professional tasks that need to be negotiatied), nursing will be a constructive force for health in society. The nursing process will then be both educative and therapeutic and the nurse and the client will be able to know and respect each other "as persons who are alike, and yet, different, as persons who share in the solution of problems" (Peplau, 1952, p. 9) and the enhancement of strengths.

REFERENCES

Blase JJ, Pajak EF: Teaching, the loss of innocence, and the psychological development of a professional self. Ed Horizons 60:65–72, 1982

Brooks JA, Kleine-Kracht AE: Evolution of a definition of nursing. Adv Nurs Sci 5:51–85, 1983

Donley R: Editorial: A community of scholars. Image 14:2, 1982

Donnelly G: How to break the handmaiden image. Nurs Life 1:50–53, 1981

Duldt BW, Giffin K, Patton BR: Interpersonal Communication in Nursing. Philadelphia, FA Davis, 1984

Erikson E: The Life Cycle Completed. New York, WW Norton, 1982

Fagin C, Diers D: Occasional notes - Nursing as metaphor. N Engl J Med: 116–117, 1983

Frame J: Faces in the Water. New York, George Braziller, 1961

Jordan B, Hearon S: Barbara Jordan - A Self Portrait. Garden City, New York, Doubleday, 1979

Kalisch BJ, Kalisch PA: Improving the image of nursing. Am J Nurs 83:48–52, 1983

Lancaster J, Lancaster W: The Nurse as Change Agent. St Louis, CV Mosby, 1982

Matejski MP: Nursing education, professionalism, and autonomy: Social constraints and the Goldmark report. Adv Nurs Sci 3:17–30, 1981

McCullers C: The Heart is a Lonely Hunter. New York, Bantam Books, 1940

Peplau HE: Interpersonal Relations in Nursing. New York, GP Putnam's Sons, 1952

Roberts SJ: Oppressed group behavior: Implications for nursing. Adv Nurs Sci 5:21–30, 1983

Rogers, ME: An Introduction to the Theoretical Basis of Nursing. Philadelphia, FA Davis, 1970

Sheehy G: Pathfinders. New York, Bantam Books, 1982

Simms LM, Lindberg J: The Nurse Person. New York, Harper & Row, 1978

Stone I: The Agony and the Ecstasy. Garden City, New York, Doubleday, 1961

Sullivan HS: The Interpersonal Theory of Psychiatry. New York, WW Norton, 1953

Uustal DB: Values clarification in nursing: Application to practice. Am J Nurs 78:2058–2063, 1978

Winstead-Fry P: The need to differentiate a nursing self. Am J Nurs 77:1452–1454, 1977

Section 2

Theoretical Bases of Professional Nursing

Chapter 5

Scientific Thought and Theory Development

THOUGHT QUESTIONS

1. What does education, practice, and research provide for the development of nursing as a science?
2. Compare the development of nursing as a science to the evolution of science in general.
3. What are the factors projected for the next two decades that will affect the scientific outlook for nursing?
4. What are six characteristics of science as a system and how does nursing presently display each of the selected characteristics?
5. What is the difference between deductive and inductive reasoning?
6. Why is theory essential to the practice of nursing?
7. What is the significance of doubt in the development of the science of nursing?
8. What are the four central concepts of nursing that identify the focus for scientific inquiry?

According to Rogers, nursing has two major dimensions: "1) the science of nursing and 2) the utilization or application of nursing's science for the betterment of man—the practice of nursing." She further states: "Without nursing science professional practice cannot exist" (Rogers, 1967, p. 7).

The science of nursing incorporates the study of relationships among nurses, clients, and environments within the context of health. Nursing's phenomena and propositions evolve from and pertain to its clinical domain—the practice setting. Nursing science will evolve theories to enable professional nurses to control nursing practice (Meleis and May, 1981, p. 33). The emergence of nursing science as an autonomous, distinctive professional discipline that is valued by society parallels the profession's and society's demand that nursing assume full responsibility for nursing's decisions, actions, and consequences (Bilitski, 1981).

Nursing science, in any of the varying models of nursing, is viewed as a dynamic system interacting with the environment. It is composed of theory, practice, research, and education. Education provides the potential practitioner with experiences to shape the belief system and to synthesize and disseminate knowledge. Theory provides the professional person with the tools to direct nursing practice. Practice provides the professional person with the setting to apply and test nursing knowledge and to develop theories. Research provides the nurse scientist with the means to test theories as they relate to the health status of clients and contribute to nursing knowledge. The movement of nursing to higher levels of organization, complexity, and functioning is dependent on continued systematic inquiry (Bilitski, 1981).

Nursing, a young science, can learn from the history of scientific development. Indeed, as one follows the emergence of present day scientific development in many disciplines, one can see how nursing in recent years has taken the same historic steps that older sciences took long ago. The following section briefly traces the evolution of scientific thought.

OVERVIEW OF THE HISTORY OF SCIENTIFIC THOUGHT

Science, which has changed the face of the earth and the boundaries of the universe, has evolved from earliest man, perhaps even prehistoric man. Science, in large degrees, accounts for the progress of mankind. Although it is not possible in the scope of this book to trace the development of science through every era of mankind's history, we have chosen to highlight three eras: Ancient Man (the beginnings of civilization), the First Scientific Revolution (1500–1700), and the Second Scientific Revolution (1900–1950) to explain the evolution of the Third Scientific Revolution, which is ongoing today in the Information Era.

Ancient Man

Early man was primarily interested in studying and improving things that were significant to his survival and suited to his conditions of life, rather than trying to discover things that could drastically change his universe. Ancient craftsmen, however, did use empirical methods. "He experimented, blindly for the most part, but with infinite patience; and in so far as he did experiment and observe his results he was fulfilling the first requirement of science" (Hawkes and Woolley, 1963, p. 666). However, when he would find the way to do something he wanted to do, he was satisfied and happy just to keep repeating the effective technique. He simply wrote down what he should do in order to repeat his initial success. He devised a cookbook. He knew that if you did things in the right order, miraculous changes occurred. He was not interested in inquiring into how or why the process worked. "How" and "why" were assumed to be the work of the gods. The universe was not rational, rather it was run by gods who were moved more by whims and passions than by reason. Throughout this early era of man, he did, in an elementary way, study and observe phenomena sufficiently to gather many isolated pieces of information. These items of empirical knowledge, however, were "treasured in isolation, each one a new fact related not so much to the accompanying facts as to the ultimate divine order," rather than "being treated collectively as a body of data from which scientific conclusions might be drawn" (Hawkes and Woolley, 1963,

p. 668). To the extent that nursing functioned primarily from protocols and proce-dures for many years, nursing exemplifies a young scientific discipline that some-what followed the methods of science that existed from 1200 BC until approximately a century ago.

In tracking the evolution of the science of mathematics, it is interesting to note that the Babylonians recorded scientific knowledge of algebra, geometry, and arith-metic, whereas the Egyptians during the same time frame possessed mathematics only in the form of simple addition. Related to mathematics, "any people whose economy is based on agriculture must needs observe the seasons, and since the farmer must plan ahead he requires something in the nature of a calendar which will give him due warning of the year's changes" (Hawkes and Woolley, 1963, p. 676). Also religious festivals had to be celebrated at special times. Farmers were not competent to draw up the calendar. That job was allotted to the leisure class, the educated, the priests, or priestly scribes. The scientific ability to move from ob-servation to prediction was really impossible for the Egyptians due to the nature of their mathematical abilities, therefore, one cannot find any reference to astronomy and related predictions of eclipses, and so forth, which they experienced. The Bab-ylonians on the other hand could make such calculations, thus, there are records of their earliest computations about the length of day and night in different seasons, the rising and setting of the moon, and the appearance and disappearance of other planets like Venus.

In terms of health and medicine, the people of the Bronze Age considered that disease, aches, and pains were caused by gods and evil spirits. Medicine therefore was associated with religion or magic. From the code of Hammurabi, which dates back to 1780 BC, it is clear that there were laws that stopped physicians from oper-ating unless they were confident of success and from prescribing for patients whom they were sure were going to die or who had an incurable disease. Although there were prescribed formulae for treating various dysfunctions of the human body, it is clear that the functions of the living body were generally misunderstood.

It was not until the time of the Greek empire that myths gave way to reason. The Greek "logos" is equivalent to empirical science. Man moved from the mytho-logical, fantastic, and poetical to the rational and concrete. Man was able to estab-lish the existence of particulars. After that man turned from particulars to universal concepts, which Plato called ideas. Mathematics and geography advanced greatly during this era.

After Confucius, around 250 BC, medicine seemed to be founded on a core of real facts. Medicine consisted of five areas: "general supervision, including the health of the emperor; health of the people; ulcers and septic treatment; supervi-sion of the imperial dietary; and veterinary service" (Pareti *et al*, 1965, p. 148). Al-though medicine and magic remained indistinguishable, India possessed some elementary knowledge of pathology and physiology. Knowledge of physiology came from embalmers. During this era, the heart was "believed to be the seat of the intellect, the blood was the source of life, and the liver the origin of its circula-tion" (Pareti *et al*, 1965, p. 149).

Serious study on the origins of the world and particulars about animals, vegeta-bles, and minerals did not appear until around the 4th century BC, the era of Greek philosophy. Medicine appeared to make scientific strides in the first century AD with the Chinese theory of the five elements (wood, fire, earth, metal, and wa-ter) and of "yang-yin (the two opposite but complementary principles of male-fe-male, positive-negative, warm-cold, etc.)" (Pareti *et al*, 1965, p. 742). In Rome, great advances were made in pharmacology, with medicines being derived from animal origin (honey, milk, and fat), from edible vegetables, herbs, roots, seeds, and from wine, other drinks, and minerals.

Sciences with beginning theoretical developments before the year 500 AD were alchemy and medicine, geology, physics, mathematics, engineering and agriculture, astronomy, architecture, philology, geography and cartography, and natural sciences like botany and zoology. Thus, well over 1,000 years ago, knowledge was beginning to be organized into systematic groupings that helped man better understand his universe.

The First Scientific Revolution: 1500–1700

The two centuries between 1500 and 1700 may be considered the most critical years in the development of civilization. During those years, the scientific method of inquiry evolved. The scientific method was the hallmark of the first great scientific revolution. In the sense that it taught men to think differently, the first scientific revolution is described as an intellectual revolution (Ware *et al*, 1966).

The Intellectual Revolution

Four basic assumptions about man and the universe evolved from the first scientific revolution and directed the thinking of men at that time and henceforth. These assumptions are defined in the principles of determinism, quantity, continuity, and impersonality. Leaving no room for uncertainty, the principle of determinism reflects the belief that "nature proceeds by a strict chain of events from cause to effect, the configuration of causes at any instant fully determining the event in the next instant, and so on forever" (Ware, *et al*, 1966, p. 127). The ability to predict comes out of this principle. Lack of predictability and the presence of uncertainty according to the principle of determinism represent ignorance. The quantitative principle expresses the exact nature of science. It reflects the belief that science consists of "measuring things and setting up precise relations between the measurements" (Ware *et al*, 1966, p. 129). In this view, man and the universe are described by numbers, for example, in spatial coordinates, time, position, amounts and locations of physical properties, and relations between these numeric characteristics. Continuity, the third principle, is concerned with the "transitions of nature from one state to another" . . . and "expressed the sense, deeply engrained in the outlook of the age, that the movements of nature are gradual" (Ware *et al*, 1966, p. 129). This principle reflects the belief that the processes of ·man and the universe are continuous.

The final principle emerging from the first scientific revolution was the principle of impersonality. The scientist was viewed as an instrument, not a person. He used observation rather than imagination, he passively found order in phenomena rather than creating it, and he did not recognize the influence of his own interaction on the phenomena under observation (Ware *et al*, 1966, p. 129).

Some of the greatest intellectuals in history influenced the first scientific revolution:

1. Descartes—Before his death in 1650, Descartes, a mathematician and physicist, concluded through rational and deductive formulations that an understanding of the universe was possible only through discovering its mathematical order. He concluded that strictly rational and deductive formulations were the only ways to study the universe. He believed that there

existed clear cause-and-effect linear relationships. Taking a mechanistic approach, he believed that man too could be explained by physical laws. Perhaps the most long-lasting effect Descartes had on man was his belief about the two distinct substances of man—mind and matter (Cartesian dualism), both of which could be explained physically. This separatist view, rather than an interactive view, between psyche and soma still influences nurses' thinking about clients (Bronowski, 1965, and Rogers, 1970).

2. Galileo—An astronomer and the founder of modern physics, Galileo lived at the same time as Descartes. He is known for establishing principles of dynamics, such as the law of falling bodies (gravity) and the discovery that the path of projectiles is a parabola. Perhaps most long-lasting was his discovery that a pendulum swinging to and fro could be used as the basis for the clock to measure time.

3. Newton—Living in the latter half of the 17th century, Newton is best known for his discoveries about light and color and gravitation. He discovered a compound character of light and discovered that color did not reside in objects, but in the light. He was perhaps best known for his work on the problem of gravitation, from which he discovered and established the ideas of mass and force. Nature was viewed as an aggregate for physical objects in motion. Many years passed before his notion that time and space had absolute values was disputed (by Einstein's theory of relativity).

4. Huygens—Living in the same era as Galileo, Newton, and Descartes, Huygens, perhaps the least well known of the scientists of the 17th century, proposed from his studies that the refraction of a beam of light resulted from a "slowing of the light waves in the denser medium" (Hempel, 1966, pp. 70–71).

Through the efforts of these early scientists, the first great revolution in science occurred. They moved mankind into a new way of thinking about nature. Although their specific deterministic views have been challenged, their contribution to mankind in terms of focusing man's intellectual pursuits on the methods of scientific inquiry has left a permanent effect on man.

The Scientific Method

The scientific investigation of phenomena was an outcome of the first scientific revolution. Defining science as the "organization of our knowledge in such a way that it commands more of the hidden potential in nature," Bronowski believed that science uses a method that finds order and meaning in our experience. He further concluded that man "masters nature not by force but by understanding" . . . and that is why science is successful and why magic fails . . . "power is the by-product of understanding" (Bronowski, 1965, pp. 14, 25, and 17–18).

The *method* of science is a particular method of reasoning known as logic. Logic encompasses principles of reasoning applicable to any branch of knowledge. Since logic is based on reason and sound judgement, it possesses a force that can be very convincing. Inquiry is a *technique* of science. It is seeking truth, information or knowledge to meet the *goal* of problem-solving. A problem is any question or matter involving doubt, uncertainty, or difficulty that needs solution. Solution is the act of solving a problem by finding the answer or explanation. The most extensive investigative process of science is research, which is the systematic inquiry or investigation into a subject in order to discover or revise facts, theories, or applications (Bronowski, 1965).

Polit and Hungler assert that the scientific method permits man to acquire knowledge in the most advanced way that has ever been developed. They declare that the scientific method creates "a system of obtaining knowledge which, though fallible, is generally more reliable than tradition, authority, experience, or inductive or deductive reasoning alone" (Polit and Hungler, 1983, p. 20). They define the scientific method as "a systematic approach to problem solving and to the expansion of knowledge" (Polit and Hungler, 1983, p. 20).

Kerlinger (1964, p. 13) defines the scientific approach as "a special systematized form of all reflective thinking and inquiry." In that process of thinking and inquiry, the scientist generally encounters an obstacle to understanding. After intellectualizing the problem and evaluating it from experience, the scientist makes observations and speculates about relationships (hypothesizes). Then the scientist deduces the consequences of the hypotheses formulated. Finally, the scientist empirically tests the hypotheses through observation, tests, and experimentation (Kerlinger, 1964, pp. 13–17).

Treece and Treece (1982, p. 51) describe the five steps of the scientific method: (1) the problem is stated, (2) an hypothesis is formulated for testing, (3) facts are gathered from observations or experimentation, (4) data are compiled and interpreted, and (5) conclusions are drawn. The scientific approach has guided scientific inquiry since the 18th century and is considered to be the most significant contribution of the first scientific revolution.

The Second Scientific Revolution: The First Half of the 20th Century

"Failure of existing rules is the prelude to a search for new ones" (Kuhn, 1962, p. 68). Emergence of a new scientific outlook occurred at the beginning of the 20th century. This new scientific outlook has been called the second scientific revolution (Ware *et al*, 1966, pp. 121–122).

Perspectives of the Physical Sciences, Mathematics, Biology, and the Social Sciences

By the 20th century, scientists realized that the physical world consisted of matter and forces between matter. Historically, the most familiar force was gravity, first conceived by Newton. Other known forces included electricity and magnetism. During the second scientific revolution, however, scientists learned a great deal more about the physical world. They found that the atom, previously considered to be indivisible, had structure and parts and that space and time was relative— "now the fast-moving electrons were found to change their mass with their speed, and a relation between mass and energy began to seem possible" (Ware *et al*, 1966, p. 131). Physical scientists also found that energy, previously assumed to be continuous and infinitely divisible, consisted of discrete units that could not be subdivided; a minimum quantity called a quantum.

The above noted changes in physics were accompanied by changes in mathematics. Very important was the move to a statistical approach. Mathematical statistics did not take the place of all judgements made by scientists, rather it provided tools "to help in restricting the area of judgment and in guiding the judgments by furnishing a quantitative basis, consistent from one occasion to another" (Ware *et al*, 1966, p. 134). Simple in its conception, statistics "divides observed phenomena into two parts, those which are random, attributable to chance, and those which are systematic, representing an effect" (Ware *et al*, 1966, p. 135). The statistical approach provided the means for the scientist to determine if the effect is real or not. In statistical measures, the effect is judged relative to the error to which the estimate is liable.

Biologic sciences were also enlightened greatly in the second scientific revolution. Genetic mechanisms were explained; the mechanism of inheritance in the genes was discovered; the structure and division of plant and animal cells was elucidated; viruses were identified; and with the discovery of substances like DNA and adenosine triphosphate (ATP), "features of organisms became apparent which substantiated at a biological level the hypothesis that all organisms are related to one another" (Ware *et al*, 1966, p. 140).

Social sciences contributed to an understanding of man that remains extremely important today. Learning, conditioning, motivation, culture, and race were explored and explained in great detail by the social scientists of the era. All of these concepts remain very important in the practice of professional nursing.

Discoveries That Necessitated Replacement of Old Theories

Whereas earlier scientists had been primarily concerned with number and measurement, after the second scientific revolution, scientists became interested in structure. The social scientist, for example, organized concepts in a way that was orderly and meaningful although their concepts were not so amenable to measurement. The relations between biologic phenomena became more important to the scientists than the number of phenomena. The concept of structure replaced the quantitative principle. Discontinuity replaced continuity as the underlying structure of the world and knowledge of the world was thus no longer viewed to be complete or exact. The principles of uncertainty and chance replaced certainty as a way of describing reality. Accepting the principle of uncertainty meant that the scientist, who viewed science as a way of describing reality, understood that they were limited by the limits of observations. "Probable" became a new word in the laws of nature. Finally, the 20th century evolved "a radically new view of the relation between the scientist and what he observes. Man came to be seen not as a detached observer but as an irremovable part of his observations" (Ware *et al*, 1966, p. 148). This concept has proven to be a cornerstone for the development of nursing theory.

Today—The Information Era—The Third Scientific Revolution

In this era of rapid scientific development, high technology permits almost instantly obsolescent discovery. Evaluation and dissemination of new facts and relationships in the world of nature raise questions about man's understanding of the human world—one's fellowman. Nursing has chosen to pursue that human understanding as its primary responsibility. Such a choice is reflected in definitions of nursing that state that nursing is the scientific study of the human's *responses* to health or health and illness.

High Technology—Outcomes of Scientific Thought

In this present era in which the silicon chip has boosted the capacity of the computer to be used inexhaustibly for scientific development and to be available to many, the technical innovations likely to occur are infinite. Indeed, this is the era of information and information processing that seems to be unlimited. The technology necessary for this rapid expansion of information and information processing has already changed the population markedly. Man has harnessed power from many sources including nuclear sources. He has learned to break down matter and recombine it in ways unthought of before. He has traveled at speeds greater than sound. He has placed satellites in orbit and survived in outer space. Medical scientists have made discoveries that have controlled many diseases and disorders and extended life dramatically.

The Scientific Outlook in the Health Professions

The health services as professional disciplines are undergoing rapid changes and are likely to change even more rapidly in the future. What are some of the profound changes occurring? Willers (1982) recorded the views of John Kralewski, director of the Center for Health Services Research, University of Minnesota, about some profound changes influencing the health professions today. They include the fact that we have a rapidly increasing aging population. Kralewski placed that fact in perspective by noting that Americans use about 1,100 hospital patient days each year for every 1,000 persons. Persons under 65 use about 600 to 700 days each year, whereas, persons over 65 use 1,800 to 2,000 days, and those over 70 use nearly 5,000 patient days per 1,000 persons. Another profound change is predicted because better technology leads to higher costs, thus overall health costs are increasing. In the organization and delivery of health services, competition between health care providers will increase. An outcome of scientific advances surpassing social advances is that for the first time in history, resource constraints will preclude the application of scientific knowledge to its fullest extent for every person. Pressing policy issues face all health professions today about the balance between scientific gains and ethical responsibilities. Perhaps nursing will play a major role in advancing ways to provide that balance. As nursing attempts to develop its scientific base in direct pursuit of its stated goal of attending to the human's responses to health process, the profession has the unique opportunity to contribute to greater understanding of man and to advance ethical decision-making in employing the gains made from technologic scientific advances.

MAJOR CONCEPTS OF THE SCIENTIFIC METHOD IN NURSING

The meaning of the term "science" is perhaps clearest if one identifies the systematic characteristics of science. Following are the characteristics of science as a system presented by Silva (1977, p. 60) on the basis of principles espoused by Van Laer:

1. "Science must show a certain coherence." That coherence needs to reflect the inter-relatedness of facts, principles, laws and theories. In nursing science, there is a further dimension of inter-relatedness that makes the process of nursing coherent, that is, the interactive phenomena of nurse, client, environment, and health.

2. "Science is concerned with definite fields of knowledge." According to Rogers, nursing, an empirical science whose purpose is to explain the phenomenon central to its concern and to make predictions about it, is focused on an abstract system which is "a matrix of concepts relevant to the life process in man" (Rogers, 1970, p. 84). She, along with other nurse theorists, have identified a common matrix of concepts inherent in nursing.

3. "Science is preferably expressed in universal statements." This suggests that nursing as a science must agree on some universal characteristics about the phenomena it proposes to investigate—man. Perhaps the most universally accepted characteristics of nursing's focus, man, are those assumed by Rogers (1970), which are:
   a. Man is a unified whole possessing his own integrity, whose innovative wholeness is reflected by his pattern and organization.
   b. Man is an open system continuously exchanging matter and energy with the environment.
   c. The direction of man's life process is unidirectional evolving irreversibly along the space-time continuum.
   d. Man is a feeling and thinking being.

4. "The statements of science must be true or probably true." Since humans are fallible, absolute truth becomes an unlikely-to-be-achieved goal. Scientists thus are asked to help mankind find reality in a trustworthy, scholarly, and systematic way. Chinn suggests that nursing needs theory in order to pursue realities significant to nursing, realities that offer a basis for validity and reliability in practice. In order to accomplish the purposes of the profession, nurse scientists must systematically abstract nursing realities. Chinn says that the abstraction process must be rigorous and systematic rather than haphazard. Such "systematically developed theory will produce a well founded basis for the continued description, explanation, prediction and control of nursing practice" (Chinn and Jacobs, 1983, p. 4).

5. "The statements of science must be logically ordered." Strict observance of the sequential steps in the scientific method are necessary for logical order. Chinn suggests that, in addition to rigorously adhering to the sequential steps in the scientific method, the nurse scientist must use the rules of logic in order to validate hypotheses for raw material from which theory is constructed. "Deductive and inductive logic represent two means by which logical interconnections among hypotheses within theory could be made" (Chinn and Jacobs, 1983, p. 59).

6. "Science must explain its investigations and arguments." If the scientist does not share his understanding and research findings, clearly he is not acting fully accountable. Feldman (1981, pp. 65–66) states, "A commitment to communicating research will help to insure quality investigations and hypothesis-testing in practice settings."

Following is a brief discussion of selected major concepts that reflect the integrity of the scientific process in nursing.

Inductive and Deductive Reasoning

Polit and Hungler (1983, pp. 19–20) assert that solutions to nursing problems are developed by means of logical thought processes. Logical reasoning combines experience and intellect. The logical reasoning process may be inductive or deductive. The process of arriving at a generalization by inference from previously collected data is inductive inference. These inferences are further described as "leading from premises about particular cases to a conclusion that has the character of a general law or principle" (Hempel, 1966, p. 10). For example, a nurse scientist may observe specific behaviors of newly diagnosed cancer patients and conclude that the diagnosis is associated with high anxiety. Deductive inference, on the other hand, demonstrates that the conclusion is "related to the premises in such a way that if the premises are true then the conclusion cannot fail to be true as well" (Hempel, 1966, p. 10). Arguments lead from the general to the particular. Stated another way, deductive reasoning "is the process of developing specific predictions from general principles" (Polit and Hungler, 1983, p. 19). To use the same example as cited above, if it is assumed that high anxiety occurs in newly diagnosed cancer patients, it would be predicted that newly diagnosed patients would exhibit symptoms of anxiety. Hempel (1966, p. 11) says that since particular cases may not react the same way in all conditions, the premises of an inductive inference might imply the conclusion only with more or less high probability, whereas, the premises of deductive inference more likely imply the conclusion with certainty. That assumption is only supported if the generalization or premise used to arrive at the conclusion is true.

Theory

Theories are generally introduced when scientists have studied a class of phenomena and have found a system of uniformities that can be expressed in the form of laws. The purpose of theories is to "explain those regularities and, generally, to afford a deeper and more accurate understanding of the phenomena in question" (Hempel, 1966, p. 70). Kerlinger states, "A theory is a set of interrelated constructs (concepts), definitions, and propositions that presents a systematic view of phenomena by specifying relations among variables, with the purpose of explaining and predicting the phenomena" (Kerlinger, 1964, p. 11). Kerlinger says further that theory is the basic aim of science. Consistent with Kerlinger's definition is Chinn's definition of theory: "A set of concepts, definitions, and propositions that projects a systematic view of phenomena by designating specific interrelationships among concepts for purposes of describing, explaining, predicting, and/or controlling phenomena" (Chinn, 1983, p. 70). Several attributes of theory are evident in this definition. There is networking of defined concepts in all theories. It has structure that gives it a systematic nature. Although the goals can take many forms, theory is goal-oriented. Finally, theory is tentative because it is based on assumptions, values, and judgments as well as empirical observations. According to Polit and Hungler, theories give scientists a method for organizing, integrating, and conceptualizing the manner in which phenomena are interrelated (Polit and Hungler, 1983, p. 22). Theories help nurses understand how and why the phenomena of nursing are associated with one another and to predict future events and relationships.

Fawcett has elaborated on the various types of theory: descriptive, explanatory, and predictive. "Descriptive theory identifies and describes specific characteristics of particular people, groups, situations, or events" (Fawcett, 1984, p. 19). Explanatory theory, more complex than descriptive theory, describes "relationships among various phenomena" (Fawcett, 1984, p. 19). Predictive theory, the most complex and powerful of all types, predicts "specific kinds of relationships among particular phenomena" (Fawcett, 1984, p. 19). To the extent that one has an understanding of nursing theories, the professional nurse can participate purposefully in the nursing process in the most effective way. Effectiveness in practice is directly related to one's ability to describe, explain, and predict the human's responses in regard to health.

Concept

The human and his interaction with the environment are extremely complex phenomena. In order to deal with this complexity, the professional nurse needs to be able to systematize. "Scientific systematization requires the establishment of diverse connections, by laws or theoretical principles, between different aspects of the empirical world, which are characterized by scientific concepts" (Hempel, 1966, p. 94). From this perspective concepts are the knots in a network of systematic interrelationships. Being more specific, Fawcett (1984, p. 2) defines concepts as "words describing mental images of phenomena." Concepts are highly abstract and general. Chinn (1983, p. 111) calls concepts the "building blocks of theory." She further explains that concepts are identified by "searching out words or groups of words that represent objects, properties, or events within the theory" (Chinn, 1983, p. 111). She states that the universe of concepts within a theory needs to be evaluated for quantity, quality, and emerging relationships between and among concepts because these concepts determine the nature, the structure, and the definition of theoretical relationships.

Fawcett (1984, pp. 5–6) and others take the position that the comprehensive nature of nursing is acknowledged when four concepts are extrapolated: the consumer person (who may be an individual, a family, group, or community), the environment (that may be alive or inanimate), health (that may include well-being and illness), and the nursing actions (that include all the interactions among nurse, client, and the environment in the pursuit of health).

Principle

"A brief statement of value and/or fundamental truth that is to be followed" in the practice of nursing is called a principle. Much of nursing practice has been based on such principles that have often been derived "from accepted facts or theoretical propositions from other disciplines without concern for testing their validity in nursing practice." Principles are generally separate entities, not integrated in a systematic way, thus they do not stimulate or validate the development of new knowledge (Chinn, 1983, pp. 204–205). In approaching nursing scientifically, the professional nurse assumes certain things to be so. "Assumptions refer to basic principles that are accepted on faith, or assumed to be true, without proof or verification" (Polit and Hungler, 1983, p. 22). Without principles, knowledgable nursing practice would be limited. Similarly to theory, principles may be descriptive, explanatory, or predictive. According to Rogers (1970, p. 95), "Principles derive from the imaginative synthesis of available data . . . and . . . are stated as hypothetical generalizations." They are provisional and symbolic and are helpful in guiding nursing practice to the extent that they reflect reality.

Law

Laws are not restricted to observational terms. They may describe the past, present, or future and may be conditional in nature. Hempel (1966, p. 55) states, "Strictly speaking, a statement asserting some uniform connection will be considered a law only if there are reasons to assume it is true." He goes on to say, however, that if this requirement were rigidly observed, many statements would not qualify as laws (examples: Galileo's and Kepler's laws). Thus, most laws hold only approximately and conditionally.

For purposes of nursing's theory development, Chinn (1983, pp. 60–61) defines law as "a highly generalizable assertion of relationship between variables." To be generalizable, the relationship proposed must consistently hold true. Generally, then, laws formulate what will happen under various sets of conditions. Since individual knowledge about humans does not serve as a basis for further generalization, it is important that nursing discover those uniform connections between events within the domain of nursing.

Types of laws, defined by content, that are as important to nursing as to all other behavioral sciences include:

1. Temporal laws—connections in which time is a real variable (*e.g.,* developmental events like aging)
2. Taxonomic laws—assertions of certain stable natural kinds of events. Kinds of events may be substances or systems to be used as units of inquiry (*e.g.,* identification of the units of inquiry in nursing that would describe, explain, and predict the human in relation to health)
3. Statistical laws—formulation of correlations between the taxonomic entities (*e.g.,* presupposed relationships between nursing behavior and client behavior). (Kaplan, 1964, pp. 109–113)

Laws offer information about what can be expected and thus form an essential element of theory on which effective nursing practice can be based.

Theoretical Framework

A theoretical framework has been called the "umbrella" encompassing concepts in interrelation (Andreoli and Thompson, 1977, p. 36). It has been defined as "a structure comprised of concepts related in some way to form a whole" (Chinn, 1983, p. 206) and as "a conceptual system . . . characterized by an interrelated set of postulates having relevance for some central phenomenon" (Rogers, 1970, p. 84). Used synonymously with theoretical framework is the term conceptual framework. Fawcett (1984, p. 2) states that the term conceptual model refers to "global ideas about individuals, groups, situations, and events of interest to a discipline" and is composed of *abstract* and *general* concepts and propositions that are linked together in a distinctive way.

Rogers (1970, p. 4) states that nursing's abstract system "is a matrix of concepts relevant to the life process in man." The general concepts of the profession, called the metaparadigm of nursing by Fawcett (1984, pp. 5–6), is a matrix of the consumer of nursing (the human client), the nurse and the nursing actions, the environment within which the nursing process occurs, and the state of health in which the person exists at the time of the nurse-client interaction. Developing the theoretical framework for nursing ensures practice that is effective in achieving the overall goal of the profession, that of improving the quality of health of all persons. With such a framework, nursing can assist people to achieve their maximum health potential. Theory offers the guiding principles that direct the practice of nursing.

Models for Nursing

Given the abstract and general concepts that are interrelated in nursing's theoretical framework, several nurse scientists have proposed their individual and distinctive ideas about the nature and process of nursing. It is accepted that "nursing models have provided a device by which assumptions can be transformed into postulates; that is, conceptualizations of reality that can be tested" and "it is clear that nursing practice is being outlined in such a way that it can be contested and corroborated—the essentials of scientific inquiry" (Andreoli and Thompson, 1977, p. 36). Each of the nurse scholars who has proposed a conceptual model has based the model on empirical observation, intuitive insights, and deductive reasoning (Fawcett, 1984, p. 4). Although they may present diverse views of nursing phenomena, each conceptual model is useful for professional nursing because of the organization it provides for thinking, observing, and interpreting in the nursing process. Each provides guidelines for practice. Fawcett (1984) reflects the thinking of herself and other nurse scholars in identifying three major categories of conceptual models of nursing: developmental, systems, and interaction models. Each category offers different approaches and different emphases in nursing process with clients although all have a common paradigm: client or patient, nurse, environment, and health. Selected conceptual models are discussed in Chapter 8, Models of Nursing.

THE SEQUENTIAL STEPS IN THE SCIENTIFIC APPROACH—A GUIDE FOR THEORY DEVELOPMENT AND PRACTICE IN NURSING

This section presents a synthesis of the scientific concepts already discussed in this chapter. The sequential steps needed for the development of theory and the implementation of professional practice are highlighted.

Doubt

Whether the professional nurse is involved in trying to build the theory base of nursing through nursing research or is involved in trying to deliver the best nursing care possible in direct relationships with consumers of nursing, the accountable professional nurse is destined to observe phenomena that raise questions. The nurse experiences moments, even long periods of not knowing how to describe, explain, or predict something about the client or the nurse-client relationship; thus, placing oneself in the position of needing further understanding to effectively carry out professional role responsibilities. That sense of question or doubt is the first step in the process of scientific inquiry.

Formulation of Problem—Using Literature and Experience of Self and Others

In addition to clearly elaborating the empirical observations that raised the doubts, the interested and accountable professional nurse reevaluates the knowledge presently possessed by self and seeks out further information from mentors, leaders, and the written literature. The nurse's guideposts for further information are the self-deduced key words that describe the phenomena or events causing doubts. In reviewing the literature and discussing with others the broad area of inquiry, the nurse critically compares her own observations with what is reported in the literature. Going through the cognitive behaviors of description, analysis, evaluation, and synthesis, the nurse crystallizes the problem that is causing the doubts and questions. Given the clear establishment of the problem, the nurse practitioner can guide the nursing process to a stage of mutually exploring the problem with the client, and then can move to the phase of operationally defining the variables involved and seeking an approach by which scientific study can be made.

Asking the Basic Question

Whether the nurse is in a researcher, practitioner, or teacher role, once the problem engendering the doubt is identified, the professional nurse uses the professional self to ask the critical question that reflects a clear identification of the problem. In the relationship with subjects, clients, or students, the professional investigator facilitates the exploration of the problem by first assessing needs and "asking the right questions."

Formulation of Hypotheses—Making Tentative Propositions

After exploring all that can be known about the problem identified and the questions raised, the nurse scientist assists those involved to explore the alternative explanations for the observed phenomena and the areas of doubt. Beyond that the nurse assists the subject, client, or student to explore several alternative solutions to the problem or alternatives that would answer the questions. Together, the scientist and the subject, client, or student, formulate their hypotheses and make the most knowledgable decision possible about the best plans for further action.

Deduction of Consequences

The "what if" dialogue that occurs between the nurse and the client in evaluating alternative proposals for the solution of a client's health problem is the same kind of dialogue that must occur with the researcher or teacher. Every potential action that is devised to solve a problem, share information, or test a proposition needs to have full discussion and evaluation in terms of potential outcomes. What is known already is the safest guide in this evaluative stage of scientific inquiry. After full exploration of the consequences of proposed actions, agreement on the best action to take is made. Detailed plans are made of what the actions are to be, how the actions will be monitored, by whom will various activities be conducted, and what will be the indicators of success—the measure of desired outcomes.

Observation and Testing

In nursing practice, research or education, proposed actions are implemented according to mutually planned strategies. Immediately, a new cycle is operative with the nurse again observing the process and outcomes of the nursing actions. In nursing practice and education, this is usually called implementation and evaluation of nursing. In nursing research, this is usually called testing the hypotheses or assessing the validity and reliability of the propositions.

Acceptance or Rejection of Proposition

After specified actions or testing have occurred, evaluation of the outcomes follows. This means that full reporting of the experiences is done, the outcomes are matched against the proposed measures of success, the critical analysis of the situation is facilitated. On the basis of these findings, the professional nurse accepts or rejects the actions or hypotheses tested in the situation. In Chapter 6 more detail is provided on this stage of research. Thus, for present purposes, it is sufficient to say that acceptance or rejection of the nursing action is based on how effective it is in achieving desired outcomes in the nursing process.

Generalization and Use in the Practice of Nursing

If the professional nurse has systematically followed the scientific process described and repeats that same process to deal with recurring questions and commonly occurring phenomena, one has a repertoire of experience and knowledge on which to generalize. Connections between phenomena have been established, findings have been replicated, and predictions can be made with acceptable degrees of accuracy. The knowledge that accrues from use of the scientific approach in nursing practice, education, and research is the basic prerequisite for nursing's meaningful contribution to society. Rogers (1970, p. 88) states the significance of nursing knowledge clearly: "Nursing's abstract system is the outgrowth of concern for human health and welfare. The science of nursing aims to provide a growing body of theoretical knowledge whereby nursing practice can achieve new levels of meaningful service to man."

THE STATUS OF NURSING AS A SCIENTIFIC DISCIPLINE

In the past 20 years, nursing has dramatically evolved as a scientific discipline. It is generally accepted that nursing has two dimensions: science and application of scientific findings in practice. Nursing has always been viewed as a practice discipline. Perhaps its greatest achievement in the past two decades is the beginning acceptance of the idea that its practice is based primarily on its own unique body of knowledge that is being scientifically derived. Given this change, nursing now has the opportunity to achieve the professional status long desired.

The Domain of Nursing—the Focus for Scientific Inquiry

It was indicated earlier in this chapter that there is growing agreement on the central concepts of the discipline of nursing. Those central concepts that could be used as parameters of the science of nursing are the client or consumer of nursing actions, the nurse and the accompanying nursing actions, the environment, and the state and process of health of the consumer. The science of nursing evolves from the descriptions, explanations, and predictions that are made of the four components and the interrelationships that keep them inseparable. Indices for measuring the phenomena and the interrelationships among the phenomena are emerging as the true scientific study of nursing evolves.

The Preparation of Nurse Scientists

To be prepared to implement fully the scientific process in nursing clearly requires professional programs organized around nursing's theoretical framework. One could argue that baccalaureate programs can develop a nurse scientist. That would mean that the nurse prepared to practice scientifically is a minority of the nursing population. For purposes of preparing the needed scientific leadership in nursing today, these authors suggest that advanced degrees in nursing are necessary. In 1980, of the 1.2 million nurses employed, less than 3,000 held doctoral degrees and only slightly more than 5% of RNs held advanced degrees including the master's degree (Institute of Medicine, 1983, pp. 36 and 215). It is evident that professional nursing must support higher education for more of its practitioners before a large impact can be felt from the benefits of scientific findings in nursing. The preparation of nurse scientists remains small, thus imposing inordinate burdens on those who do exist. It is perceived however, that nursing has begun to experience some gratification from the efforts of its few nurse scientists. That perception is the basis for optimism that nursing will develop into the scientific discipline envisioned by its leaders for over a century.

REFERENCES

Andreoli KG, Thompson CE: The nature of science in nursing. Image 9:32–37, 1977
Bilitski JS: Nursing science and the laws of health: The test of substance as a step in the process of theory development. Adv Nurs Sci 4:15–29, 1981
Bronowski J: Science and Human Values, rev ed. New York, Harper Torchbooks, 1965
Chinn PL, Jacobs MK: Theory and Nursing—A Systematic Approach. St Louis, CV Mosby, 1983
Fawcett J: Analysis and Evaluation of Conceptual Models of Nursing. Philadelphia, FA Davis, 1984
Feldman HR: Commentary: A science of nursing—to be or not to be. Image 13:63–66, 1981
Hawkes J, Woolley L: History of Mankind, Cultural and Scientific Development, vol 1, Prehistory and the Beginnings of Civilization. New York, Harper & Row, 1963
Hempel CG: Philosophy of Natural Science. Englewood Cliffs, New Jersey, Prentice-Hall, 1966
Institute of Medicine, Division of Health Care Services: Nursing and Nursing Education: Public Policies and Private Actions. Washington, DC, Nat Academy, 1983
Kaplan A: The Conduct of Inquiry, San Francisco, Chandler, 1964

Kerlinger FN: Foundations of Behavioral Research. New York, Holt, Rinehart & Winston, 1964

Kuhn TS: The Structure of Scientific Revolutions. Chicago, University of Chicago, Press 1962

Meleis A, May K: Nursing theory and scholarliness in the doctoral program. Adv Nurs Sci 4:32–33, 1981

Pareti L assisted by Brezzi P, Petech L: History of Mankind, Cultural and Scientific Development, vol II, The Ancient World. New York, Harper & Row, 1965

Polit DF, Hungler BP: Nursing Research: Principles and Methods, ed 2. Philadelphia, JB Lippincott, 1983

Rogers ME: An Introduction to the Theoretical Basis of Nursing. Philadelphia, FA Davis, 1970

Rogers ME: Nursing: Today's happening. Paper presented at Annual Alumnae Day, University of North Carolina, School of Nursing, June 2, 1967

Silva MC: Philosophy, science, theory: Interrelationships and implications for nursing research. Image 9:59–63, 1977

Treece EW, Treece JM Jr: Elements of Research in Nursing, ed 3. St Louis, CV Mosby, 1982

Ware CF, Panikkar KM, Romein JM: History of Mankind, Cultural and Scientific Development, vol VI, The Twentieth Century. New York, Harper & Row, 1966

Willers L: Health care 2000. Health Sciences, pp 6–9. University of Minnesota Press, 1982

Chapter 6

The Research Process

THOUGHT QUESTIONS

1. What are the purposes for research in nursing?

2. In your opinion, what kind of research is needed the most today for the advancement of nursing?

3. What are ways that professional nurses can contribute to research in nursing?

4. How does the nurse researcher go about developing a research problem?

5. What are the sequential steps in nursing research?

6. Why does the researcher need an understanding of ethics in order to conduct research?

7. How should the increase in nursing research and researchers affect the public image of nursing?

Research could be considered the most extensive investigative process of science. Kerlinger's (1964, p. 13) definition of scientific research, proposed some 20 years ago, is that "Scientific research is systematic, controlled, empirical, and critical investigation of hypothetical propositions about the presumed relations among natural phenomena." Chinn and Jacobs (1983, p. 147) more simply state that "research is the rigorous application of the methods of science in order to obtain reliable and valid knowledge about reality." They explain that research is conducted for two purposes: to test theoretical relationships and to generate concepts or relationships for the construction of theory. Fawcett (1982, p. 57) states that research in nursing "generates the knowledge that is used in practice, while practice generates ideas for research." Synthesizing what research is, Dempsey and Dempsey (1981, pp. 4–5) note: "Research is a scientific process of inquiry and/or experimentation that involves purposeful, systematic and rigorous collection of data. Analysis and interpretation of the data are then made in order to gain new knowledge or add to existing knowledge. Research has the ultimate aim of developing an organized body of scientific knowledge." From their perspective, research has several purposes: finding answers to questions, finding solutions to problems, discovering and interpreting

93

new facts, testing theories in order to revise presently accepted theories/laws in light of new conditions or facts, and formulating new theories. In the profession of nursing, achievement of all these purposes of scientific research are needed in order to practice accountably.

THE NEED FOR NURSING RESEARCH

Serious efforts to conduct nursing research and develop the theory to guide practice began some 20 to 25 years ago. The statements of nurse researchers of the early 1960s are still appropriate today. In 1965, Downs, now a well-known nurse researcher, speaking at the Upsilon Chapter, Sigma Theta Tau, Research Conference, New York University, Dec. 10, 1965, called for scholars in nursing to conduct research: "One of the greatest needs in nursing today is the development of a respectable body of basic research that can advance the theoretical foundations of nursing practice." Two years later, Rogers, now a leading nurse theoretician, described research as one of the most prestigious words in the English language at the time and warned nurses of the necessity to understand research as legitimate scientific inquiry. She challenged nurses to accept the professional criterion that states: "A given body of theoretical or abstract knowledge is specific to a given discipline and encompasses the discipline's descriptive, explanatory, and predictive principles which guide its practitioners" (Speaking on "Nursing Science: Research and Researcher" at the Annual Conference on Research and Nursing, Teachers College, Columbia University, N.Y., Feb. 3, 1967). Thus, nursing research was viewed as professional responsibility, without which, professional practice could not exist. In expounding on the complexity of knowledge and skill required to safeguard the recipients of nursing in a highly technologically advanced era, at that same research conference, Rogers stated and has often repeated her now internationally known view: "Only the most uninformed and those endeavoring to maintain a long obsolete hierarchal control would propose that in today's world society is better served by ignorance than by knowledge." Responses like this from nursing leaders of two decades ago engendered scholars in nursing to accept the challenge to participate in nursing research in pursuit of the professional goal of basing the practice of nursing on theory and fact rather than opinion and prescribed protocols from other disciplines.

The Need for Knowledge of the Process of Nursing

Nursing is a process between the nurse and the client that is composed of two equally important elements, cognitions and interpersonal relationships. It is based on critical thinking and interaction. Therefore, if nurses are to understand the process of nursing, the nursing knowledge must be based on research that describes and measures the cognitive and interpersonal elements of the nurse, the client, and, most importantly, the interaction of the nurse and the client in their mutual effort to maximize health.

Historically, research focused on understanding the nurse better. Most of the earliest nursing research were really "nurse" studies. Although the emphasis has shifted away from studying the nurse, some important studies of the nurse continue to add to the knowledge base for the nurse component of the nursing process. Most "nurse" studies today address the nurse in relation to the client or employer, or other environmental factors. An example of such a study is Hanson and Chater's (1983, pp. 48–52) investigation of roles selected by nurses as they relate to the managerial interests and personal attributes of the nurse. Such studies assist the profession in understanding the needs of nurses and in using that understanding in recruiting and retention.

Tinkle and Beaton, (1983, p. 31) who conclude that the profession exists by virtue of a commitment to provide care for people, state: "If the concerns and perceptions of the recipients of nursing services are considered unimportant factors in nursing research, then nurses may indeed be providing nursing care that is more meaningful to themselves than to patients." This idea could be expanded to conclude that nursing studies that fail to consider the interactional elements between the nurse and the client may lack validity.

Evidence that the profession values the interactional process between the nurse and the client is the fact that nursing literature has discussed the process of empathy in the helping process for over 35 years (Gagan, 1983, p. 65). Gagan (1983, p. 66) further points out that nurses have not necessarily ranked high in empathic abilities and that the methodologies used in past research on empathy warrant scrutiny, thus, there is needed "reassessment of empathic measurement in the nursing arena." In a recent editorial, Steel (1984, p. 4) emphasized the value of the nurse-consumer relationship in the profession and declared that the inseparable relationship between nursing and society keeps the focus on those nursing serves and "elevates us to a partnership with the people we serve rather than a partnership solely with other health care providers."

Thinking of the nursing process as a partnership suggests that the dynamics and outcomes of that partnership need to be a central focus in nursing research. In all nursing models, the nurse is viewed as a helper in some way. Cronenwett and Brickman (1983, pp. 84–88) validate the need to evaluate models of helping in the nurse-consumer partnership. They suggest the need to evaluate the effectiveness of at least four models of helping:

1. The moral model, in which the nurse would not feel obligated to help, rather would feel obligated to compel persons to take action on their own behalf.
2. The compensatory model, in which the nurse would not blame clients for their health problem, but would hold them responsible for their solution.
3. The medical model, in which the nurse would not hold clients responsible for the origin or solution for their health problem—they would be supported in adopting the sick role.
4. The enlightenment model, in which the client is blamed for causing the problem, but is not responsible for the solution, rather, the client puts self in the hands of the helper. (Cronenwett and Brickman, 1983, pp. 84–88)

Although one could argue that evidence in nursing already exists that suggests that some of these models are not appropriate for the nursing process, one could also argue more effectively if one had data to support the thesis that one model was correlated more positively with effective outcomes in the nursing process.

Specific interventions used in the nursing process need to be measured and evaluated for effectiveness in meeting the client's needs. Although little of nursing's practice has been investigated and measured systematically in a controlled way, much of the nursing research that has occurred recently has focused on interventions used by nurses in the nursing process. Examples of such studies are:

1. Nurses have studied the effectiveness of four different treatment techniques in preventing and controlling breast pain and engorgement in nonnursing mothers (Brooten *et al* 1983, pp. 225–229).
2. Communication patterns used in health teaching have been studied in relation to the information recall of the client (Kishi, 1983, pp. 230–235).
3. The intervention of "childbirth preparation" has been measured in terms of its effectiveness in promoting marital satisfaction during the antepartum and postpartum period (Moore, 1983, pp. 73–79).

Critical to developing the theory base on which nursing is practiced is the continued support for nursing researchers to describe, explain, and predict phenomena associated with the process of nursing, that is, to value and implement studies that are focused on the cognitive and interpersonal aspects of the nurse-client relationship. Cognitive and interpersonal processes that are understood and validated to be helpful can then be more purposefully implemented. Such development will greatly aid the professional nurse in influencing the client to achieve greater health. Donaldson and Crowley (1978, pp. 113–120) identified such processes as one central theme of inquiry for nursing. Nursing investigators have begun to provide structures for nursing researchers to study the process of nursing according to particular conceptual models. For example, Melnyk (1983, pp. 170–174) has elaborated a process for examining Orem's nursing theory and Derdiarian (1983, pp. 196–201) has developed an instrument for research development using the behavioral systems model for nursing. In order to intervene purposefully, nurses must have knowledge about the processes that are positive in promoting change toward greater health. The beginning structure of inquiry in any of the major conceptual models of nursing should be helpful to the practicing nurse who accepts the responsibility for measuring the effectiveness of the nursing process with clients.

The Need for Knowledge of the Client Systems in Nursing

In all models of nursing described today, the central focus for the nurse is the human, sometimes referred to as man, or the human system, or client, or patient, among other possibilities. Sometimes the nurse practices in an environment in which the client system is an individual human. At other times the client system toward whom professional efforts are directed is the family or a small group related by some significant support process or structure between or among the various individual members. At other times, the nurse directs professional efforts toward a larger group, a community. That client system is characterized by one or more common bonds between individuals that has some impact on health. Most of the nursing research to date has studied the individual as client. For many years survey studies have been done to project the health service needs of communities. Regardless of the level of the client system, what is important is the fact that nurses are accepting the professional responsibility for systematically gathering data about the client. That information increases understanding, enabling the nurse to deliver effective services to clients. For example, Miles and Crandall (1983, pp. 19–23) have conducted multiple studies of bereaved parents that help nurses understand the client system better. In each of their studies they sought clues, through self-descriptions, to the positive and negative resolutions following the death of a child.

Perhaps the client system that has been researched the least in nursing is the family, although certain family member relationships have been investigated (*e.g.*, the mother-child relationship). Gilliss (1983, p. 50), acknowledging the growing interest of nurses in studying the family as a unit of health behavior and health service, has pointed out the complexity of nursing research in which one tries to examine the family as an aggregate. Since the family is viewed as greater than or different from the sum of its parts, the nurse researcher needs "consensus about *what* should be evaluated and how selected methods might access the data that make the family unit more than the sum of its parts" (Gilliss, 1983, p. 50). Gilliss (1983, p. 56) categorizes nursing's concern with the family: (1) the family as a context for human behavior—concerned with the impact of the family unit on the health of individuals; (2) the family as a unit of health and illness—concerned with the impact of the health of individuals on the family unit. To study either of these concerns and hold the view of the family as the client, the nurse must focus the study on the *family process,* not on individual members independently. Nursing has begun to address research needs of family nursing—to conceptualize what the family unit is, to validate procedures for studying the family process, and to use statistical measures appropriate to measuring aggregate behavior in the analysis of *family* data.

Regardless of the size or complexity of the client system, one needs to understand the relevant characteristics of that human system that are related to the life process and health. Donaldson and Crowley (1978, pp. 113–120) identified the exploration, description, and classification of the life process in humans as a significant theme for nursing research. Understanding the life process is basic to the further understanding of the human system that is central to nursing (i.e., identification of what constitutes health, well-being, or the optimum functioning of the human). Gortner (1983, p. 5) has stated: "There appears to be a growing consensus on the nature of the research paradigms as representing human responses in health and illness."

The Need for Knowledge of the Interaction Between Client Systems and the Environment

Another focus for nursing research is the interaction between the client and the environment. Nurses need to understand what kinds of client-environmental relationships contribute to greater or lesser well-being. Part of nursing's responsibilities is to promote environmental supports of health. A review of the literature indicates that nurses do value environmental relationships and the climate that exists in the environment in which the client exists. For example, there are repeated studies that indicate the positive factors associated with an environment that promotes mother-infant interaction upon delivery and during the period early after delivery. Curry (1982, p. 73) has studied the effect of early skin-to-skin contact between mother and newborn on the maternal attachment behavior and the mother's self-concept and found no significant difference from the contact on the early attachment behaviors; however, there appeared to be a positive effect on the mother's self-concept. Others have investigated the effects of holding the newborn at delivery on bonding and paternal-fetal attachment behavior (Toney, 1983, pp. 16–19, and Weaver *et al,* 1983, pp. 68–72). The environment associated with diagnostic surgical procedures has also been studied. For example, Scott conducted an investigation of anxiety, critical thinking, and information processing during and after breast biopsy (Scott,

1983, pp. 24–28). Stressful environments have also begun to be studied by nurses. For example, Hurley (1983, pp. 164–169) has studied communication variables and marital conflict stress through voice analysis, and Patterson and McCubbin (1983, pp. 255–264) have studied cumulative life stress and its effect on changes in the health of children with a chronic illness. Upshur (1983, pp. 13–20) has studied four major environmental approaches to providing respite care, a support service for families with disabled members. The environments investigated were homes, group day care, group residential care and adjunct residential programs. Hirschfeld (1983, pp. 23–32), studying home care versus institutionalization of the person with senile brain disease, found that mutuality was a critical factor in the environment for families to be able to give home care. All of these studies contribute to the enlightenment of the nurse about environmental factors and their relationship to client needs in the nursing process. That increased knowledge can then be applied to nursing practice. In addition, such understanding provides data the nurse can use to influence policies and other decisions associated with planning and implementing health care delivery services for the present and future generations.

The Need for Knowledge of Health and Healthy Lifestyles

Newman (1982, p. 87) states: "Health is the least developed component of nursing science and yet the most crucial, since health is designated as the pivotal point of the profession." The phenomena of nursing are the phenomena of health. Dependent on one's view of health, the nurse uses theory to guide actions. Thus, it is important for every individual nurse to make explicit her values about health and to begin to search for the identification of those behaviors that contribute to well-being. Once the assumption is clear about the way one views health, studies will emerge that classify behaviors and life-styles that contribute to greater health. Newman (1982, p. 87) says, ". . . if health were viewed as adaptation to internal and external stimuli, then theory, which guides action to bring about such a state, would differ considerably from that which guides action to promote health if health were viewed as growth, or expanding consciousness."

THE CONTRIBUTION OF NURSING RESEARCH TO THE HEALTH CARE DELIVERY SYSTEM

The quantity of nurses and the qualities of the nursing process make it imperative that the health care delivery system both encourage and acknowledge the value of nursing research. For many years, nurses have been the largest component of the health care delivery system. That factor alone gives them the opportunity to investigate the health care needs and explore the significance and value of nursing care. However, quantity of nurses alone does not lead to a valid assumption that great numbers of nurses are prepared to contribute to improved health care through nursing research. In citing the low number of nurses adequately prepared to do research, Paletta (1980, pp. 4–6) offers a model to enhance the state of nursing research. She suggests that the accomplishment of three objectives are necessary for nursing to fulfill its professional obligations in the delivery of health care:

1. Nursing education will develop programs to educate practitioners skilled in scientific inquiry at all levels of practice.

2. Nursing research will be an integral part of nursing education and nursing practice.
3. Nursing practice will establish an environment receptive to inquiry and professional practice. (Paletta, 1980, pp. 5–6)

It is believed that all three of these objectives are beginning to be achieved in nursing. Although nursing research has been truly recognized for only 20 to 25 years, the cadre of nurses prepared to conduct research is growing, and, perhaps more importantly, many nurses are beginning to value the need for research and the positive outcomes that research data yield. Nurses are beginning to recognize the power that comes from data-based information rather than opinion. That power can be seen in the emerging influence that nursing plays in shaping the policy decisions about health care delivery at the local, state, federal, and even international levels. Research is providing that necessary data base, which not only is vital to policy decisions, but also to nursing practice outcomes.

Recent evidence of support for nursing research is shown in the recommendations of the Institute of Medicine to Congress about support for funding of nursing. Based on the survey data about the proportion of the nursing population prepared to conduct research, the lack of research to inform nursing practice and to enhance nursing education, and the great need for research, the Institute of Medicine strongly supported increased funding for preparation of nurse researchers and the conduct of nursing research (Institute of Medicine, 1983).

Client Needs for Nursing Services

A profession offers the public a needed service. In times of limited resources it is particularly critical that the need for the service offered be clearly documented with data about clients and potential clients that substantiates that nursing is needed in order to promote, maintain, or restore health. Data that direct planning and policy-makers about which nursing services are needed must also be gathered. The more data a profession has to support that some particular nursing service is needed, the more likely it is that service will be funded. Opinions based on the values and stereotypes of the professional rather than actual data about the recipients are likely to be less effective arguments for funding a service. It is critical that nursing's commitment of resources and nursing's service to clients be based on data systematically collected in a controlled way. Much nursing research is needed that substantiates the important roles the nurse plays in offering services that improve the health status of the public. It is generally accepted that until nursing documents its significance in the delivery of care to clients, nursing will not be fully supported for the accomplishment of its professional goals, will not be viewed by the public as a vital member of the health care team, and will not gain control over its work policies, protocols, work environment, and/or reimbursement. To the extent that nurses can gather data through the research process, they increase the likelihood of an improved image for nursing held by clients, other health care delivery team members, and by nursing itself. Such client data build a strong case for nursing meeting the professional criterion of providing a needed human service.

Oda (1983, p. 10) reminds nurse researchers that they need the voluntary cooperation of subjects, that they need "to have empathy for the research subjects and be aware of the demands or effects that participation will have on them." In conducting research to establish client needs, the nurse researcher has the opportunity to establish mutually agreed-upon goals. The nurse presents the significance of the study of client needs in terms of what it has the potential to do for them, that is, that the findings reflect sincere interest in understanding them (clients) better and that the establishment of a clear picture of their (clients') needs is done for the purpose of offering better nursing care so that the health needs of the public can be better served. In addition to providing a data base on which decisions can be made, such nursing research could serve to enhance the image of nursing in the eyes of the subjects. That image-building activity with the public it serves can enhance the potential for nursing to practice in a way more acceptable to its practitioners, in a way that is responsible for and accountable to its constituency, and in a way in which nursing has control of decisions, policies, and protocols.

An example of nurses trying to use research strategies to demonstrate client needs for nursing services is the collaborative research of nurses in five eastern states and Washington, D.C. for purposes of studying the implications of "governmental budget cuts on access to maternity care and on perinatal morbidity" (The American Nurse, 1983, p. 1). Legislators and policy-makers are influenced more by information provided by data than by requests based on professional opinion.

Cost-Effectiveness of Professional Nursing Activities in Primary, Secondary, and Tertiary Health Care Delivery Systems

Perhaps the most influential data that professional nursing can provide through nursing research today is that obtained about costs. After a long era of continually spiraling health costs, the public now demands more accountability for the spending of health care dollars. If nursing is to act responsibly for the health care dollar, nurses must know the cost-effectiveness of nursing care in all kinds of health care delivery systems: primary, secondary, and tertiary. A spokesperson for the profession on the economic value of nursing research, Fagin (1982, p. 1) emphasizes, "There is no question that improved quality of care carries an economic value." She urges nurse researchers to measure economic dimensions along with the dimension of improvement of the quality of care. She suggests that the profession's research on economic value can be categorized into four areas: the organization of nursing services, the testing of specific nursing interventions (including roles, procedures, and technology), the comparison of effectiveness of nurses to other providers of health care, and alternate or nontraditional models of practice.

Brooten reported on past studies of nursing that addressed the continuing needs for the care of low birthweight infants. She concludes that the rate of low birthweight infants is unlikely to change in the near future and that "efforts to improve their outcomes and to control the costs of their care will continue" (Brooten, 1983, p. 83). She validates the importance of nursing research that examines "alternative models of care that are efficacious, that justify their costs, and that promote the image and self-determination of the profession in advancing its practice" (Brooten, 1983, p. 83).

Intensive care units, which have grown rapidly in the past two decades, have become significant work environments for hospital nurses today. Draper reports that intensive care is three times more costly than regular hospital care and that large investments have been made in that form of delivery although the "efficacy of intensive care has yet to be firmly substantiated" (Draper, 1983, pp. 90–91). Nurses are concerned with the questions of improved survival and quality of life as well as the temporary efficacy of physiologic ICU treatments. Nurses have begun to address these concerns through research. For example, Draper (1983, pp. 90–94) reports on her work with colleagues at the ICU Research Center at George Washington University. They are studying the types of clients that are admitted to ICUs, what kinds of services ICU clients are receiving, and the client benefits of their ICU services. Costs of such forms of care continue to be evaluated against the benefits of such care for ICU clients. Nursing must continue to systematically assess its value in every setting in which care is delivered. Costs outcomes could provide directions to the policy-makers and resource allocators, who, in turn, could assist nurses to practice in the most cost-effective modes of delivery. That, no doubt, would serve the public most in improving its health status.

The need for nursing research is evident. The contribution that nursing research makes to the delivery of health care is substantiated. The baccalaureate-prepared nurse can contribute to nursing research in several ways:

1. Use nursing research findings to guide nursing practice.
2. Value a sense of inquiry about the phenomenon of nursing.
3. Participate in research projects if opportunity is provided.
4. Refine abilities to collect, organize, categorize, and analyze data.
5. Suggest nursing research questions that need to be addressed to improve practice.

In order to participate in the above ways, one must have an understanding of the research process.

OVERVIEW OF THE RESEARCH PROCESS IN NURSING

The objective of this section is to assist the student in understanding the components of the research process to the extent that the logical steps of inquiry can be described and pursued in greater detail as she continues to develop abilities as a researcher in nursing. This section serves only as an overview for the process. "Remember, conducting a study using the research process is a systematic, planned activity that can be thought of as a chain of reasoning" (Dempsey and Dempsey, 1981, p. 22). Beginning with the nurse's query about some aspect of nursing, the research process structures the systematic investigation of that question and the reporting of the answers and new questions about that aspect of nursing. The research process follows the methods of science, which essentially means that the process has an identifiable order, includes controls over factors not being investigated, includes the gathering of evidence about the question, is built on a theoretical framework, and operates for the purpose of applying results to improve the practice of nursing.

Sensitivity to the Need to Raise Questions about the Domain of Nursing

The most significant step in the nursing process may be the first one, that is, the nurse's articulation of a question that needs to be answered for the purpose of increasing professional understanding to better serve the public. Nurses are accountable for asking questions that reflect sensitivity to the need to better understand all that is within the domain of nursing. These domains include the client in terms of his response to his health status, the nurse in terms of professional characteristics and responsibilities, the environment in which both exist, the dynamics of health, and the interactions among all these factors in the nursing domain.

Knowledge of the following steps of research will facilitate the nurse's use of findings in practice.

Focus on the Problem Area

From where do the questions that need to be answered about nursing arise? From these questions, which ones require research for adequate response? Which ones have sufficient data already for effective problem-solving? Polit and Hungler (1983, p. 62) suggest that the experience of the professional person can be used to raise questions because that experience calls on the nurse to make decisions, some of which have little support in theory or research findings. The integrity and efficacy of the nursing process depend on the nurse's ability to systematically explore the questions raised. Fuller (1982, p. 61) suggests that the nurse can use professional experience as a basis for questions needing investigation. She also encourages nurses to specify the focus on a problem area by reviewing the current research and other information on a topic of interest. Polit and Hungler (1983, pp. 63–64) suggest that another source of problem questions can be elaborated from the theoretical basis or conceptual model used to guide practice, research, and education in nursing.

The development of the research problem, according to Polit and Hungler (1983) incorporates the following sequential steps:

1. Note a general area of interest about which you have some questions.
2. Narrow the topic through critical evaluation of ideas with mentor or expert. That evaluation must address feasibility and worth.
3. Establish the benefit of the investigation of the selected problem to nursing by addressing who will benefit, what are the applications, what is the potential for the results to be relevant to theoretical basis of practice, and does anyone care about the potential findings (how important is it to nursing practice or education?).
4. Establish that the problem selected is amenable to scientific methodology and is not chiefly a moral issue.
5. Critique the feasibility of the problem in terms of time factors, availability of subjects, cooperation required, necessary facilities and equipment, and costs.

The initial review of the literature will help to accomplish these steps in the early development of the problem.

Initial Review of the Literature

Once the researcher has raised a question, an initial review of the literature is helpful in identifying the major variables in the area of interest, finding out what is already known, gathering feasibility data on the needs for investigation of that question, and refining the focus of the problem to be investigated.

Fawcett states that a review of the literature should be used to evaluate scientific merit. She points out the need for replication of studies: "Repeated study of the same research question in different settings using different samples or populations and conducted by different investigators helps to establish the generalizability of research findings" (Fawcett, 1982, p. 57). In light of the need for generalizability that increases scientific merit, nursing researchers perhaps need to more vigorously use the literature as a source for developing a nursing research problem—to look for studies that need replication. Fawcett (1982, p. 57) reported that she found only five replication studies in a review of two major nursing research journals over an 18-month period encompassing the reports of 145 studies. Beginning nursing researchers could be assisted in developing research skills by conducting replication studies. The contribution to the scientific base of nursing from replication studies could be enormous.

The review of the literature should serve to make the researcher aware of all the possible relevant material available about a problem of interest. Materials helpful to the location of the resource material are indexes from nursing, related disciplines, and popular literature; abstracting services from nursing and related disciplines; computer searches; dictionaries; encyclopedias; guides; and directories (Fox, 1982, pp. 100–104). Reference librarians in most libraries are able to help the beginning nurse researcher with all these materials.

In summary, the initial review of the literature should serve the purpose of answering some questions about the topic of interest, describing other peoples' interests in the topic, and developing a strong knowledge base of what has been written and reported on the topic (Gunter, 1981, p. 11). Such a knowledge base makes it possible for the researcher to move on to the next stage of research, that is, specifying the problem and defining the variables.

Specification of Problems and Defining Variables

Once the initial review of the literature is completed and the researcher has gained an understanding of the research topic in general and possesses a sense of what kinds of studies exist about the area of interest, the researcher is able to more clearly delineate the problem to be investigated. A decision is made about exactly what is to be investigated, that is, what part of the domain of nursing is to be studied. The nurse researcher may be investigating some aspect of the client that is clearly important to understand in the nursing process, some health phenomenon of the client, some client outcomes associated with particular nursing interventions, some aspect of the nurse-client relationship, some aspect of the delivery of nursing care services, some aspect of the environment that affects the health status, or any combination of these factors in the nursing domain.

The clear articulation of the problem incorporates the identification of the phenomenon to be investigated. Generally, this research phenomenon is called a *variable*. A variable is a characteristic, a trait, a property, or a condition. If the variable is purposefully manipulated by the researcher in order to observe and measure another variable, it is called an *independent variable*. The variable that is observed and measured and is presumed to be influenced by or related in some special way to the independent variable is called the *dependent variable*. An example of a problem to be investigated that has one variable that is manipulated and another that is observed and measured is: What is the relationship between specific parenting guidance by the professional nurse and the development of positive nutritional habits of the toddler? The independent variable in this investigation is the specific parenting guidance and the dependent variable is the nutritional habits of the toddler.

In order to make these variables measurable, the researcher must determine exactly what is meant by each of the variables—what constitutes parenting guidance and what constitutes positive nutritional habits in the toddler. The statement of the problem may be in the form of a question or a declaration. In both cases, the problem statement must also clearly identify who is to be studied as well as what is to be studied. In order for a problem to be appropriate for research in nursing, Diers (1979, pp. 13–15) suggests that it should meet three criteria: (1) It should reflect a difference that matters to nursing, that is, it should be significant to the domain of nursing; (2) It should show a relationship to general and conceptual issues, that is, it has the potential of contributing to nursing knowledge; (3) The investigator must have access to and control of the phenomenon to be studied, that is, measurement must be possible.

Establishment of Tentative Propositions—Hypotheses and the Second Review of the Literature

After the nurse researcher has clarified the problem under investigation, studied the data available, and recalled observations from professional experiences, the investigator may formulate a hypothesis. All studies do not require that the researcher state hypotheses. For example, surveys, historical studies, and studies that are exploratory in nature do not require hypotheses. The purpose of such studies is to identify or describe variables that are significant to nursing. If, however, the researcher designs a study that requires the manipulation of an independent variable and the measurement of a dependent variable, hypotheses must be stated and tested. "A hypothesis is a conjectural statement, a tentative proposition, about the relation between two or more . . . variables" (Kerlinger, 1964, p. 15). Nurses have excellent opportunities to form some hunches about the relationships between variables they observe in practice. Thought of as bridges, hypotheses connect theory with observation and are derived from observations, reasoning, and theory. "Hypotheses are the only scientific means today by which conjectured relations between and among variables can be tested" (Trussell, *et al,* 1981, p. 107).

Since the hypothesis can be viewed as an "untested proposition about a population" (Armstrong, 1981, p. 31), the researcher writes it to reflect accurately the testing to be done. Armstrong suggests the following points in developing and writing hypotheses:

1. They are neutral in tone rather than biased by the investigator.
2. They are parsimonius in wording.
3. They are written in present tense.
4. All variables are precisely defined.
5. The dependent and independent variables are precisely identified.
6. The means of measuring the dependent variable is disclosed. (Armstrong, 1981, p. 37)

Hypotheses are tested statistically in relation to the laws of chance, thus are based on statistical probability and incur an element of risk. How much risk can be afforded is a judgement of the investigator. When permanent or serious consequences are involved the investigator cannot afford to take too many risks (Trussell *et al,* 1981, p. 107). Since hypotheses sometimes force the investigator to infer the findings on the sample to the population, the researcher uses probability statistics for testing. The degree of risks one takes is called the *level of significance* (Trussell *et al*, 1981, p. 108). Significance means that the relationship between variables comes out of something other than chance. At the stage in research when the researcher is determining hypotheses, further review of the literature is used to evaluate testing procedures and to project a research design appropriate for the investigation of the variable(s). Fox advises that the researcher specifically uses this review of the literature to learn what investigative methods have been used, how data has been collected and analyzed, and "what has and has not been successful in previous research" (Fox, 1982, p. 35).

In summary, hypotheses are stated in order to declare the researcher's proposition about the relationship between variables and serve as the means for testing the proposed relationship.

Determination of the Type of Research Design that is Suitable

The nurse researcher selects the type of research design suitable for the study on the basis of the appropriate approach to inquiry, either descriptive, experimental, or historical. In the descriptive approach, the design is based on describing the on-going events of the present. In the experimental approach, the design is based on the need to manipulate a specific variable in order to measure the effect on other variables. In the historic approach, the design is based on the desire to describe and/or evaluate past events (Dempsey and Dempsey, 1981, p. 10).

Development of Measurement Methods and Instruments

After the approach is selected for a particular study, the researcher must decide on the appropriate method for gathering the data on the variables. Although there is a wide variety of techniques for collecting data, all techniques are a variation of three methods: observation, questioning, and measurement (Fox, 1982, p. 194). The method selected for a particular research project is based on the purpose for data-gathering. Fox (1982, pp. 194–195) classifies purposes as:

1. Information seeking. The purpose is to gain knowledge about a phenomenon.
2. Ordering. The purpose is to learn how the subject orders a set of items in terms of some criterion.
3. Evaluation or appraisal. The purpose is to evaluate some phenomenon.
4. Behavioral description. The purpose is to describe specific behavior(s) in nursing context.
5. Provide the basis for inference or prediction. The purpose is to investigate the dynamics that motivate human behavior in order to infer or predict behavior.

Depending on the purpose of the research, the investigator selects instruments for the collection of data. As noted earlier, those instruments generally are categorized under three methods: observation, questioning, and measurement. Examples of data collection instruments from these categories are critical incidents, tests, interviews, questionnaires, checklists, records, scales, and physical measurement techniques. It is suggested that an effective way to select an instrument is to try out instrument(s) in trial testing, that is, run a pilot study for purposes of selecting and adapting instruments to measure variables (Ackerman and Lohnes, 1981, p. 70; Fox and Ventura, 1983, pp. 122–125). The researcher strives to select a measurement tool that is appropriate to answer the research question, is not biased, and has precision in measuring the variables under study. The beginning researcher is encouraged to use data collection tools that are already in existence. Sometimes, however, no tools exist. Hymovich (1981, p. 71), for example, reported that no tool was available for assessing the impact of chronic illness on family development nor for assessing the outcome of interventions, thus, she and her colleagues developed the chronicity impact and coping instrument in the form of a parent questionnaire.

What is important about the data collection technique is that it must provide the researcher with reliability and validity. *Reliability* is that attribute of the instrument that means that it will produce accurate, stable data over time. *Validity* is the characteristic of the instrument that means that the instrument actually measures what it purports to measure (Fox, 1982, pp. 259–260).

In addition to selecting the instruments for data collection during this stage of research, the nurse must also determine the composition of the sample, establish a process for collecting data from the sample, and prepare a format for the collection of data, classification of data, and storage of data for later analysis. The sample of subjects must be clearly described and the method for choosing the subjects must be appropriate. The number in the sample selected must meet statistical requirements in order to appropriately draw conclusions about the findings.

Assurance of an Ethical Process

Essential to the conduct of scientific inquiry in any discipline is the assurance of an ethical process for the subjects. Protection of human rights must be assured (Dempsey and Dempsey, 1981, p. 256). That protection is provided primarily by the provision of informed consent and freedom from harm. Informed consent means that the subject is provided with a clear description of what the study is about and how he fits into the study. The subject must understand and consent to the particular role he plays in the study. Having given informed consent does not prohibit the subject from changing his mind any time during the study and withdrawing from the study. Protection from harm means just that—the investigator will not knowingly do anything that will harm or abuse the subject.

Collection of Data

After protection for human rights is assured for all subjects, the data can be collected. Before subjects can even be approached, however, the investigator must have approval from appropriate agency personnel if subjects are associated with an institution. The researcher or a specified data collector then orients each subject clearly and concisely to the method of data collection. Then the data collection instrument is administered to each subject in the same manner. Throughout this implementation stage of the research process, the investigator follows the written proposal (in the methodology) as closely as possible. In the process of collecting data, the researcher records the data on the prepared forms developed earlier. Then the data are ready to be classified and organized to be ready for analysis.

Analysis of Data and Report of Findings

Data are organized in a manner that makes it amenable to analysis. If the researcher's goal is simply to display the data that is found, no analysis other than the narrative description of the displayed data is needed. If, however, the researcher aims to infer some characteristics about a population or to evaluate some relationship between variables, the organized data must be subjected to statistical analysis. Computations are done. If hypotheses have been stated, statistical testing of those hypotheses must be done. Electronic data processing is usually available for such analyses (Mason, 1981, pp. 108–109).

On the basis of accurate analysis of the data, the researcher must report the findings exactly as they occurred. Summaries of the data must reflect the individual subject's findings exactly. All data that has been collected for purposes of testing the hypotheses must be reported. Tables, charts, and graphs are commonly used to present data. They need to be pertinent, clear, and well labeled, and they need to be discussed in the text of the research report (Dempsey and Dempsey, 1981, p. 257). The reports of the findings are then used to draw conclusions.

Conclusions and Implications

Using the theoretical framework on which the study is based and the analysis of the data collected, the researcher must then determine the meaning of those findings and their value to nursing. Findings are analyzed first by inspection of the statistical tests performed to test the hypotheses or evaluate data. Then the researcher must interpret what the numerical analysis means. Abbott proposes that the researcher generally interprets the findings in one of four ways: positive, which means the findings supported the predicted relationship and demonstrated statistical significance, that is, findings were not due to chance alone; negative, which means the results were not in the predicted direction; contradictory, which means that part of the findings were positive and part were negative; and unanticipated findings, which means that an unpredicted relationship was discovered (Abbott, 1981, p. 132).

Based on the analysis and interpretation of data, generalizations might be made about "the meaning of the data and its relevance to groups different from the sample" (Abbott, 1981, p. 132). Generalizations should emerge only from the findings and the researcher should not go beyond the data as a result of the excitement generated by scientific discovery. The inferences on which the generalizations are based are the product of tested and untested concepts and specific findings in a given population, thus, it is not appropriate or accurate to generalize to great extents. The generalizations that are made are influential in nursing practice, education, and research. The more valid those generalizations are, the more useful they are in application to the practice of professional nursing as well as to the development of the theory base for nursing.

The implications of the study are usually related to one of the three aspects of professional nursing: practice with clients, education of the professional, and further research in nursing. Implications are generally reported in the section of a research study called recommendations. The implications are spelled out for practice, that is, how it affects the nursing process with clients. Recommendations are usually given for the impact that the findings should have on the education of its practitioners and on future research that needs to be conducted. If the recommendations are clearly and concisely stated and are derived logically, they are the power of the study. Indeed, nursing practice based on research findings and recommendations is a primary goal of the science of nursing (Abbott, 1981, pp. 133–134).

The Written Report

Research completed but not written up is wasted. It can be argued that the research process is really not complete until it is shared in writing or some other public medium. Abbott (1981, p. 135) clearly states the purpose of a research report: "The purpose of a research report is to present in an organized fashion a research project that has been designed, implemented, and analyzed." Characteristics of an effective research report are brevity, clarity, and complete objectivity. Although there are variations on the form of the report that may be determined by faculty, the style manual used, or other institutional requirements, the usual report follows the outline of the research process presented in this chapter. Most outlines develop the areas of the problem statement, the review of literature, the methods of investigation, the presentation of findings, the discussion of the analyses and conclusions, the bibliographic data, and the appendixes. The reader is directed to either a nursing research book or a writing style manual for specific guidance in developing each of these parts of the written research report.

THE RICHNESS OF POTENTIAL FOR NURSING RESEARCH TODAY

A visit to a college or university today reveals the strides that nursing has made in developing research and researchers. Among the many nursing journals one can find at least six major research journals. These journals reflect important strengths of an emerging profession. However, according to Smith (1979, p. 75), who reviewed theses, doctoral dissertations, journals, newsletters, and textbooks, the research is primarily limited to individual efforts and there is no obvious, structured, coherent system in developing the theoretical base for nursing. As the profession emerges from its scientific childhood characterized by individual efforts, it moves into an era marked by cooperative and later collaborative efforts. This developmental principle suggests that the future for nursing research holds not only critical responsibilities for the development of a scientific identity for the profession, but also the significant rewards that go with the maturing process.

RECOMMENDATIONS FOR NURSING RESEARCH—PROFESSIONAL ACCOUNTABILITY

Central to the growth and development of any profession is research to develop and validate the theory on which the profession is built. Also essential to any practice discipline is research to validate principles and techniques of practice. Nursing, which is viewed as a practice discipline, thus critically needs nursing research for purposes of the establishment of the theoretical base for the profession and nursing research that is concerned with the direct application of knowledge in nursing practice. Further, it is imperative that this practice research not only focus on the outcomes of nursing practice in terms of the human's health, but also must measure cost-effectiveness in the delivery of professional nursing practice as part of the broader system of health care delivery.

Recommendations

In 1983, two major documents were published that reflected the urgent and comprehensive need, as well as support, for research in nursing: the National Commission on Nursing's *Summary Report and Recommendations* and the Institute of Medicine's report *Nursing and Nursing Education: Public Policies and Private Actions.* See Chapter 18 and Appendix A for more information on the Institute of Medicine study.

Citing the great need for doctorally prepared nurses to lead in research and theory development for the profession, the Institute of Medicine reported that in 1980 there were approximately 4,000 doctorally prepared nurses, 50% of whom were in faculty positions; however, only 6% of those indicated that research was their major activity; thus, the greatest need for doctorally prepared nurses in the next 5 years is in the area of research and theory development, where it is projected that 371 more persons are needed. The second greatest need for doctorally prepared nurses was for leadership preparation in clinical practice, where that need was projected to be 359 persons. Comparing the proportion of nursing faculty with doctorates in programs of nursing where doctoral degrees are offered, the study showed that 35% of such programs' nursing faculty possessed earned doctorates, whereas, 90% of engineering and science faculties held earned doctorates (Institute of Medicine, 1983, pp. 136–137).

The Institute of Medicine study (IOM study) suggested that the nurses prepared for advanced clinical practice could make great impact by translating research into practice. "The advanced degree nurse prepared to remain current in a specialty can use research findings to develop appropriate nursing interventions and, acting as a teacher and role model can ensure that the most efficacious regimens are followed by the staff" (Institute of Medicine, 1983, p. 140). The IOM group recommended that Congress should expand federal support to increase fellowships, loans, and program support at the graduate level, both masters and doctoral, in order to increase the population's access to education to prepare for research among other needs. Another recommendation was, "The federal government should establish an organizational entity to place nursing research in the mainstream of scientific investigation" (Institute of Medicine, 1983, p. 19). They believed that a national focal point was needed to promote research, inform nursing and other health care workers of such research, and increase the potential for discovery and application of methods to improve patient outcomes. Research specifically to provide "scientifically valid measurements of the knowledge and performance competencies of nurses with various levels and types of educational preparation and experience" was indicated to be an area of great need, thus, this study recommended federal and private funding to support such research. To properly plan for financial support to prepare nursing's manpower, real evidence of performance differences among graduates from different types of preparatory programs is needed. Other research needs indicated for manpower planning and decision-making were the needs for the systematic collection and analysis of data on nurse supply and demand. Finally, in relation to research, the IOM group called for research to evaluate promising management approaches. Guidelines are needed that reflect the most useful management approaches in achieving the goals of professional nurse retention and higher quality client care (Institute of Medicine, 1983, p. 216).

The National Commission on Nursing recommendations that reflect the need for and significance of nursing research were:

1. Nursing Practice. "High priority should be given to nursing research and to preparation of nurse researchers. Through research, nurses can test, refine, and advance the knowledge base on which improved education and practice must rest." (National Commission on Nursing, 1983, p. 11)
2. Nursing Education
   a. "Current trends in nursing toward pursuit of . . . advanced degrees for clinical specialization, administration, teaching, and research should be facilitated.
   b. To assist these trends toward baccalaureate and higher degree preparation, the profession must outline the common body of knowledge . . . essential for nursing practice . . ." (National Commission on Nursing, 1983, p. 15)

The Commission envisioned that the current trends in the profession will influence the health care providers to experiment with new ways to deliver cost-effective quality patient care (National Commission on Nursing, 1983, p. 22). Since nursing constitutes the largest professional group in the delivery system, it must assume a leadership role in conducting research to measure cost-effective quality care outcomes for the consumers. In order to provide competent practitioners who can assume full professional responsibility for the practice of nursing, nursing education must reflect research based practice in its programs.

For each of nursing's key relationships, the Commission suggested action plans and research projects that could be used to enhance the future effectiveness of nursing care (Table 6–1).

Inherent in all of the recent recommendations for nursing research is the belief that progress in achieving the goals of the profession can best be made if nursing education and practice decisions, plans, and policies are based on verified data rather than opinion and bias. That process of verification occurs only if the controls of scientific research are employed.

The Researcher in "The Information Era"

High technology offers great support for the researcher today. The storage, retrieval, and analysis of data afforded by computer support makes the time factor much more appealing and possible for many nurses to conduct research. In most of the educational and practice settings in the immediate future, one should not have to manually manage data. Another great help to research that the computer offers is that its ability to "crunch numbers" opens up almost unlimited analysis of data. Thus, one can use one's findings to a fuller capacity. It is anticipated that the word-processing supports offered by computers should be helpful in getting more research findings shared with more people. Thus, nursing is moving into a period of valuing and conducting research at a time when technology is greatly supportive to many aspects of the research process.

The Nurse as Scholar-Researcher: The Essential Element in Changing the Public Image of Nurses and Nursing

Traditionally nurses have not been viewed as scholars. As a result, their higher education and research productivity have been extremely limited. What the public has seen is a group of nurses in which 70% or more have less than a bachelor's de-

TABLE 6–1.   Research Projects Needed to Enhance Future Effectiveness in
              Nursing Care

Relationships	Research Projects
Nurses/Physicians/Health care administrators/Hospital trustees	Research to determine under what conditions multidisciplinary health care teams function efficiently and effectively.
Nurses/Health Care institutions	Career ladder programs—evaluation research to determine: 1. Which features promote excellence in clinical patient care and desired advancement of nurses in clinical, management, education, and research roles 2. The effects of these features on the quality and cost of patient care and nurse retention and turnover rates 3. Factors that influence nurse advancement, such as education, experience, tenure, and personal and other factors Studies of nursing in rural areas are needed to evaluate: 1. Patient needs 2. Needed knowledge, skills, and composition of registered nurses. 3. Data base to establish special programs for RNs desiring graduate study in rural nursing.
Nurses/Nursing profession	Nurse researchers, clinical specialists, nurse educators, and nurse administrators could engage in research to develop and test the knowledge base used in clinical nursing care and identify ways to use nurses' patient care experiences to identify areas for nursing research that can be practically applied.
Nursing profession/Nursing education	Research to evaluate variables in effective arrangements to retain and expand existing educational resources and to develop new types of educational programs that result in quality nursing education and accessibility to students.
Nursing education/Nursing practice	Research to determine features that influence the effectiveness of health care institutions that successfully assimilate nurses following graduation and promote development of clinical knowledge and skill. Research to evaluate and define features that promote or hinder cooperation be-

(*Table continues on p. 112*)

TABLE 6–1.   Research Projects Needed to Enhance Future Effectiveness in Nursing Care (*Continued*)

Relationships	Research Projects
	tween nursing education and practice, such as evaluation of linkages that should be in place to promote cooperation of universities and health care agencies.
	Research about theory and organizational designs for effective integration of education and practice and mechanisms and conditions that more fully develop nursing's clinical roles.
Nursing/Public	Data base gathered through nursing research should be shared by nurses who act as participants in state and regional planning. Such participation should ensure adequacy, availability, and appropriateness of educational programs for nurses.

(Modified from: National Commission on Nursing: Summary Report and Recommendations. Chicago, The Hospital Research and Educational Trust, 1983)

gree. That lack of credentialing alone probably explains the very tiny proportion of researchers in nursing. However, as nursing has developed its own theory base in the last quarter-century, nurses have begun to value the scholarship role of the nurse. Most nurses today would probably agree that a practice based on research is desirable. Capitalizing on that agreement the profession could begin to present a different image to the public. In order to actualize the motivation to base nursing practice on research, educational programs need to prepare students in scientific inquiry while preparing them to apply theory in the conduct of professional roles.

Matejski (1979, p. 80) supports the idea that nursing activities focus on assisting man to maintain, attain, and/or regain health and that, to do this, the nurse must possess knowledge about the influence of culture, social attitudes, and economics on health as well as the sciences that develop understanding of man and his environment. As the profession begins to educate more nurses in these areas, it is more likely that the public will begin to see a scholarly side of nursing. It is also likely to help nurses feel like scholars and react like scholars. If the profession nourishes this scholarship in nurses, it will undoubtedly help change the image of the nurse. Because scholars accept that research is a vital component of nursing, the development of scholars will increase the supply of researchers and the profession and the public will be better served.

The 1960s and the 1970s represented the era in which many researchers and scholars provided a beginning theory base for nursing. The 1980s and 1990s represent an era in which researchers and scholars will be more significant to the emergence of nursing as an autonomous profession and to the provision of better nursing services to the public.

REFERENCES

Abbott NK: The research report. *In* Krampitz S, Pavlovich N (eds): Readings for Nursing Research. St Louis, CV Mosby, 1981

Ackerman WB, Lohnes PR: Research Methods for Nurses. New York, McGraw Hill, 1981

American Association of Colleges of Nursing: Nursing Research Position Statement. Washington, DC, American Association of Colleges of Nursing, 1981

Armstrong RL: Hypothesis formulation. *In* Krampitz S, Pavlovich N (eds): Readings for Nursing Research. St Louis, CV Mosby, 1981

Brooten D: Issues for research on alternative patterns of care for low birthweight infants. Image 15:80–83, 1983

Brooten DA, Brown LP, Hollingsworth AO et al: A comparison of four treatments to prevent and control breast pain and engorgement in nonnursing mothers. Nurs Res 32:225–229, 1983

Chinn PL, Jacobs MK: Theory and Nursing—A Systematic Approach. St Louis, CV Mosby, 1983

Cronenwett LR, Brickman P: Models of helping and coping in childbirth. Nurs Res 32:84–88, 1983

Curry MA: Maternal attachment behavior and the mother's self concept: The effect of early skin-to-skin contact. Nurs Res 31:73, 1982

Dempsey PA, Dempsey AD: The Research Process in Nursing. New York, D Van Nostrand, 1981

Derdiarian AK: An instrument for theory and research development using the behavioral systems model for nursing. I. Nurs Res 32:196–201, 1983

Diers D: Research in Nursing Practice. Philadelphia, JB Lippincott, 1979

Donaldson S, Crowley D: The discipline of nursing. Nurs Outlook 26:113–120, 1978

Draper EA: Benefits and costs of intensive care. Image 15:90–94, 1983

Fagin CM: The economic value of nursing research. Paper presented at Council of Nurse Researchers Meeting, American Nurses Association, Washington, DC, June 27, 1982

Fawcett J: Utilization of nursing research findings. Image 14:57–59, 1982

Fox DJ: Fundamentals of Research in Nursing, ed 4. Norwalk, Conn, Appleton-Century-Crofts, 1982

Fox RN, Ventura MR: Small-scale administration of instruments and procedures. Nurs Res 32:122–125, 1983

Fuller EO: Selecting a Clinical Problem for Research. Image 14:60–61, 1982

Gagan JM: Methodological notes on empathy. Adv Nurs Sci 5:65–72, 1983

Gilliss CL: The family as a unit of analysis: Strategies for the nurse researcher. Adv Nurs Sci 5:50–59, 1983

Gortner S: The history and philosophy of nursing science and research. Adv Nurs Sci 5:1–8, 1983

Gunter L: Literature review. *In* Kramptiz S, Pavlovich N (eds): Readings for Nursing Research. St Louis, CV Mosby, 1981

Hanson HA, Chater S: Role selection by nurses: Managerial interests and personal attributes. Nurs Res 32:48–52, 1983

Hirschfeld M: Homecare versus institutionalization: Family care-giving and senile brain disease. Int J Nurs Study 20:23–32, 1983

Hurley PM: Communication variables and voice analysis of marital conflict stress. Nurs Res 32:164–169, 1983

Hymovich DM: Assessing the impact of chronic childhood illness on the family and parent coping. Image 13:71–74, 1981

Institute of Medicine, Division of Health Care Services: Nursing and Nursing Education: Public Policies and Private Actions. Washington, DC, National Academy Press, 1983

Kerlinger FN: Foundations of Behavioral Research. New York, Holt, Rinehart & Winston, 1964

Kishi KI: Communication patterns of health teaching and information recall. Nurs Res 32:230–235, 1983

Mason D: Data analysis: Introduction. *In* Krampitz S, Pavlovich N (eds): Readings for Nursing Research. St Louis, CV Mosby, 1981

Matejski MP: Humanities: The nurse and historical research. Image 11:80–85, 1979

Melnyk KAM: The process of theory analysis: An examination of the theory of Dorothea E. Orem. Nurs Res 32:170–174, 1983

Miles MS, Crandall EKB: The search for meaning and its potential for affecting growth in bereaved parents. Health Values: Achieving High Level Wellness 7:19–23, 1983

Moore D: Preprared childbirth and marital satisfaction during the antepartum and post partum periods. Nurs Res 32:73–79, 1983

National Commission on Nursing: Summary Report and Recommendations. Chicago, The Hospital Research and Educational Trust, 1983

Newman MA: What differentiates clinical research? Image 14:86–88, 1982

Oda DS: Social and political facilitation of research. Adv Nurs Sci 5:9–15, 1983

Paletta JL: Nursing research: An integral part of professional nursing. Image 12:3–6, 1980

Patterson JM, McCubbin HI: The impact of family life events and changes on the health of a chronically ill child. Fam Rel 32:255–264, 1983

Polit DF, Hungler B: Nursing Research: Principles and Methods. Philadelphia, JB Lippincott, 1983

Scott D: Anxiety, critical thinking and information processing during and after breast biopsy. Nurs Res 32:24–28, 1983

Smith MC: Proposed metaparadigm for nursing research and theory development. Image 11:75–79, 1979

Steel J: Editorial: Statement moves us to focus on what nurses fix. Am Nurs 16:4, January 1984

Tinkle MB, Beaton JL: Toward a new view of science: Implications for nursing research. Adv Nurs Sci 5:27–36, 1983

Toney L: The effects of holding the newborn at delivery on paternal bonding. Nurs Res 32:16–19, 1983

Trussell P, Brandt A, Knapp S: Using Nursing Research: Discovery, Analysis, and Interpretation. Wakefield, Mass, Nursing Resources, 1981

Upshur CC: Developing respite care: A support service for families with disabled members. Fam Rel 32:13–20, 1983

Weaver RH, Harding R, Cranley MS: An exploration of paternal-fetal attachment behavior. Nurs Res 32:68–72, 1983

Chapter 7

Theories as a Basis for Practice

THOUGHT QUESTIONS

1. Does any type of theory seem "the best," or might any of the theories be applied in particular situations?
2. What are the strengths and weaknesses of each of the theories?
3. How would each theory affect the nature of nursing intervention?

Nurses have traditionally based their practice on intuition, experience, or "the way I was taught." These methods lead to rote and stereotypic practice. The value of theories is that they provide bases for hypotheses about practice that make it possible to derive a rationale for nursing actions. Theories that are testable will provide a knowledge base for the science of nursing. As the science of nursing develops, nurses will be able to more accurately understand and explain past events, and provide a basis for prediction and control of future events. In addition, practice based on science will support the image of nursing as a professional discipline.

A theory is a "logically interconnected set of propositions used to describe, explain, and predict, a part of the empirical world" (Riehl and Roy, 1980, p. 5). By taking individual concepts, such as man, society, health, and nursing, and developing statements of possible relationships between them, a theory makes it possible "to systematically explain approaches to nursing care and to predict outcomes" (Torres, 1980, p. 4).

Torres (1980, pp. 5–7) suggested the following characteristics of theories:

1. "Theories can interrelate concepts in such a way as to create a different way of looking at a particular phenomenon.
2. Theories must be logical in nature.
3. Theories can be the bases for hypotheses that can be tested.
4. Theories contribute to and assist in increasing the general body of knowledge within the discipline through the research implemented to validate them.
5. Theories can be utilized by practitioners to guide and improve their practice.

115

6. Theories must be consistent with other validated theories, laws and principles."

It has been suggested that different levels of theory are appropriate to serve different purposes (Dickoff and James, 1968 and Walker and Avant, 1983), as listed in Table 7–1. The lowest level, theory for the purpose of *description* (factor isolating theory), requires that the factors, or variables, that are involved be identified and defined. For example, to describe a situation involving a nurse and a client, the variables nurse and client would need to be defined, in addition to significant elements in the situation. Thus, the nurse may be a senior student, and the client a hospitalized post-myocardial infarction patient. A clear description of the situation depends on the identification of accurate and essential details about each of the variables, in terms that are commonly understood.

The purpose of the next level of theory is the *explanation* of a situation (factor relating theory). This requires identification of the possible relationships between the variables. In the example above, the nurse may be trying for the second time to teach the client about a low sodium diet. There are possible relationships between the diet and the diagnosis, between the nurse and the client, and between the diagnosis and the client. Situational variables that may affect these relationships help to clarify explanation. Thus, possible explanations for the previously unsuccessful teaching might include lack of concentration on the part of the client, related to chest pain or anxiety, or lack of trust in the nurse with whom the client has had no previous relationship.

The third level of theory aims to *predict* the outcomes when variables are manipulated (situation relating theory). For example, it might be predicted that recall of what was taught concerning diet will be increased if teaching is done when the client's pain and anxiety are decreased or absent. And at the fourth and highest level of practice theory, the purpose is *control* of the situation (situation producing theory). This level of theory makes it possible to prescribe actions that will bring about desired goals. Thus, the variables that lead to successful teaching about diet are known and have been supported through research. At this level of theory, nursing intervention has a high probability of accomplishing the desired goals.

Stevens (1979) on the other hand, suggests two levels of theory. The first level is labeled descriptive theory because it makes it possible to look at a phenomenon and identify its major elements or events. This level of theory does not identify why the elements are present, nor why and how they relate to each other; that is the function of the second level, explanatory theory, which may deal with cause and effect, correlations, or the rules that regulate interactions among the variables.

TABLE 7–1.   Levels of Theory Development

Dickoff and James		Walker and Avant
Factor isolating theory	=	Description
Factor relating theory	=	Explanation
Situation relating theory	=	Prediction
Situation producing theory	=	Control

Explanatory theory can also be used to control the outcomes of nursing intervention.

Following is a description of four kinds of theories about the nature of change: systems theory, stress and adaptation theories, growth and development theories, and rhythm theory. All of these theories, which were developed outside of nursing, have been applied in nursing to offer different explanations of the changes due to interrelationships between humans, health, environment, and nursing, and to therefore guide the application of the nursing process. The principles of systems theory have also been used as the theoretical framework for this book.

SYSTEMS THEORY

Systems theory is concerned with changes due to interactions between all the various factors (variables) in a situation. In humans, interactions between the person and environment occur continuously. Thus, the situation is complex and constantly changing. Systems theory provides a way to understand the many influences on the whole person, and the possible impact of change of any part on the whole. This theory can be very useful in nursing to understand, predict, and control the possible effects of nursing care on the client system and the concurrent effects of the interaction on the nurse system.

A system is defined as "a whole with interrelated parts, in which the parts have a function and the system as a totality has a function" (Auger, 1976, p. 21). Systems are organized into hierarchical levels of complexity. Single systems may be *subsystems* of more complex systems, while each system also has a *suprasystem.*

An individual is composed of cells, organs, and physiologic systems, the subsystems of man. These subsystems are continuously interacting and changing. For example, as a person eats, the blood supply to the gastrointestinal organs increases. Absorption of carbohydrate increases the blood glucose level, which results in increased secretion of insulin. Simultaneously, changes in the blood circulation and level of glucose affect the level of attention and "hunger." The person may feel "satisfied" and "contented." The gastrointestinal, endocrine, cardiovascular, and/or emotional systems are subsystems of the person, and the whole person is the suprasystem for each of the physiologic or psychologic systems. The interaction of subsystems comprise the *internal environment* of the person.

The person is a subsystem of the family system (family is a suprasystem of the individual), which is a subsystem of the community system, and so on. Subsystems may be isolated for study, but humans are more than and different from the sum of their parts (Rogers, 1970, p. 46). Thus, a person cannot be characterized by describing physiologic, psychologic, and sociocultural subsystems. A person's behavior is holistic, a reflection of the person as a whole. The focus is on interaction among the various parts of the system rather than on a description of the function of the parts themselves (Auger, 1976, p. 20).

All living systems are *open systems,* which means that they exchange matter, energy, and information across their boundaries with the environment (Sills and Hall, 1977, p. 20). The internal environment is in constant interaction with a changing environment external to the person. As changes occur in one, the other is affected. For example, walking into a cold room (change in the external environment) affects a variety of physiologic and psychologic subsystems of the internal environment that will change the person's blood flow, ability to concentrate, feeling of comfort, and so on. Similarly, an angry outburst (change in the internal environment) has a demonstrable effect on the mood of others. It is this openness of human systems that makes nursing intervention possible.

> A general systems approach allows for consideration of man at his subsystems levels, as a total human being, and as a social creature who networks himself with others in hierarchically arranged human systems of increasing complexity. Thus man, from the level of the individual to the level of society, can be conceptualized as client and become the target system for nursing intervention. (Sills and Hall, 1977, pp. 24–25)

Energy, or information, or matter provide *input* for the system. The system "transforms, creates, and organizes input in the process known as 'throughput' which results in a reorganization of the input" (Sills and Hall, 1977, p. 21). Thus, each system modifies its input. Simultaneously, energy, information, and/or matter is given off into the environment as output. When output is returned to the system as input, the process is known as *feedback*. For example, when a nurse gives a client information about a therapeutic diet, this is system input (for the client system). What the client eats is one type of system output (based on the throughput related to assimilation and acceptance of the information originally given). The nurse, using the client's reported food intake as feedback, can help to either reinforce or modify the client's future behavior (Fig. 7–1).

Humans can be viewed as "an interrelated, interdependent, interacting, complex organism, constantly influencing and being influenced by his environment" (Sills and Hall, 1977, p. 24). At any time, since the person is in constant interaction with the environment, a number of interrelated factors, including the influence of the nurse, will affect the client's health status. The person's response, in turn, will then result in change of the environment. Because of these interactions, a change in any part affects the whole human-environment system.

Use of systems theory to guide nursing process directs assessment of the relationships between of all the variables that impact the client-environment interaction, including the influence of the nurse. In intervention the nurse must anticipate the system-wide impact from change in any part of the system, and appreciate the simultaneous rather than cause-and-effect nature of change in open systems.

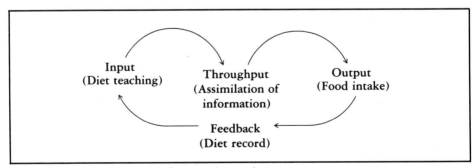

Figure 7–1. An example of systems interaction.

STRESS AND ADAPTATION THEORIES

Stress and adaptation theories view change due to person-environment interaction in terms of cause and effect. The person certainly has to adjust to changes in order to avoid disturbance of a balanced existence. The adaptation theory provides a way to understand how the balance is maintained, and the possible effects of disturbed equilibrium. This theory has been widely applied to explain, predict, and control biologic (physiologic and psychologic) responses of the person. It is the basis for much current medical therapy.

The human body functions as a whole. All body cells are affected by the activities of other cells. This communication is made possible because all cells are surrounded by the same fluids (*e.g.,* blood, lymph, interstitial fluid), which form an *internal environment* for the entire body. The internal environment provides a medium for the exchange of nutrients and wastes, and provides a stable physiochemical environment for cell function.

Normal physiologic function of cells requires that the constancy of the internal environment be maintained within relatively narrow boundaries even though the body is constantly changing in response to interactions between the internal and external environment. The needed stability of the internal environment is maintained through feedback between regulatory mechanisms. As changes occur in the internal environment, regulatory systems such as the nervous system and/or the endocrine system respond to keep the change within well-defined limits. The word *homeostasis* (homeo—like, similar; stasis—stay) was originally used by Cannon (1929) to describe constancy of the internal environment due to the action of regulatory mechanisms. Constancy does not mean that the internal environment is static. It is constantly changing, but a relative equilibrium is maintained.

The regulatory systems operate by way of *compensation.* Any change in the internal environment automatically initiates a response that will minimize or counteract the change. For example, when the blood sugar drops, the endocrine system responds with an increased secretion of cortisol, which decreases the rate of glucose use by cells and stimulates the conversion of amino acids into glucose. These compensatory actions cause the blood sugar to rise. If it should increase above acceptable limits, insulin secretion would increase the rate of glucose uptake by cells tending to reduce the blood glucose level.

Compensation occurs constantly as the body adjusts to stimuli that tend to disturb equilibrium. These forces are called *stressors.* A stressor may be anything that creates change in the internal environment and thus places demands on the body to compensate. A change in temperature of the external environment, hunger, joy, infection, and change in sleep pattern are all potential stressors. Thus, stressors may be beneficial or harmful, but they all require the body to respond. The response of the body is called *adaptation.* The ability to adapt to changes in life events may be synonomous with health, or may be a major factor in determining a person's potential for health or disease.

One way that a person adapts is by means of coping mechanisms that "refer to efforts to master conditions of harm, threat, or challenge when a routine or automatic response is not readily available" (Monat and Lazarus, 1977, p. 8). Some people regard coping methods primarily as psychologic barriers when a stressor is perceived as a threat. Thus, a person's reaction to stress would involve cognitive appraisal and psychologic coping methods, in addition to physiologic reactions.

Selye's Stress Theory

Hans Selye's theory of stress, developed in the 1940s, focuses on physiologic responses to acute stressors. Many kinds of different variables can be stressors. When various tissues are affected by stressors, they send signals by way of the nervous and/or endocrine systems to the brain. Selye defines *stress* as "the state manifested by a specific syndrome which consists of all the non-specifically induced changes within a biologic system" (Selye, 1976, p. 64). Regardless of which specific stressors are involved, the body responds with the same generalized changes, which Selye labeled the general adaptation syndrome (G.A.S.). The purpose of the G.A.S. is "the confinement of stress to the smallest area capable of meeting the requirements of a situation" (Selye, 1976, p. 162).

The G.A.S. occurs in three stages. The first to occur is the alarm reaction during which mechanisms are mobilized to maintain life. Next is the stage of resistance during which the most appropriate specific channel of defense is mobilized. If the body response is not sufficient to control the stressors, the body enters the stage of exhaustion. The reaction spreads, and since the defenses are exhausted, death occurs. If resistance is sufficient, the body returns to a state of balance, although residual damage may remain. For example, when bacteria enter the body in sufficient numbers, an alarm reaction is set off. Resistance may result in confining and killing the organisms, but scar tissue may remain; or resistance may not confine the organisms and systemic infection ensues. If resistance is sufficiently exhausted, the person may die of the infection.

Selye also suggests that the bodies' own defensive adaptative reactions cause diseases of adaptation. If the stressor is a microorganism, then inflammatory responses to localize and destroy the stressor are appropriate and helpful. But if, for example, the stressor is anxiety about taking a test, then the inflammatory response is not helpful, and may cause physiologic damage (such as digestion of the lining of the stomach, which if prolonged, could result in a stomach ulcer. Thus, if the stress response is excessive or inappropriate, disease may result.

Recently however, Selye's theory has been challenged. Researchers such as Lazarus (Monat and Lazarus, 1977) believe that the mind must consider a stressor to be threatening before the body responds with hormonal changes. This integration of mind *and* body is consistent with the development of systems theory. In addition, it appears that "there may be specific as well as general causes of distinct stress-related disease patterns" (Monat and Lazarus, 1977, p. 7), and that "different individuals respond to the same conditions in different ways" (Appley and Trumbull, 1977, p. 66). In addition, where Selye's theory is based on a specific syndrome in response to any nonspecific stressor, there is a growing body of evidence that supports the concept of different patterns of hormonal response to different stressors in the same person.

A more general theory of stress would begin with activation of the system by a stressor or potential stressor. This would lead to subjective or cognitive appraisal of the threat involved. This step is at least partially unconscious, and involves consideration of the intensity, extent, and context of the activation and available emotional and physiologic resources for coping. Based on this appraisal, the person may react with physiologic and/or behavioral outcomes, which could be associated with symptoms. Appraisal of the situation would continue, including the effectiveness of coping responses.

This stress model recognizes potential differences in response between individuals as well as differences in the same person at different times. Intra-individual differences may be due to a number of influences such as past experience, variation in time, the amount of control the individual can exert in the situation, the predictability of the activator, and the ability of the individual to learn new ways of coping. Some of the variables that can modify the responses of different people to the same activator are the degree of threat the activator represents, the amount of social support the individual can obtain, and the effects of prior learning and adaptation. In this model, stressors lead to coping, which results in growth and change of the person (Scott *et al*, 1980; Bieliauskas, 1982; Ziemer, 1982).

Use of Selye's stress theory to guide nursing process is most applicable in relation to assessment of physiologic stressors and adaptation responses. The goal of intervention is the support of body defenses with reduction of additional stress. This theory has been widely used in medicine. A holistic stress-coping model is consistent with nursing intervention and is the basis for at least one widely used nursing model (see Chapter 8, Models of Nursing). Crisis theory, which follows, has been viewed by medicine within a disease-oriented stress framework. However, crisis theory can be viewed within a health-oriented stress-coping model as described above.

Crisis Theory

The crisis theory has developed within psychiatry in order to guide intervention for people experiencing acute "peak periods" or "turning points" that seem to occur "with any change in which the demands upon a system are greater than the resources" (Menke, 1977, p. 56). The theory is based on the assumption that "all systems require some stability and predictability to function and promote growth; otherwise chaos, disorganization, and dysfunction occur" (Menke, 1977, p. 61). It is proposed that periods of acute change are superimposed on this basic pattern of stability. If the individual is unable to adapt to the change and cope, crisis occurs. Fitzpatrick (1982, p. 25) has summarized current perspectives in crisis theory:

1. The life process includes a succession of crisis experiences.
2. A crisis poses a threat to the individual which places equilibrium and sense of self in jeopardy.
3. The goal of crisis resolution is the return to the pre-crisis level of functioning i.e., the restoration of equilibrium.
4. Crises possess the potential for opportunity, i.e., they can be growth experiences.
5. A crisis is by definition time limited; as such it is a transitional point in the person's experiences of life.
6. Specific phases of the crisis experience can be identified and described.
7. Crises are more accessible to intervention at their peak.
8. Precipitating events may be identified in relation to the occurrence of crises.
9. Previous experiences with crises increase the ability to function in current crises.
10. The crisis experience includes a constellation of feelings associated with the upset state.
11. Resolution of crises may be directly linked to mental health and illness; crises may be resolved in positive or negative ways."

Caplan (1964, pp. 40–41) initially described the phase within a crisis experience. In phase one, a stimulus (the change) causes a rise in the person's anxiety and causes the person to use his usual problem-solving methods to reduce his discomfort. In phase two, the stimulus continues, but, since the usual methods to resolve the situation fail, anxiety continues to increase. In phase three, the individual mobilizes additional internal and external resources, and the anxiety may be resolved. If, however, these resources are not sufficient, phase four occurs, and the person enters active crisis. As Caplan (1964, p. 41) says, "If the problem continues and can neither be solved with need satisfaction nor avoided by need resignation or perceptual distortion, the tension mounts to a breaking point and results in major disorganization with drastic results."

There are two types of crisis: developmental and situational. A developmental, or maturational crisis, may have a gradual onset and occur during a transitional period between developmental phases. A situational crisis is a sudden, unexpected event. All crises "involve actual loss or the threat of loss" (Menke, 1977, p. 58), and "present an individual both with an opportunity for personality growth and with the danger of increased vulnerability to mental disorder" (Caplan, 1964, p. 36).

There are distinct differences between medicine and nursing in the way that crisis theory has been interpreted. Medicine considers crisis as a period of disequilibrium "which presents a threat to the individual's homeostasis" (Fitzpatrick, 1982, p. 23), while nursing considers crisis to offer the individual an opportunity for goal achievement, problem resolution, and growth.

The use of crisis theory to guide nursing process directs the assessment of the client's history as well as factors directly involved in the onset of the heightened anxiety. Also needed is an assessment of the individual's strengths, supports, and coping mechanisms available for dealing with the situation. Intervention strategies are influenced by the goal of helping the individual to use the experience to foster personal growth.

GROWTH AND DEVELOPMENT THEORIES

Developmental theories assume linear growth or change that has predictable, irreversible direction, occurs in degrees (stages), and progresses toward a maximum potential (Chin, 1980). Developmental theory facilitates the planning of future-oriented interventions, since "the direction, sequence of stages, form of progress from stage to stage, causative forces, and desired end points are known and predictable" (Thibodeau, 1983 p. 47). The application of this type of theory to interpersonal, psychosocial, psychosexual, cognitive, and moral development is discussed in the following sections. Nursing intervention based on developmental theory is heavily influenced by predictable and generalizable expectations of all people, interpreted in terms of the client's specific history.

Growth is defined as an increase in physical size and shape to some point of optimal maturity (Billingham, 1982, p. 4). Growth is constant change, which involves the entire person through patterns of organization and regulation. Since no change is isolated, each modifies the individual as a whole. Thus, assessment of growth requires data about all aspects of the individual.

Growth is continuous and orderly with regular trends in direction. For example, the direction of motor growth is from the head to the extremities (cephalocaudal sequence), and from the central part of the body toward the periphery (proxidistal sequence). As a result, a child sits before he stands, and has control of shoulder movements before those of the fingers. However, although growth is patterned and continuous, it is not always smooth and gradual. Different aspects develop at different rates.

Each person grows in a unique pattern, influenced by intrinsic factors (e.g., genetic), extrinsic factors (*e.g.,* nutrition), and the interplay between the person and his environment (*e.g.,* emotional responses). The age at which milestones such as the tripling of birth weight are reached vary greatly. While there are critical periods for some types of growth (*e.g.,* gross structural differentiation in the first trimester of gestation), in general, a growth trend is much more important than the age at which milestones are reached.

Development is related to functional changes that are usually qualitative. As with growth, multiple factors influence development, although there is disagreement about the relative importance of maturational (biologic) versus environmental influences. All aspects of human development are interrelated and integrated. Because development proceeds in a sequential pattern, realistic expectations for behavior can be predicted.

There are a number of theories about how development occurs. The classical approach is what is called *stage theory.* It is believed that all people pass through a number of levels (stages). The stages differ in quality, but the order is fixed and a person cannot skip or reorder a stage or stages. Mastering the tasks of one stage forms the basis for mastering the tasks of the next. People do differ in how fast they move through these stages and in the level of development they finally reach.

Theorists vary in their beliefs about whether certain stages are critical for development. Those who believe that development is primarily determined by genetic factors warn of irreversible unfavorable effects if there is a lack of appropriate development in each stage. Thus, Freud would relate chain smoking in an adult to unfulfilled oral gratification as an infant. Piaget believed certain stages were preferable for development. But, since he also believed in the interaction of intrinsic and environmental influences, he would have expected that development would continue even if it were hindered. Age limits have been developed by which a person is expected to have moved on to the next stage.

Various stage theorists have described components of development. Six theorists whose theories have had wide applicability to nursing will be examined: Sullivan, Piaget, Kohlberg, Freud, Erikson, and Maslow. It is important to remember however, that although each stage has characteristic traits and developmental tasks, each individual demonstrates uniqueness of style and behavior. It should also be remembered that each of these theories explores only one subsystem in development.

Sullivan's Interpersonal Theory

Harry Stack Sullivan's interpersonal theory is based on the belief that human behavior and personality develop as a result of interpersonal relationships with significant others. He said, "psychiatry seeks to study the biologically and culturally conditioned . . . interpersonal processes occurring in the interpersonal situations in which the observant psychiatrist does his work" (Sullivan, 1953, p. 20).

Sullivan believed that personality development is divided into periods of growth. Stages occur universally but are not rigidly fixed. They are strongly influenced, especially in the later stages, by cultural differences. The stages are infancy, childhood, juvenile era, preadolescence, early adolescence, midadolescence, late adolescence, and mature adulthood. In each stage the person strives to achieve satisfaction and security in interpersonal relationships with significant others. Satisfaction occurs when biologic tensions are relieved, and thus, satisfaction needs are met. Security is achieved by reflected appraisals of worth by significant others. When security needs are met, anxiety is relieved.

Satisfaction and security needs are inextricably intertwined in the infant. The meeting of satisfaction needs through "tenderness" behaviors on the part of significant others is perceived by the infant as gratification of both the biologic tension state and the need for security. Ministering to physical needs results in satisfaction. In the infant, these ministrations also carry an empathized message of security to relieve the tensions of anxiety. For example, feeding by a mother who feels very positively about the infant results in relief of the tensions of hunger and anxiety. The "mothering one" has the capacity to induce satisfaction and security or to induce anxiety and increase biologic tensions. The "mothering one" is also affected by the infant's state. These kinds of emotional communications, which allow for transmission of anxiety or satisfaction from mother to infant and from infant to mother, are termed empathy.

Sullivan viewed the infant as alternating between periods of satisfaction and security or anxiety as increased tension states resulting from interpersonal experiences primarily with his mother. He labeled these experiences as occurring in the prototaxic mode, meaning that they occurred before the infant was able to use symbols. The attainment of satisfaction caused a profound sense of well-being and security. This power, or feeling of ability, was considered to be an accomplishment with (rather than over) others. If the infant recurrently experienced a lack of satisfaction and security, it was proposed that he developed a power drive, due to a lack of a positive image. In other words, a person needs to have a feeling of ability, which Sullivan termed power. If that need is thwarted, a "drive for power" develops. Sullivan believed that "the manner in which (the power motive) is satisfied and fulfilled mainly determines the growth and characteristics of personality" (Mullahy, 1953, p. 243).

With the transition from infancy to childhood, there is a change in the significant other from solely the caring person to include other close associates (*e.g.,* friends, teachers). In addition, the child begins to use language. At this time, the deliberate acculturation process accelerates, since the child is beginning to use symbols. These types of experiences occur in the parataxic mode suggesting that the child uses symbols in a very individual and private way. Sullivan specifically termed verbal parataxic experiences as autistic. The child is now able to discriminate experience into separate unrelated parts. Thus, anxiety can be discriminated and associated with specific experiences. In response to anxiety, if it is strong enough, the child may apply selective inattention and barely notice certain experiences. If anxiety is strong enough experiences may be dissociated. Dissociated processes are not accessible to the individual, and profound changes in personality occur if they are reintegrated in psychiatric therapy. Sullivan believed that "anxiety is the chief disruptive force in interpersonal relations and the main factor in the development of serious difficulties in living" (Cohen, 1953, p. xv).

The impact of interpersonal relationships on the formation of the self-system is emphasized in all of Sullivan's writing. He believed that the person learns who he is through reflected appraisals of others, communicated through relationships. He believed that personality could only be studied through the participation of a trained observer in interpersonal communications. The person's behavior in these interpersonal relationships was believed to mirror the person's self-concept developed early in life, called "good me," "bad me," and "not me." He believed that the basic tendency of the personality is toward mental health, and that there is a great resistance to change of the personality.

The juvenile era, which follows childhood, is often associated with beginning of school, and another change in significant others. There is a tendency toward cooperation with friends, in contrast to the previous efforts to please parents. This is a time for learning the meaning of competition and compromise. Experiences, which now occur in the syntaxic mode, can be conceptualized in symbols that have a common meaning, and can readily be communicated from one person to another. Experiences in the syntaxic mode are strongly influenced by anticipation based on previous experiences.

Preadolescence, between the ages of 8 and 12, is associated with development of the capacity to love. This emotion means that the satisfactions and security of a loved one assume as much significance as one's own. Frequently, the first love relationships are developed with friends of the same sex, manifested in activities mostly with peers of the same sex.

Sullivan divided adolescence into three phases: early adolescence from the first evidence of puberty to completion of voice changes; midadolescence, involving patterning of genital behavior; and late adolescence, with the beginnings of sexual intimacy. In western cultures, with the relative postponement of sexual intimacy, a great deal of anxiety is generated during adolescence. Ways of dealing with anxiety largely reflect the self-image the person has developed in infancy and childhood.

Mature adulthood is characterized by self-respect, respect for others, a feeling of dignity, and the ability to exert appropriate initiative. This stage does not necessarily reflect chronologic age, and Sullivan believed that many people do not achieve their full potential.

In summary, Sullivan believed that personality develops as a result of interpersonal communication, and in fact can only be assessed within an interpersonal relationship. He believed that anxiety interferes with communication, and causes a large part of mental disorders. He conceptualized personality growth occurring in stages, with the early stages exerting the primary influences on development of the self-system. Use of Sullivan's theory to guide nursing process involves development of a therapeutic interpersonal relationship with the client to facilitate assessment of factors associated with client anxiety as well as to intervene to reduce anxiety. Appreciation of the stages of personality growth can help the nurse to understand possible reasons for client problems, and suggest possible intervention strategies. For example, the nurse would anticipate that diagnosis of a chronic disease (*e.g.,* diabetes) in an adolescent might lead to rejection of treatment because it makes him "different" from his significant others, his friends. Appreciation for the underlying conflict might lead to teaching by the nurse of how to modify the diet and activity plan to permit "normal" activities when in the company of friends.

Piaget's Theory of Cognitive Development

Jean Piaget developed a theory to explain the processes involved in thinking or cognition. His theory deals with ways in which the mind acquires and uses knowledge. In other words, he deals with how intelligence is developed.

Piaget believed that cognition is similar to other biologic systems; that it is structured, but also maintains adaptability with the environment. These characteristics are found in people of all ages. According to his theory, the mind constantly experiences sensory stimuli. These bits of information are first taken in (assimilation) and organized by the mind. But then the cognitive structure must be modified (accommodation) in order to accept the new information. For example, the first time a young child sees a dog, the color, size, and behavior of the animal are assimilated into the child's mind as "dog." However, when other dogs are seen, the child's mind must permit differences of size, color, and behavior in "dog." Thus, the mind adapts and "dog" becomes generalized. Piaget believed that there must always be a balance, or an equilibrium, between assimilation and accommodation. The balance however is short-lived, since assimilation of new information continues cognitive development cyclically toward increasingly complex thought (Fig. 7–2).

In addition to these general characteristics of intellectual growth, Piaget also believed in a universal pattern of development of cognition through well-defined stages. These stages are described briefly below.

In the sensorimotor stage, from birth to about 2 years of age, the infant develops the concept that objects have permanence even when they are not seen (representational ability), learns to differentiate between self and everything else (overcomes egocentrism), and through repetition, discovers cause and effect. Toward the end of this stage, symbolic thought documents that the child can understand the results of actions before they are performed.

The preoperational stage, which lasts from about 2 through 6 years of age, is characterized mainly by the development of symbolic functioning, including imagery and language. By the end of this period the child develops the ability to conserve, or to conceptualize a variety of aspects of an object as permanent and reversible. If any aspect, such as shape or size of an object changes, the child is able to understand that other qualities remain the same. Thus, a lump of clay remains the same size even if the shape is changed.

Reversibility of thought is essential to the concrete operational stage, which lasts from about 6 to about 11 or 12 years of age. At this stage the child is able to think about actions wihout actually experiencing them. However, he is unable to consider what is not concrete reality (*e.g.,* rabbits are not purple), and is unable to differentiate between what is thought and what is reality. Thus, hypothetical answers are viewed as arbitrary solutions. The concepts of classification (*e.g.,* grouping all of one size, shape, color), seriation (ordering in size), and number are developed. True hypothetical thought characterizes the formal operational stage, which begins about the age of 11 or 12. The adolescent is able to think beyond the reality of the present and to project the possibilities of the future.

The use of Piaget's theory in the application of the nursing process should include modification of intervention strategies based on assessment of a client's level of cognitive development. For example, explanations to a young child about what will happen in surgery should be concrete and simple, and take into consideration the level of the child's development of symbolic thought.

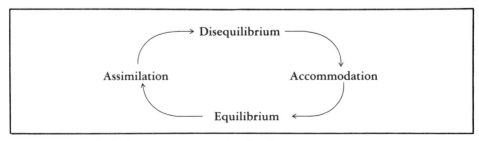

Figure 7–2. Cyclical processes in cognitive development.

Kohlberg's Theory of Moral Reasoning

Lawrence Kohlberg (1981) attempts to explain the development of the reasoning processes that underlie morality rather than simply determine whether behavior is moral. He believes that the various levels of moral reasoning always occur in the same sequence, but that people vary in how far and how fast they develop. Since development is a gradual process, at any given point a person may be functioning at more than one level.

In level one, *preconventional moral reasoning,* what is considered right is literal obedience to rules and authority, avoiding punishment, and not doing physical harm to others. Early in this level an act is considered right or wrong depending on whether or not it is associated with punishment. The superior power of authorities is a major incentive. Later in this level an act is considered right if it meets the person's needs or the needs of someone close to the person. Right is also what is fair, meaning a deal or an equal exchange. As the person begins to consider the needs of others, he moves toward the next level of reasoning.

Level two, *conventional moral reasoning,* involves acting as others expect. Early in this level the person acts in order to win approval. Thus, right is playing a good (nice) role, being concerned about other people and their feelings, and keeping loyalty and trust with partners. Later in this level, rules have become ends in themselves. The person acts to maintain the established authority. The right is doing one's duty and upholding the social order. However, when the person begins to think about what society should do in return, there is a transition to the next reasoning level.

Kohlberg suggests that some people may pass through a transitional level at this point. Choice is viewed as personal and based on subjective emotions. Conscience is seen as arbitrary and relative, as are such ideas as "duty" and what is "morally right." If a person moves into the third level, that of *postconvention,* moral decisions are generated from rights, values, and principles. Early in this level the person considers the relationship between himself and society to be reciprocal. It is right to uphold the basic rights, values, and legal contracts of society. Thus, legal contracts determine behavior arbitrarily. One may have difficulty integrating the conflicts between the moral view and the legal view. But, by the final stage in level three, the ultimate appeal is to an internalized conscience. It is acceptable to interpret rules subjectively within universal principles of morality. The most basic universal principle of justice is the equality of human rights and respect for the dignity of humans as individuals.

More advanced levels of moral reasoning have been found to be associated with higher critical thinking, more adequate moral behavior, and professional rather than technical education in nursing (Ketefian, 1981). Kohlberg's theory can help the nurse to better understand the basis for moral judgments by clients and colleagues, as well as to better understand what may underlie her own ethical choices.

Freud's Theory of Psychosexual Development

Sigmund Freud believed that the mind is composed of three parts. First in development is the id, which unconsciously represents the influence of heredity. "It contains everything that is inherited, that is present at birth, that is laid down in the constitution—above all, therefore, the instincts" (Freud, 1949, p. 2). The ego is a special organization in the brain that acts as an intermediary between the id and the external world. By gaining control over the demands of the instincts, the ego maintains the person's self-preservation by dealing in reality with the world. The super-ego is a special organization in the ego that maintains the rules and customs of society. The constant interaction among these three areas of the mind, in Freud's view, provides the unconscious basis for much of a person's behavior.

Freud's theory of psychosexual development is built on the concept of libido, or human mental energy. He believed that libido caused tension in localized areas of the body that could only be released through stimulation. Thus, "libidinal gratification" was a reduction of tension through stimulation of the appropriate body areas. Freud believed that the libido changed its area of localization (or erogenous zone) in stages. His view was that the sequence of the stages was the same for everyone, and was primarily maturational, but that the effects could be modified by a person's experience.

The first stage, which occurs during the first year of life, is the oral stage, and is focused on repeated sucking and biting experiences involving the mouth. From the end of the first year through the third year is the anal stage, which is focused on retention or release of feces. From the third to the fifth year is the phallic stage that leads to resolution of the oedipus or electra complex and identification with the parent of the same sex as that of the child. From the fifth year until adolescence, Freud believed that the libido was latent, focusing eventually on reproductive functions in the genital stage.

Freud's stages of psychosexual development have been used to describe adult behaviors. A person who is "always attempting to take in" wealth, power, or food, who smokes or makes biting remarks may be releasing oral libidinal energy. Behavior related to anal libidinal gratification might be messy or wasteful ("letting everything hang out"), or excessively neat and orderly and "uptight" about showing emotions.

Freud believed that the phallic stage was associated with the development of conscience. For the male child, the father is the ego ideal, which Freud related to the development of a strong super ego and conscience. However, since the female child identifies with the mother, Freud believed that the result was an incomplete formation of conscience in women. As one might expect, these ideas have received much criticism in recent years.

The concept of anxiety is very important in Freud's theory. Anxiety serves a useful purpose as a warning of impending danger, but it is painful, and thus the individual attempts to cope with the anxiety. Often the ego can cope with the anxiety by rational measures, but, if these are not effective, the ego resorts to irrational protective measures, which are referred to as ego-defense mechanisms, because they serve to protect the self from hurt and devaluation. These defense mechanisms reduce the painful anxiety, but they do so at the expense of distorting reality, and thus the ego does not deal directly with the stressful situation.

Freud also assumed that objectionable memories, wishes, and impulses are less painful for the ego and arouse less anxiety when they have been repressed and thus excluded from consciousness. The individual is unaware of these unconscious desires although they may be reflected in fantasies and dreams. The implication is that people are often unaware of the "real" motivation behind their behavior.

Freud's major contribution was the concept of the unconscious mind. His work was the basis for psychoanalytic theory, and led to a ferment of activity in psychologic theory. His theory can guide the nurse in the assessment of defense mechanisms against anxiety (in the client and the nurse), and can suggest interventions based on an appreciation of the possible meaning of client behavior.

Erikson's Theory of Psychosocial Development

Erik Erikson expanded on Freud's psychosexual theories to propose a psychosocial theory that stresses the interrelationships between personality (the ego) and social forces that affect its development. Healthy development proceeds as the personality develops the capability to deal with the changing demands of reality.

Erikson believed that certain parts of the personality developed at (and only at) critical stages of development. In defining the epigenetic principle, he stated that "anything that grows has a ground plan from which parts arise, each part having a time of special ascendancy, until all parts have arisen to form a functioning whole" (Erikson, 1968, p. 92). In other words, there is a sequence of stages in which development of a certain part of the personality becomes most critical. The individual must pass through all these stages before a complete sense of identity can be developed, but these stages are governed by a maturational timetable. If in any stage the specific capability of the personality is not developed, it will remain underdeveloped forever, as there are no "second chances." The remainder of personality development will be altered, resulting in neuroses or ineffective ways of dealing with reality.

Erikson's stages of psychosocial development (Erikson, 1959) begin with the oral sensory stage. The infant is bombarded with stimulation. If the infant perceives sensory input as relatively pleasant and benign, he will begin to develop a sense of basic trust. If, however, the world is perceived as painful or dangerous, a sense of mistrust will develop. The emotional crisis, then, is between trust versus mistrust (Lerner, 1976, p. 202). Trust, like all emotional outcomes, is viewed on a continuum, where the healthiest feelings fall toward (but not at) the positive outcome on the continuum. For example, a person with absolute trust will not recognize danger. Also unhealthy is a person who has developed a basic sense of mistrust. The goal is the development of a sense of trust that is positive yet retains appropriate caution.

The second stage is the anal-musculature stage. During this stage the child needs to develop control of all his muscles by learning when to hold on and when to let go. If the child develops control of his body (bowel movements, feedings), he will develop a sense of autonomy. If his lack of control means that others have to do things for him that are expected of him, he will develop a sense of shame and doubt. Thus, the second psychosocial crisis is between autonomy and shame and doubt.

The third stage, the genital-locomotor stage, corresponds to Freud's phallic stage. As the child's psychosocial conflicts are resolved, he needs to be able to distance himself from his parents. If he is able to move away on his own, he will develop a sense of initiative and purpose. If, on the other hand, the child is unable to "break the apron strings," he will develop a sense of guilt. The crisis is between initiative versus guilt.

In the fourth stage, latency, the child learns skills especially needed for adulthood. If he learns what to do and how to do it, he will develop a sense of industry and competence. If others have learned to perform tasks while the child meets repeated failures, he will develop a sense of inferiority. The crisis is between industry versus inferiority.

The stage of puberty and adolescence corresponds to Freud's genital stage. At this time major physical, emotional, and cognitive changes occur in the adolescent that bring about an identity crisis. The adolescent needs to be able to develop a role-defining identity, so he knows who he is and what he believes. Otherwise, he will feel a sense of role confusion or identity diffusion. So, the crisis is between identity versus role confusion.

In stage six, young adulthood, societal expectations are oriented toward marriage or other close emotional relationships. If the young adult is able to give of himself in a total sharing relationship, he will feel a sense of intimacy. If, however, he had not earlier developed a sense of self, he will feel a sense of isolation and a feeling of being alone. Thus, the crisis is between intimacy versus isolation.

If the adult has successfully achieved intimacy, he can attempt to become a productive, contributing member of society. If he is successful, he will have a sense of generativity. If his output is below his expectations, he will feel a sense of stagnation. For some time societal roles assumed that men achieved a sense of generativity through income-producing work, while women were expected to produce and rear children. There is increasing acceptance, however, of a wider role for women (if not for men) in our current society.

In stage eight, maturity, the individual is reaching the end of his life span. If he has successfully progressed through the previous stages of development, he will feel a sense of ego integrity and wisdom. He will feel that he has led a full and complete life. If, however, he feels that he has not gained everything from life that he feels he needed, he will feel a sense of despair, that "time was running out." The crisis is between ego integrity versus despair.

Erikson's theory broadens the understanding of factors involved in personality development to include social forces. An understanding of possible influences on the formation of personality can assist the nurse to intervene with a better understanding of the basis for client behavior. Erikson's stages have also been used in this book to describe the development of the professional self-concept (see Chapter 4, Development of the Professional Self-Concept).

Maslow's Theory of Psychosocial Development

Abraham Maslow (1968, p. 33) conceptualized growth as "a continued, more or less steady upward or forward development." He believed that in the process of growth, a person has to gratify basic needs before the person can be motivated toward self-actualization (becoming all the person is capable of becoming).

Thus, Maslow proposed a hierarchy of basic needs. Highest on the hierarchy are physiologic needs that are essential for survival. These needs include food, water, air, sleep, and sex. Next are the needs for safety, which include security, stability, protection, freedom from anxiety, and some degree of routine and predictability in daily living. When physiologic and safety needs have been sufficiently met, belonging and love in a caring relationship assumes a primary importance. Gratification of this need is an essential prerequisite to meeting esteem needs, which include reputation, status, prestige, and a feeling of self-esteem built on confidence and individual self-worth. Only after (1) physiologic, (2) safety, (3) belonging and love, and (4) esteem needs have been satisfied to a sufficient degree can the person focus on the need for fulfillment of his potential and capacities. Maslow believed that the tasks of self-actualization were basically intrapersonal, and included the discovery of self and the development of a positive outlook toward life.

Maslow hypothesized that people who have met their basic needs, and become self-actualizing people, are then motivated by a new set of needs, which he labeled B-values (being values) or metaneeds. Examples of such B-values are truth, goodness, beauty, perfection, and order. When B-values are deprived, the person may develop "metapathologies" characterized by such symptoms as alienation, loss of zest in life, apathy, despair, and "metagrumbles" (Maslow, 1971), which prevent full growth and development of the person.

Maslow's theory of a hierarchy in the order of needs and his development of the concept of actualization as a need beyond basic needs, provide a rationale for the organization of assessment data and determination of priorities for intervention, and thus, have been widely applied to nursing curricula and practice. For example, in meeting the needs of a young adult who has just broken her leg skiing, the nurse would medicate for pain (physiologic need) before addressing anxiety (safety need) and concern about how to maintain activities of daily living (esteem need).

RHYTHM THEORY

Rhythm theories consider cyclical, and thus predictable, change. Patterns are composed of reoccurring cycles of phenomena or behavior, which permits the nurse to anticipate particular patterning at certain times, and to adapt intervention accordingly.

Humans are characterized by distinctive patterning, and by continuous repatterning in rhythmic waves. Many biologic rhythms complete a cycle every 24 hours. This is called a *circadian period* (circa; diem). Those rhythms that complete more than one cycle in a 24-hour period are known as *ultradian rhythms*. For example, sleep consists of four stages that reoccur every 90 minutes in an orderly sequence (Kleitman, 1963). There is also evidence that there are ultradian cycles in activity and oral activity during wakefulness (Kleitman, 1969). There are also monthly rhythms such as the menstrual cycle, which are labeled infradian since they are cycles of more than 24 hours but less than a year, and annual rhythms. As knowledge about rhythms increases, it is also becoming obvious that there are many other less familiar rhythmicities such as the circaseptan rhythm of one cycle in 7 plus or minus 3 days!

Biologic rhythms are composed of waves that have a high and a low point, or a peak and a trough. The peaks of many circadian rhythms occur very close together in clock time, and normally maintain that phase relationship (Mills, 1966). It is widely believed that the environment, in a process known as synchonization, maintains a customary relationship of the rhythm with clock time (Halberg, 1960). In humans, it is assumed that societal routine is the dominant synchronizer in external timing. However, another view is that the internal integration and coordination of rhythms may not be controlled by a clock but by another internal rhythm (Mills, 1966). It has been shown that when external time is shifted (*e.g.*, by way of plane travel across time zones), the usual phase relationships are disturbed while the individual rhythms are resynchronized. The amount of time needed for individual rhythms to resynchronize with clock time varies. So, the usual phase relationships will be disturbed for a period—certainly days—and possibly weeks or months. In fact, studies of nurses working a night shift for years showed that usual phase relationships had never become established (Weitzman and Pollack, 1979).

What is the significance of biologic rhythmicity for nursing? It has been assumed (but not yet demonstrated) that the maintenance of phase relationships is associated with health, and that disturbed phase relationships among rhythms is associated with disturbed function and possibly the incidence of illness symptoms (Leddy, 1973). More information is needed about factors that could be manipulated to encourage faster resynchronization of an individual rhythm, or possibly prevent desynchronization in the first place. People vary in the time of day that they are most alert, able to concentrate, most susceptible to pain, have greater muscle strength, are most fearful, and so forth. In addition, various medications act differently depending on when they are administered. Duration and strength of action can vary significantly (Halberg *et al*, 1980). Knowledge of a client's rhythm patterning would enable interventions to be timed for the greatest effectiveness.

Knowledge by the nurse of her own patterning could help her to schedule activities at a time of greatest effectiveness, or at least encourage greater vigilance against error. If a change from day to night shift is necessary, it should be realized that many phase relationships will be disturbed for at least 2 weeks (the resynchronization of body temperature is a good indicator).

Time needs to be considered in the collection, recording, and sampling of data. For example, urinary output is normally much lower during midnight to 8 AM (Reinberg and Ghata, 1964). If the output during the night is as high as during the day, this is an indication of abnormality, even if the total amount appears normal.

Rhythm theory is in an early developmental stage and much is still unknown. The basic assumption however, that human rhythmicity is fundamental to life and affects every facet of functioning, is well documented. Use of this theory in the nursing process mandates consideration of the timing of rhythms in relation to each other, external time, and therapeutic intervention modalities. It also implies the

TABLE 7–2. Comparison of Concepts in Selected Theories

Theory	Man	Man-Environment Interaction	Health	Example of Nursing Implication
Systems	Multiple interacting subsystems that form the human system	Simultaneous change in both systems	Tendency toward increased complexity	Nurse system and client system are mutually affected
Stress and Adaptation	Multiple subsystems that share an internal environment	Man copes and compensates for environmental change	Constancy of the internal environment within "normal" parameters	Support coping mechanisms of client
Growth and Development	Intrinsic potential leads to change in stages	Linear and irreversible. Affect change when applied at appropriate time	Predictable change toward maximal potential	Monitor appropriateness of development
Rhythm	Changing in cycles toward increased complexity	Environment modifies internal rhythms	Synchrony of phase relationships	Restore phase relationships by manipulating synchronizers

need for consideration of the interrelationships in the open system between the client's rhythms and the nurse's rhythms. The theory has much potential for practice and for research in nursing.

SUMMARY

A number of theories with a potential impact on practice have been discussed in this chapter and are compared in Table 7-2. However, the way that theories are used to predict and explain events that affect nursing practice, depends on the particular conception or model of nursing that is used for a framework. In the next chapter, a number of different models of nursing are explored and contrasted.

REFERENCES

Appley M, Trumbull R: On the concept of psychological stress. *In* Monat A, Lazarus R (eds): Stress and Coping: An Anthology, pp 58–66. New York, Columbia University Press, 1977

Auger JR: Behavioral Systems and Nursing. Englewood Cliffs, Prentice-Hall, 1976

Bieliauskas LA: Stress and Its Relationship to Health and Illness. Boulder, Westview Press, 1982

Billingham KA: Developmental Psychology for the Health Care Professions. Boulder, Westview Press, 1982

Cannon WB: The sympathetic division of the autonomic system in relation to homeostasis. Arch Neurol Psych 22:282–294, 1929

Caplan G: Principles of Preventive Psychiatry. New York, Basic Books, 1964

Chin R: The utility of systems models and developmental models for practitioners. *In* Riehl JP, Roy C (eds): Conceptual Models for Nursing Practice, ed 2, pp 21–37. New York, Appleton-Century-Crofts, 1980

Cohen MB: Introduction. *In* Sullivan HS: The Interpersonal Theory of Psychiatry. New York, WW Norton, 1953

Dickoff J, James P: A theory of theories: A position paper. Nurs Res 17:197–203, 1968

Erikson EH: Identity, Youth and Crisis. New York, WW Norton, 1968

Erikson EH: Growth and Crisis of the Health Personality. Identity and the Life Cycle. Monograph 1:1, Psych Issues, New York, International Universities Press, 1959

Fitzpatrick J: The crisis perspective: Relationship to nursing. *In* Fitzpatrick JJ, Whall AL, Johnston RL et al: Nursing Models and their Psychiatric Mental Health Applications, pp 19–35. Bowie, Robert J. Brady, 1982

Freud S: An Outline of Psychoanalysis. New York, WW Norton, 1949

Halberg F: The 24-hour scale: A time dimension of adaptive functional organization. Persp Biol Med III:491–527, Summer 1960

Halberg F, Kabat HF, Klein P: Chronopharmacology: A therapeutic frontier. Am J Hosp Pharm 37:101–106, January 1980

Helmore GA: Piaget—A Practical Consideration. Oxford, Pergamon Press, 1969

Ketefian S: Moral reasoning and moral behavior. Nurs Res 30:171–176, May-June 1981

Kleitman N: Sleep and Wakefulness. Chicago, University of Chicago Press, 1963

Kleitman N: Basic Rest-Activity Cycle in Relation to Sleep and Wakefulness. Sleep Physiology and Pathology, pp 33–38. Philadelphia, JB Lippincott, 1969

Kohlberg L: The Philosophy of Moral Development. Moral Stages and the Idea of Justice. San Francisco, Harper & Row, 1981

Leddy S: Sleep and Phase Shifting of Biological Rhythms. Unpublished dissertation, New York University, 1973

Lerner RM: Concepts and Theories of Human Development. Boston, Addison-Wesley, 1976

Maslow AH: Toward A Psychology of Being, ed 2. New York, Van Nostrand Reinhold, 1968

Maslow AH: The Farther Reaches of Human Nature, pp 318–319. New York, Viking Press, 1971

Menke EM: Persistence, change and crisis. *In* Hall JE, Weaver BR (eds): Distributive Nursing Practice: A Systems Approach to Community Health, pp 51–64. Philadelphia, JB Lippincott, 1977

Mills JN: Human circadian rhythms. Physiol Rev 46:128–171, 1966

Monat A, Lazarus R (eds): Stress and Coping: An Anthology. New York, Columbia University Press, 1977

Mullahy P: A theory of interpersonal relations and the evolution of personality. *In* Sullivan HS: The Collected Works. New York, WW Norton, 1953

Riehl JP, Roy C: Conceptual models for Nursing Practice, ed 2. New York, Appleton-Century-Crofts, 1980

Reinberg A, Ghata J: Biological Rhythms. New York, Walker, 1964

Rogers ME: An Introduction to the Theoretical Basis of Nursing. Philadelphia, FA Davis Co. 1970

Selye H: The Stress of Life, rev ed. New York, McGraw-Hill, 1976

Scott DW, Oberst MT, Dropkin MJ: A stress-coping model. Adv Nurs Sci:9–23, 1980

Sills GM, Hall JE: A general systems perspective for nursing. *In* Hall JE, Weaver BR (eds): Distributive Nursing Practice: A System Approach to Community Health. Philadelphia, JB Lippincott, 1977

Stevens BJ: Nursing Theory: Analysis, Application, Evaluation. Boston, Little, Brown, 1979

Sullivan HS: The Collected Works. New York, WW Norton, 1953

Thibodeau JA: Nursing Models: Analysis and Evaluation. Monterey, Wadsworth Health Science Division, 1983

Torres G: The Place of Concepts and Theories Within Nursing. *In* George JB (Chairperson, The Nursing Theories Conference Group): Nursing Theories. The Base for Professional Nursing Practice. Englewood Cliffs, Prentice-Hall, 1980

Walker LO, Avant KC: Strategies for Theory Construction in Nursing. Norwalk, Appleton-Century-Crofts, 1983

Weitzman ED, Pollack CP: Disorders of the circadian sleep-wake cycle. Med Times 107:83–94, June 1979

Ziemer MM: Coping Behavior: A Response to Stress. Adv Nurs Sci:4–12, July 1982

Chapter 8

Models of Nursing

THOUGHT QUESTIONS

1. Does the human strive toward stability and balance, or toward variety and continuous change?
2. Is human behavior reflective of an indivisible entity, or a composite of a variety of components?
3. What are the roles of innovation and change in the determination of health? Are they disruptive or necessary?
4. How does the rate of change affect coping?
5. Does the person affect the environment or is he only affected by it?
6. Are interactions between the person and the environment cause and effect (linear) or continuous and simultaneous (multidimensional)?
7. Does nursing foster becoming or being (future or present)?
8. Is nursing done with, for, or to the person?

Until fairly recently, "nursing science" was derived principally from social, biologic, and medical science theories. However, from the 1950s to the present, an increasing number of nursing theorists have developed models of nursing that provide bases for the development of nursing theories and nursing knowledge.

A model, as an abstraction of reality, provides a way to visualize reality to simplify thinking. For example, an airplane model provides a representation of a "real" airplane. A model shows how various concepts are interrelated, and applies theories to predict or evaluate consequences of various alternative actions. "A conceptual model for nursing practice is a systematically constructed, scientifically based, and logically related set of concepts that identify the essential components of nursing practice together with the theoretical bases for these concepts and the values required in their use by the practitioner" (Johnson, as quoted by Riehl and Roy, 1980, p. 6).

A model describes the concepts that make up its composition. Thus, a nursing model includes (1) a description of the person who receives nursing care (the patient or client), (2) a view of the nature of the environment, and (3) a description of the nature of nursing. The articulating concept between the others is (4) the view of what comprises health.

In the following section, six models of nursing developed by Peplau, Johnson, Neuman, Orem, Roy, and Rogers, which are currently being applied and tested in education and practice settings, are described and compared. All of the models describe the same four concepts: (1) the person who receives nursing care (man, patient, client, person); (2) the environment (society); (3) health (or health-illness, or health and illness); and (4) nursing and the nurse (goals, roles, functions). However, the models vary in the amount of emphasis given to each of these concepts, as well as in the kinds of theories used to explain the interrelationships between the concepts.

The presentations, roughly in the order of their chronologic development, present the essence of each of the models so that the reader can appreciate the similiarities and differences between them. The intent is to clarify, rather than to analyze strengths or weaknesses, or to select the "best." Applications of the nursing process based on these models are found in Chapter 12, The Nursing Process.

HILDEGARD PEPLAU INTERPERSONAL RELATIONS MODEL

Terms

Tension—results from needs and leads to behavior to meet the needs and reduce discomfort.

Therapeutic relationship—interpersonal communication between a client and a nurse to solve the health problems of the client.

The essence of the Peplau model, which is a process organized model, is the human relationship between "an individual who is sick, or in need of health services, and a nurse especially educated to recognize and to respond to the need for help" (Peplau, 1952, pp. 5–6). This model, first published in 1952, "initiated a move from intrapsychic emphasis within psychiatric mental health nursing, and a dominant focus on physical care within general nursing to an interpersonal focus in both" (Reed and Johnston, 1983, p. 28).

Peplau views the *person* as "an organism that lives in an unstable equilibrium (i.e. physiological, psychological, and social fluidity) and life is the process of striving in the direction of stable equilibrium, i.e. a fixed pattern that is never reached except in death" (Peplau, 1952, p. 82). The person has needs that result in tension. Tension leads to behavior intended to reduce the tension and meet the needs.

In this model, the nurse is concerned with the health needs of individuals and groups in communities. *Health* "implies forward movement of personality and other ongoing human processes in the direction of creative, constructive, productive, personal, and community living" (Peplau, 1952, p. 12). Thus, according to Peplau, health requires that physiologic and personality needs have been met, and that the person is able to express his capabilities in a productive way (Peplau, 1952, pp. 14–15).

Nursing helps people to meet their present needs. When they are met, more mature needs can emerge and the personality moves forward.

Nursing is a significant, *therapeutic, interpersonal* process. It functions cooperatively with other human processes that make health possible for individuals in communities . . . Nursing is an educative instrument, a maturing force, that aims to promote forward movement of personality. (Peplau, 1952, p. 16)

In Peplau's model, the relationship between the nurse and the patient is the critical aspect of the therapeutic process. Initially, the two strangers have separate goals and interests. However, as the relationship progresses, the nurse and the patient develop a mutual understanding of health goals for the client, which leads to collaborative efforts to solve any health problems. The relationship, then, provides the means to resolve frustration, conflict, and/or anxiety, in order to meet patient needs (Peplau, 1952, p. 86).

Peplau describes four phases in the nurse-patient relationship: orientation, identification, exploitation, and resolution. In the orientation phase, the individual has a felt need and seeks professional assistance. The nurse in participation with the patient and all members of the professional team, focuses on gathering data, reinforcing and clarifying what others have communicated to the patient, and identifying problems.

As the relationship shifts into the identification phase, the patient begins to respond selectively to persons who seem to offer the help needed. At this time the patient may explore and express the feelings associated with his perception of the problem. The nurse's observations can develop clarity about the patient's expectations of the nurse, and can also clarify the nurse's expectations of the ability of a particular patient to handle his problem.

The phase of exploitation overlaps with the phases of identification and resolution. The "exploitation" is of the relationship, and refers to use of the relationship to the fullest possible extent in order to derive the greatest amount of benefit through change. The patient fully uses the services offered to him, but as convalescence begins there may be conflicts between dependence and independence, with shifts in behavior associated with the rapidly changing needs. The nurse should try to meet the patient's needs as they emerge, rather than assuming needs on the basis of preconceptions. As recovery proceeds, the patient can be assisted toward identifying and orienting toward new goals with a gradual decreasing of the identification with the helping person.

The phase of resolution is a freeing process that, for success, depends on the preceding chain of events. The patient's needs for psychologic dependency and sustaining relationships must have been worked through in order to strengthen his ability to stand more or less alone. Medical recovery may not coincide with readiness to terminate the nurse-patient relationship. If the patient is capable of resuming independence, the nurse may need to help him to work through his reluctance to separate. If problems continue despite medical "cure," termination of the relationship is premature.

Peplau describes a number of roles a nurse may assume within the various phases of the nurse-patient relationship. In the role of stranger, emphasis should be on respect and positive interest. The nurse should accept the patient as he is, as an emotionally able person, and should make an effort to say what she wants the patient to hear. As a resource person, the nurse should give specific answers to questions, but needs to be sensitive to questions that involve feelings or relate to larger problems. The nurse also may function in the roles of teacher and leader, helping the patient to learn through active participation in experiences. She may function as a counselor, and as a surrogate, helping the patient to see her as an individual, rather than in a relationship colored by reactivated past feelings. All of these roles help to promote nursing as an educative, therapeutic, and maturing force.

TABLE 8–1.   Major Concepts as Defined in the Peplau Model

Person:	Striving toward equilibrium Self-system in physiologic, psychologic, and social fluidity
Health:	Meeting physiologic and personality needs so that capabilities can be met in a productive way
Illness:	Symptoms from anxiety bound energy
Environment:	Significant others with whom the person interacts
Nursing:	Therapeutic interpersonal process carried out through the relationship between the person and the nurse

This conceptual model emphasizes the therapeutic nature of the nurse–patient relationship. The use of self by way of communication strategies has had wide applicability to the use of the nursing process to promote change and advocacy. The major concepts as defined in the Peplau model are summarized in Table 8–1.

DOROTHY JOHNSON BEHAVIORAL SYSTEM MODEL FOR NURSING

Terms

Behavioral system—the person, composed of interaction among and between seven subsystems

The essence of the behavioral system model for nursing, which is organized around behavioral systems of the person, is Johnson's conceptualization of man as a behavioral system made up of interrelated subsystems. The person attempts to maintain a balanced system, but environmental interaction can cause instability and health problems. Nursing intervention aims to assist the person to regain equilibrium.

The emphasis in Johnson's model is on the *person* as a behavioral system. The system is identified by actions and behaviors that are regulated and controlled by biologic, psychologic, and sociologic factors. The system is composed of seven interacting subsystems that carry out specialized functions for the system as a whole (Johnson, 1980, pp. 212–214). These seven subsystems are as follows:

1. The attachment or *affiliative* subsystem serves the function of security, and makes possible social inclusion, intimacy, and the formation and maintenance of a strong social bond.
2. The *dependency* subsystem calls for a response of nurturance. It has as its consequence, approval, attention or recognition, and physical assistance.
3. The *ingestive* subsystem serves the broad function of appetite satisfaction.
4. The *eliminative* subsystem involves learned behavior in the excretion of wastes.
5. The *sexual* subsystem is involved in procreation and gratification, and covers the broad range of behaviors dependent on biologic sex, including but not limited to courting and mating.

6. The *aggressive* subsystem is related to self-protection and preservation.
7. The *achievement* subsystem functions for mastery or control of some aspect of the self or environment measured against some standard of excellence.

Each subsystem has structural elements and functional requirements (Johnson, 1980, pp. 210–212). The *structural elements* are (1) the drive or goal being sought; (2) the set, or the person's predisposition to act; (3) the choices, or scope of alternatives for action; and (4) the person's behavior. The *functional* requirements include (1) protection from harmful (noxious) influences; (2) nurturance through the input of appropriate supplies; and (3) stimulation to enhance growth and prevent stagnation. These requirements must be met through the individual's own efforts or through outside assistance (the nurse) "for each to grow, develop and remain viable" (Johnson, 1980, p. 212).

While the emphasis is on the subsystems comprising the behavioral system (man), it is assumed that each person has a unique pattern of interactions that distinguish him as a total entity. The system attempts to maintain balance, while environmental forces (everything external to the interacting subsystems) influence the system and may cause a lack of balance or health problems.

Health-illness is not specifically defined in the Johnson model. However, clearly *health* is associated with system equilibrium. Illness is associated with a lack of functional or structural balance within or unbalanced interaction between the subsystems. The major causes of instability are (1) inadequate or inappropriate development of the system or its parts; (2) breakdown in internal regulatory or control mechanisms; (3) exposure to noxious influences; (4) inadequate stimulation of the system; or (5) lack of adequate environmental input (Loveland-Cherry and Wilkerson, 1983, p. 120).

Nursing is only implicated when there is disruption of system balance. "A state of imbalance or instability in the behavioral system results in the need for nursing actions; and appropriate nursing actions results in the maintenance or restoration of behavioral system balance and stability" (Loveland-Cherry and Wilkerson, 1983, p. 129). There is no defined role for nursing in relation to health maintenance or promotion. "Nursing is an external regulatory force which acts to preserve the organization and integration of the patient's behavior at an optimal level under those conditions in which the behavior constitutes a threat to physical or social health, or in which illness is found" (Johnson, 1980, p. 214). Thus, "unless there is instability or less than optimal functioning in the behavioral system, nursing has no identified goal" (Loveland-Cherry and Wilkerson, 1983, p. 128).

Nursing can impose external regulatory or control mechanisms (*e.g.*, setting limits on behavior), change structural units in a desirable direction (*e.g.*, teaching), fulfill the functional requirements of the subsystems (*e.g.*, providing essential environmental conditions or resources), or help regulate balance between subsystems (*e.g.*, modify diet to promote elimination). There is no indication of potential for active decision-making on the part of the patient.

In summary, the Johnson behavioral system model emphasizes "reactive relationships within an illness focus" (Loveland-Cherry and Wilkerson, 1983, p. 131). As the interacting subsystems attempt to maintain balance, they are affected by environmental forces that may result in disequilibrium. The nurse may intervene in order to "restore, maintain or attain behavioral system balance and stability at the highest possible level for the individual" (Johnson, 1980, p. 214). A summary of the major concepts as they are defined in the Johnson model appears in Table 8–2.

TABLE 8–2.   Major Concepts as Defined in the Johnson Model

Person:	Attempting to maintain balance. Interrelated subsystems that form a behavioral system
Health:	System equilibrium
Illness:	Lack of balance between the subsystems
Environment:	Input from sources outside the person
Nursing:	External force to restore system stability

DOROTHEA OREM SELF-CARE NURSING MODEL

Terms

Self-care—activities that a person performs for himself (when able) that contribute to health

Self-care deficit—lack of ability of the person to perform all the activities needed for healthy functioning

Self-care requisites—needs that are universal or associated with development or deviation from health

Self-care demand—therapeutic actions to meet needs

The essence of Orem's model of nursing, which is organized around the goal of nursing, is the concept of self-care. Self-care is the individual's own "action that has pattern and sequence and when it is effectively performed contributes in specific ways to human structural integrity, human functioning, and human development" (Orem, 1980, p. 37). Self-care activities are learned as the individual matures, and are affected by the cultural beliefs, habits, and customs of the family and the society. A person's age, developmental state, and/or state of health can affect the ability to perform self-care activities. For example, a parent or guardian must maintain continuous therapeutic care for a child.

Nursing is concerned with the *individual's* need for self-care action in order to help the patient to "sustain life and health, recover from disease or injury, and cope with their effects" (Orem, 1980, p. 6). In Orem's view, nursing care may be offered to "individual and multiperson units," but only individuals have self-care requisites. The nurse cares for, assists or does something for the patient to achieve the health results that the patient desires (Orem, 1980, p. 126).

Orem implies that *health* is related to normal structure and function, since "any deviation from normal structure or functioning is properly referred to as an absence of health in the sense of wholeness or integrity" (Orem, 1980, p. 118). She refers to the physical, psychologic, interpersonal, and social aspects of health, but indicates that they are inseparable in the individual. "A human being is a unity that can be viewed as functioning biologically, symbolically and socially" (Orem, 1980, p. 120). There may be a variety of states of "well-being or health," and a person may move from one state to another, but, constancy of "internal and external conditions" is associated with health.

Orem suggests that some people may have self-care requisites (needs) associated with development or with deviation from health. All people have the following universal self-care requisites:

1. Maintenance of a sufficient intake of air, water, and food.
2. Provision of care associated with elimination processes and excrements.
3. Maintenance of a balance between activity and rest and between solitude and social interaction.
4. Prevention of hazards to life, functioning, and well-being.
5. Promotion of human functioning and development within social groups in accord with potential, known limitations, and the desire to be normal. (Orem, 1980, p. 42)

Identified needs (self-care requisites) require actions known as the therapeutic self-care demand. Universal and developmental self-care requisites lead to maintenance and promotion of health and prevention of specific diseases. This is termed primary prevention self-care demand. Health deviation self-care requisites lead to prevention of complications and prolonged disability after illness. This is termed secondary prevention self-care demand. Tertiary prevention self-care demand brings about effective and satisfying function in accord with existing powers. The therapeutic self-care demand can be determined by identifying all existing or possible self-care requisites, identifying methods for meeting self-care requisites, and designing, implementing, and evaluating a plan of action. This is the *nursing* process.

Orem describes three stages in the nursing process. The first stage involves the determination of "why a person should be under nursing care." This stage primarily involves assessment of the patient's therapeutic self-care demand, any deficits for performing self-care activities, and what future goals are appropriate. The second stage involves designing a system of nursing that will lead to achievement of health goals. This stage primarily involves planning methods to meet self-care requisites in view of existing limitations. The third stage involves implementation and evaluation of actions to overcome self-care limitations, provide therapeutic self-care, and prevent the development of new self-care limitations.

Thus, candidates for nursing are patients who have insufficient current or projected capability for providing self-care. "It is the need for compensatory action (to overcome an inability or limited ability to engage in care) or for action to help in the development or regulation of self-care abilities that is the basis for a nursing relationship" (Orem, 1980, p. 58).

To help project the scope of nursing responsibility and the roles and actions of patients and nurses, Orem has designed three types of nursing systems. In the wholly compensatory system, the patient is either unable to perform any deliberate action (*e.g.,* coma), or may be unable to ambulate, manipulate, or make reasoned judgements. In these cases, nurses provide and manage self-care and make judgements and decisions about self-care requisites. In a partly compensatory system, both the patient and the nurse perform care measures, while in the supportive-educative system, the patient is able to perform or can and should learn to perform required measures of therapeutic self-care but cannot do so without assistance.

This model emphasizes a role for the nurse only when the patient is unable to provide for his own self-care requisites. Nursing intervention may be aimed at maintaining health, preventing illness, or restoring health, and may involve actions for or with the patient. The model is widely used in practice and education, and is

TABLE 8–3.	Major Concepts as Defined in Orem's Model
Person:	Inseparable physical, psychologic, interpersonal, and social aspects
Health:	Constancy of internal and external conditions that permits self-care needs to be met
Illness:	Deviation from normal structure or function resulting in self-care deficits
Environment:	Factors external to the person
Nursing:	Actions to overcome or prevent the development of self-care limitations or provide therapeutic self-care for an individual who is unable to do so

the basis for some beginning research. Major concepts as they are defined in Orem's model are summarized in Table 8-3.

SISTER CALLISTA ROY'S ADAPTATION MODEL

Terms

Stressors—stimuli from the environment that require the person to adapt

Adaptive modes—ways that the person adapts (e.g., through physiologic needs, self-concept, role function, or interdependence relations)

Classes of stimuli—focal (immediately confronting the person), contextual (all other stimuli present), and residual (nonspecific stimuli such as beliefs or attitudes)

Adaptation level—range of a person's ability to respond to and cope with stimuli

Coping—ways of responding to stressors

The essence of the Roy model, organized around adaptive behaviors of the person, is the set of processes by which a person adapts to environmental stressors. In the Roy model, the person as a unified system is viewed from the perspective of a bio-psycho-social being. The person is in constant interaction with a changing environment. The transaction between the environmental demand of adaptation and the person's response is stress (Roy and Roberts, 1981, p. 56).

The *person* is affected by stressors that are described as focal stimuli. The focal stimulus is a change immediately confronting the person that requires an adaptive response. Contextual (all other stimuli present) and residual stimuli (other relevant factors) mediate and contribute to the effect of the stressor to produce the interaction called stress. The pooled effect of the three classes of stimuli result in the adaptation level. The person's adaptation level determines a zone that indicates the range of further stimulation that will have a positive or adaptive response. If further stimuli fall outside of the zone, the person cannot respond positively, and ineffective coping occurs.

"Coping refers to routine, accustomed patterns of behaviors to deal with daily situations as well as to the production of new ways of behaving when drastic changes defy the familiar responses" (Roy and Roberts, 1981, p. 56). The two major coping mechanisms are the regulator and the cognator. The regulator subsystem is composed mainly of neural, endocrine, and perception-psychomotor components. The cognator subsystem includes psychosocial pathways and provides for perceptual/information processing, learning, judgement, and emotion.

Persons are conceptualized by Roy as having four modes or methods of adaptation: physiologic, self-concept, role function, and interdependence relations. The desired end result is a state where conditions promote the goals of the person including survival, growth, reproduction, and mastery.

Thus, in the Roy model, adaptation is both a process of coping with stressors and an end state produced by the process. When coping mechanisms are effective in dealing with stress, a dynamic state of equilibrium results that fosters the goals of the person. When unusual stresses or weakened coping mechanisms make the person's usual attempts to cope ineffective, then nursing care is needed (Roy and Roberts, 1981, p. 45). The client may be a family, community or society, but Roy emphasizes adaptation of the individual (Roy and Roberts, 1981, p. 42).

"Health is a state of human functioning whereby the person continually adapts to change" (Galbreath, 1980, p. 201). *Health* can be viewed on a continuum from death to extremely poor health to poor health to normal health to good health to high-level wellness to peak wellness (Fig. 8-1).

The goal of *nursing* is the person's adaptation through the four adaptive modes. "The criterion for judging when the goal has been reached is generally any positive response made by the recipient to the stimuli present that frees energy for responses to other stimuli" (Riehl and Roy, 1980, p. 183). The goal of adaptation is fostered through nursing assessment and intervention, with the patient as an active participant.

Using the Roy model, assessment would focus first on identification of patient behaviors in each of the adaptive modes and recognition of the person's position on a health-illness continuum. Second level assessments would include identification of focal, contextual, and residual factors that may be affecting the patient. The nurse thus makes a nursing diagnosis of deficits or excesses of basic needs that are the cause of ineffective patient behaviors (Roy and Roberts, 1980, p. 47).

Nursing intervention involves increasing, decreasing or maintaining focal, contextual, and/or residual stimuli so that the patient can cope. Roy emphasizes that in intervening, the nurse "should be constantly aware of the active responsibility of the patient to participate in his own care when he is able to do so" (Roy and Roberts, 1981, p. 47).

This model provides a classification system for stressors that may affect adaptation, as well as a system for classifying nursing assessments. A widely used model, it is the basis for a growing body of research. Major concepts as defined in Roy's model are summarized in Table 8-4.

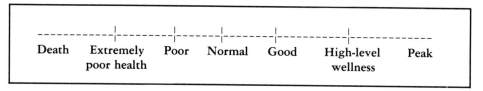

Figure 8-1. Health continuum in Roy's model. (Roy SC: Introduction to Nursing: An adaptation Model, p 18, 1976. Reprinted by permission of Prentice-Hall, Englewood Cliffs, NJ)

TABLE 8–4. Major Concepts as Defined in Roy's Model

Person:	Bio-psycho-social being forming a unified system that seeks equilibrium
Health:	Adaptation resulting from successful coping with stressors
Illness:	Ineffective coping on a continuum from death toward adaptation
Environment:	External conditions and influences that affect the development of the person
Nursing:	Manipulation of stimuli to foster successful coping

BETTY NEUMAN HEALTH-CARE SYSTEMS MODEL

Terms

Lines of defense—ways in which an individual deals with stressors in order to maintain equilibrium of the system

Lines of resistance—protection from stressors

The Neuman model, organized around stress reduction, is primarily concerned with the effects of stress and reactions to stress on the development and maintenance of health. The person is described as an open system that interacts with the environment to order to promote "harmony and balance between his internal and external environment" (Neuman, 1982, p. 14). The person is a composite of physiologic, psychologic, sociocultural, and developmental variables that are viewed as a whole. "No one part can be looked at in isolation . . . just as the single part influences perception of the whole, the patterns of the whole influence awareness of the part" (Neuman, 1982, p. 14). Thus, the functioning of any subsystem or part of a system must be evaluated in the context of the entire system.

The *person* is constantly affected by stressors. Stressors are tension producing stimuli that have the potential of disturbing a person's equilibrium or normal line of defense. This normal line of defense is the person's "usual steady state." It is the way in which an individual usually deals with stressors. Stressors may be (1) intrapersonal, that is, forces occurring from within the individual; (2) interpersonal, that is, forces occurring between individuals; or (3) extrapersonal, that is, forces occurring from outside the individual. Resistance to stressors are provided by the flexible line of defense, which is a dynamic protective buffer made up of all variables affecting an individual at any point in time. For example, these variables may include a person's physiologic structure and condition, sociocultural background, developmental state, cognitive skills, age, sex, and so forth. The interrelationships between these variables determine the amount of resistance an individual has to any stressor or stressors.

If the flexible line of defense is no longer able to protect the person against a stressor, the stressor breaks through the normal line of defense. In other words, the person's equilibrium is disturbed and there is a reaction. The reaction may lead toward restoration of balance or toward death, depending on the internal lines of resistance that attempt to restore balance (return the person to the normal line of defense). The reaction to the stressor and the prognosis are influenced by the number and strength of the stressors affecting the person, the length of time that the person is affected, and the meaningfulness of the stressor to the individual.

Neuman intends the model to "assist individuals, families and groups to attain and maintain a maximum level of total wellness by purposeful interventions" (Neuman, 1982, p. 11). It is not clear what "total wellness" means in this model. *Wellness* is defined as "a state of saturation—one of inertness free of disrupting needs" (Neuman, 1982, p. 10). Wellness seems to be related to dynamic equilibrium of the normal line of defense, where stressors are successfully overcome or avoided by the flexible line of defense. Neuman defines illness as "a state of insufficiency—disrupting needs are yet to be satisfied" (Neuman, 1982, p. 10). Illness appears to be a separate state when a stressor or stressors have broken through the normal line of defense and have caused a reaction with the person's lines of resistance.

Nursing intervention is "aimed at reduction of stress factors and adverse conditions which either affect or could affect optimal functioning in a given client situation" (Neuman, 1980, p. 119). Nursing intervention is accomplished through primary, secondary, or tertiary prevention. Primary prevention is appropriate before the person comes in contact with a stressor. "The goal of primary prevention is to prevent the stressor from penetrating the normal line of defense or to lessen the degree of reaction by reducing the possibility of encounter with the stressor, reducing its strength, and/or strengthening the flexible line of defense" (Venable, 1980, p. 136). This is primarily accomplished by assessment of individual patients to identify and decrease possible risk factors associated with stressors. Planning, intervention, and evaluation of strategies to strengthen the normal line of defense may also be appropriate. Secondary prevention is appropriate after the stressor has penetrated the normal line of defense. Care involves early case finding, and planning and evaluations of interventions related to symptoms. Tertiary prevention accompanies restoration of balance, moving in a circular manner toward primary prevention. The focus is on "reeducation to prevent future occurrences, readaptation, and maintenance of stability" (Venable, 1980, p. 136).

This recently developed model suggests various primary, secondary, and tertiary prevention nursing activities to reduce stress factors and strengthen the individual's resistance. It has many possible applications to nursing process. The major concepts as defined in the Neuman model are summarized in Table 8-5.

TABLE 8–5.	Major Concepts as Defined in the Neuman Model
Person:	Open system seeking balance and harmony. Composite of physiologic, psychologic, sociocultural, and developmental variables viewed as a whole
Health:	Dynamic equilibrium of the normal line of defense
Illness:	Due to reaction of stressors with lines of resistance
Environment:	Internal and external stressors and resistance factors
Nursing:	Reduction of stressors through primary, secondary, or tertiary prevention

MARTHA ROGERS' SCIENCE OF UNITARY MAN _____

Terms

Space-time continuum–a four-dimensional combination of both elements

The essence of the Rogerian model, organized around person-environmental interaction, is a conceptual system built on an assumption of the person as a unified energy field that is continuously exchanging matter and energy with the environment. Rogers proposes that "man is a unified whole possessing his own integrity and manifesting characteristics that are more than and different from the sum of his parts" (Rogers, 1970, p. 47). Physical, biologic, psychologic, social, cultural, and spiritual attributes are merged into behavior that reflects the total person as an indivisible whole. Rogers believes that it is not possible to describe man by combining attributes of each of the parts. Only as the parts lose their particular identity is it possible to describe the person.

The *person* is an organized energy field that has a unique pattern. The energy field that is the person is continuously exchanging matter and energy with the environmental energy field resulting in continuous repatterning of both the person and the environment (Rogers, 1970, p. 53). These exchanges of energy result in increasing complexity and innovativeness of the person. Rogers believes that this life process "evolves irreversibly and unidirectionally along the space-time continuum" (Rogers, 1970, p. 59). She conceptualizes this unidirectionality as a spiral, with self-regulation "directed toward achieving increasing complexity of organization—not toward achieving equilibrium and stability" (Rogers, 1970, p. 64). The person is also characterized by "the capacity for abstraction and imagery, language and thought, sensation and emotion" (Rogers, 1970, p. 73).

Rogers deals with normal and pathologic processes equally. She does not view *health* and illness as separate states, nor in a linear relationship. "Ease and dis-ease are dichotomous notions that cannot be used to account for the dynamic complexity and uncertain fulfillment of man's unfolding" (Rogers, 1970, p. 42).

Nursing intervention is aimed toward repatterning of man and environment in order to achieve maximum health potential of the person (Rogers, 1970, pp. 86, 127). "People must be informed and active participants in the search for health. Intervention should be directed toward assisting individuals to mobilize their resources, consciously and unconsciously, so that the man-environment relationship may be strengthened and the integrity of the individual heightened" (Rogers, 1970, p. 134). "Maintenance and promotion of health, prevention of disease, nursing diagnosis, intervention, and rehabilitation encompass the scope of nursing's goals" (Rogers, 1970, p. 86).

Rogers has described three principles that explain the life process in man and predict its evolution (Rogers, 1980, p. 333). The principle of *complementarity* emphasizes that man's energy field and the environmental energy field must be perceived at the same time. The relationship is one of constant interaction and mutual simultaneous change. In other words, "they are reciprocal systems in which molding and being molded are taking place at the same time" (Rogers, 1970, p. 97). The principle of *helicy* predicts that the nature and direction of change occurs "along a spiraling longitudinal axis bound in space-time" (Rogers, 1970, p. 101). The human field becomes increasingly diverse with time. As the person ages, be-

TABLE 8–6.	Major Concepts as Defined in the Rogerian Model
Person:	Unified and patterned energy field
Health:	Increasing complexity and innovativeness of patterning
Environment:	Energy field continuously interacting with the energy field that is the person.
Nursing:	Repatterning of person and environment to achieve maximum health potential of the person

havior is not repeated, but may reoccur at ever more complex levels. The principle of *resonancy* indicates that change in pattern and organization toward increased complexity of the field occurs by way of waves, "manifesting continuous change from lower frequency, longer wave patterns to higher-frequency, shorter wave patterns" (Rogers, 1980, p. 333).

Rogers believes that an understanding of the mechanisms that affect the life process in man make it possible for the nurse to purposefully intervene to affect repatterning of the person in a desired direction. In the process, the nurse is also changed. Her emphasis on holistic man and on the simultaneous and continuous interaction between man and environment are concepts that are now widely accepted in nursing. Major concepts as defined in the Rogerian model are summarized in Table 8-6.

RESEARCH RELATED TO MODELS OF NURSING

Three kinds of research related to models of nursing are currently being conducted. One approach is to test the relationships predicted by the model. For example, Floyd predicted changes in sleep-wakefulness rhythms based on the Rogerian principles of resonancy and helicy. She found evidence that workers undergoing shift rotation (change in the environmental field) manifested increased total wakefulness time and frequency of sleep-wakefulness cycles (indicators of diversity and complexity of sleep-wakefulness cycles). However, these data have not been replicated, and Floyd discusses a number of limitations of control in the study that might have affected the findings (Floyd, 1983).

Another approach is the use of a model as a framework for descriptive analysis. For example, Derdiarian and Forsythe used the perspective of Johnson's behavioral systems model to measure and describe the perceived behavioral changes of the cancer patient. They developed an instrument to describe the existence, direction, quality, importance, and effects of the "imbalance in the patient's behavioral system" (Derdiarian and Forsythe, 1983, p. 260) that were believed to be associated with the illness process. It has been suggested that these kind of data can form a basis for problem definition and nursing intervention. The tool is in early stages of testing for construct validity and replication of findings.

A few studies attempt to modify nursing care through use of a model. One example of such a study is Ziemer's (1983) giving of information preoperatively (increasing lines of defense) in order to reduce pain symptoms postoperatively.

TABLE 8–7. Similarities and Differences of Conceptualization in Six Selected Nursing Models

	Goal	Person Composition	Health	Environment	Nursing
Peplau	Equilibrium	System with physiologic, psychologic, and social components	Meeting needs	Significant others	Therapeutic interpersonal process
Johnson	Balance	Behavioral system with seven subsystems	Equilibrium	External inputs	External force to restore stability
Orem	Constancy	Whole with physical, psychologic, interpersonal, social aspects	Meeting self-care needs	External forces	Actions to limit self-care deficits
Roy	Equilibrium	System with bio-psycho-social components	Adaptation	External conditions	Manipulation of stimuli to foster coping
Neuman	Balance	Composite of physiologic, psychological, sociocultural, developmental variables	Equilibrium	Internal and external stressors	Reduction of stressors
Rogers	Increased complexity of pattern	Indivisible energy field	Increasing innovativeness of patterning	Contiguous, continuously interacting energy field	Repatterning to facilitate potential

Unfortunately, in this study hypotheses based on Neuman's model were not supported.

The issue of the usefulness of nursing models has been raised. A model does provide a useful system for classification of data during the nursing process. A model also proposes theoretical relationships that can be tested through research. But are the differences in terms between models simply a semantic shell game? Does the model used to organize data make any real difference in the nursing care given the client? What difference does it make if the cause of a problem is labeled a "noxious influence" affecting a behavioral subsystem, a "self-care deficit" leading to a "self-care demand," or a "focal stimulus," which is a stressor? How is care given any differently if its purpose is labeled to limit self-care deficits, reduce stressors, or foster coping?

Nursing science is in an early stage of development. There has been a great deal of discussion about whether there should be a model for nursing. The controversy, however, and the popularity of several models document that there is no agreement about how nursing can be described or how its goals can best be achieved. Is the controversy about the relative merits of different models irrelevant or premature and thus diversionary? In the absence of consensus, perhaps research might more productively be focused on testing relationships predicted by theory and on the implications of the findings for improving practice.

SUMMARY

In this early stage of the development of nursing science, a number of nursing theorists have published models of nursing. Six of the best known have been summarized and compared in this chapter (Table 8-7). The implications of various models for application of the nursing process will be demonstrated in Chapter 12, The Nursing Process.

REFERENCES

Derdiarian AK, Forsythe AB: An instrument for theory and research development using the behavioral systems model for nursing: The cancer patient. Nurs Res 32:260–266, September–October 1983

Floyd J: Research using Rogers' conceptual system: Development of a testable theorem. Adv Nurs Sci: 37–48, January 1983

Galbreath JG: Sister Callista Roy. In George JB (ed): Nursing Theories: The Base for Professinal Nursing Practice, pp 199–212. Englewood Cliffs, Prentice-Hall, 1980

George JB (Chairperson, The Nursing Theories Conference Group): Nursing Theories: The Base for Professional Nursing Practice. Englewood Cliffs, Prentice-Hall, 1980

Johnson DE: The behavioral system model for nursing. In Riehl JP, Roy SC (eds): Conceptual Models for Nursing Practice, ed 2, pp 207–216. New York, Appleton-Century-Crofts, 1980

Lippitt GL: Visualizing Change. Model Building and the Change Process. San Diego, University Associates, 1973

Loveland-Cherry C, Wilkerson SA: Dorothy Johnson's behavioral system model. In Fitzpatrick JJ, Whall AL (eds): Conceptual Models of Nursing: Analysis and Application, pp 117–135. Bowie, Robert J. Brady, 1983

Neuman B: The Neuman Systems Model. Application to Nursing Education and Practice. Norwalk, Appleton-Century Crofts, 1982

Neuman B: The Betty Neuman health-care systems model: A total person approach to patient problems. *In* Riehl JP, Roy SC (eds): Conceptual Models for Nursing Practice, ed 2, pp 119–131. New York, Appleton-Century-Crofts, 1980

Orem DE: Nursing: Concepts of Practice, 2nd. New York, McGraw-Hill, 1980

Peplau HE: Interpersonal Relations in Nursing. New York, GP Putnam's Sons, 1952

Reed PG, Johnston RL: Peplau's nursing model: The interpersonal process. In Fitzpatrick JJ, Whall Al (eds): Conceptual Models of Nursing: Analysis and Application, pp 27–46. Bowie, Robert J Brady, 1983

Riehl JP, Roy SC: Conceptual Models for Nursing Practice. New York, Appleton-Century-Crofts, 1980

Rogers ME: An Introduction To The Theoretical Basis of Nursing. Philadelphia, FA Davis, 1970

Rogers ME: Nursing: A science of unitary man. *In* Riehl JP, Roy SC (eds): Conceptual Models for Nursing Practice, pp 329–337. New York, Appleton-Century-Crofts, 1980

Roy SC, Roberts SL: Theory Construction in Nursing: An Adaptation Model. Englewood Cliffs, Prentice-Hall, 1981

Venable JF: The Neuman health-care systems model: An analysis. *In* Riehl JP, Roy SC (eds): Conceptual Models for Nursing Practice, ed 2, pp 135–150. New York, Appleton-Century-Crofts, 1980

Ziemer MM: Effect of information on post-surgical coping. Nurs Res 32:282–287, September–October 1983

Section 3

Delivery of Professional Nursing

Chapter 9

The Health Process

Thought Questions

1. How does well-being differ from health? Illness from disease?
2. What factors cause individual variability in well-being?
3. What are the beliefs and norms of the "provider culture"? Why might these be important for the nurse to understand?
4. How can the nurse foster health-promoting behavior in clients and herself?

When asked why they went into nursing, many nurses answer, "to help people." By this they usually mean to help sick people get better. Nursing, in the minds of many people, is associated with medicine and hospitals, since most nurses work for hospitals caring for sick people.

The major purpose of the hospital is to support the medical regimen to treat disease and dysfunction. The public image of what nursing is and what nurses do has been influenced by the medical definition of health as the absence of disease. The association of nursing with disease and sickness is at the heart of the traditional characterization of the nurse as the so-called physician's handmaiden. This issue is discussed in Chapter 17, "The Contributor to the Profession Role."

Cure of disease is the major purpose of medicine, but "health care" delivery aimed predominantly at cure of disease is wasteful of resources and very costly. Increasingly, the public is becoming aware of the need to prevent illness and promote and maintain well-being. Nurses care for the responses of people to threats to well-being and/or illness. Thus, the nursing profession has the potential to make a major impact on our society's philosophy and delivery of health care through roles designed to promote health.

In this chapter, the concepts disease, illness, sickness, health, well-being, and wellness are defined. Several alternate conceptual models of their interrelationships are presented. A number of factors (multideterminants) that may influence a person's well-being status are explored in depth. The final section of the chapter considers nursing interventions for prevention of illness and promotion of well-being and health.

WELL-BEING–ILLNESS RELATIONSHIPS

Both laymen and health professionals often define good health as the absence of the clinical signs of disease. Are health and illness poles on a continuum, qualitatively different phenomena, or even on the same level of discourse? After a definition of concepts, these philosophical questions are addressed.

Definitions

Disease

Disease is a medical term. It is a process of alteration of body functions resulting in a reduction of capacities or a shortening of the normal life span (Twaddle, 1977, p. 97). The objective of the physician is to classify observable changes in structure and/or function of the body (signs) into a recognizable clinical syndrome. A correct label, or diagnosis, implies course and duration, communicability, prognosis, and appropriate treatment. Medical intervention is aimed at curing the disease. Part of nursing intervention supports and promotes the medical regimen through, among other things, administration of treatments, encouragement of rest, and evaluation of the effectiveness of intervention.

Historically, diseases were believed to be due to one agent, which, in a sufficient dose, caused certain predictable signs and symptoms. Increasingly, however, a variety of factors related to the person (host), agent, and environment have been viewed as being interrelated in the cause, and the effectiveness of the treatment of disease. All of these multideterminants and their interactions must be considered in determining a plan of care.

Illness

Illness is a subjective feeling of being unhealthy that may or may not be related to disease. A person may have a disease without feeling ill, and may feel ill in the absence of disease. For example, a person may have hypertension (a disease) controlled with medication, and have no symptoms (no illness). Or the person may have pain, and thus feel ill, but not have an identifiable disease. What is important is how the person feels and what he does because of those feelings. Nursing intervention aims to identify a cause for and decrease the symptoms if possible, while medical care focuses on efforts to label and treat disease. When a person's illness is accepted by society, and thus given legitimacy, it is considered sickness.

Sickness

Sickness is a status, a social entity that is usually associated with disease or illness although it may occur independently of them (Twaddle, 1977, p. 97). Once the person is defined as sick, a variety of dependent behaviors are condoned that otherwise might be considered unacceptable. The nurse's role is to assist the person until he is able to reassume responsibility for decision-making.

Health

Health is very difficult to define. Health is described in various sources as a value judgement, a subjective state, a relative concept, a spectrum, a cycle, a process, and as an abstraction that cannot be measured objectively (Siegel, 1973, pp. 282–283). In many definitions, physiologic and psychologic components of health are dichotomized. Other subconcepts that might be included in definitions of health include environmental and social influences, freedom from pain and/or disease, optimum capability, ability to adapt, purposeful direction and meaning in life, and harmony, balance, or sense of well-being (Keller, 1981, p. 49).

Smith (1981) presents four models of health that "can be viewed as forming a scale—a progressive expansion of the idea of health" (Smith, 1981, p. 47). The *clinical model* is the most narrow view. People are seen as physiologic systems with interrelated functions. Health is identified as the absence of signs and symptoms of disease or disability as identified by medical science. Thus, health might be defined as "a state of not being sick" (Ardell, 1979, p. 18), or "a relatively passive state of freedom from illness . . . a condition of relative homeostasis" (Dunn, 1977, p. 9). Much of our present health care delivery system is set up to deal with disease and illness after it occurs, based on this model of "health." In the clinical model of health, the opposite end of the continuum from health is disease.

Next on the scale is the idea of health as *role-performance.* This model adds social and psychologic standards to the concept of health. The critical criterion of health is the ability of individuals to fulfill their roles in society with the maximum (*e.g.,* best, highest) expected performance. If a person is unable to perform his expected roles, it can mean illness even if he appears clinically healthy. An example of this type of definition is "somatic health is . . . the state of optimum capacity for the effective performance of valued tasks" (Parsons, 1958, p. 168). In the role-performance model of health, the opposite end of the continuum from health is sickness.

Incorporating the clinical and role-performance models is the *adaptive model.* Health is perceived as a condition in which the individual can engage in effective interaction with the physical and social environment. There is an indication of growth and change in this model. For example, Murray and Zentner (1979, pp. 5–6) define health as "a purposeful, adaptive response, physically, mentally, emotionally, and socially, to internal and external stimuli in order to maintain stability and comfort." Siegel (1973, p. 286) describes health as "an outcome of interplay between the internal environment and external multi-environments." In the adaptive model of health, the opposite end of the continuum from health is illness.

Smith considers the *eudaimonistic model* to be the most comprehensive conception of health. In this model, health is a condition of actualization or realization of the potential of the individual. For example, human health "is a process of becoming; a dynamic movement toward a full realization of latent possibilities, not only in the human body, but in human feeling, minds, and spirits" (Greifinger, 1977, p. 207). "Health transcends biological fitness. It is primarily a measure of each person's ability to do what he wants to do and become what he wants to become" (Dubos, 1978, p. 74). In the eudaimonistic model of health, health is consistent with "high level wellness," and at the opposite end of the continuum from disabling illness.

Mallick suggests that definitions of health fall into two categories: open ended and functional. The open ended definitions suggest, like the eudaimonistic model above, "an ideal on the horizon that can be approached but never reached" (Wylie, 1970, p. 100). Functional definitions, like the role-performance classification of Smith, relate health to the ability to function despite the presence of sickness (Mallick, 1979, p. 30). Wylie adds a possible third category, elastic, which like the adaptive classification "picture a positive interaction between the person or community and the environment" (Wylie, 1970, p. 101). This view incorporates the concept that maximum health requires choice and conscious participation of the individual (Dubos, 1978 p. 80; Hollen, 1981, p. 27). Figure 9-1 compares Mallick's categories with those of Smith.

Well-Being

Well-being, as defined in this book, is a subjective perception of balance, harmony, and vitality. It is a state that can be described objectively. It occurs in degrees. At the lowest levels, the individual would be labeled "ill." At the highest levels, an individual would perceive maximum satisfaction and feeling of contribution. Thus, well-being status can be plotted on a continuum such as diagrammed in Figure 9-2.

Health is a goal and an everchanging process, while well-being is a variable state that is contiguous with illness. It is our contention that the current inability to quantify health is due to confusion of the *process* of health with the well-being *status*. Well-being can be described and measured. Health, on the other hand, encompasses well-being and illness, and is an evolving potential that cannot be quantified.

Nurses try to help people to move toward well-being by focusing on strengths as well as weaknesses, and by collaborating with clients to promote growth toward the client's potential for health. The client's goals and feelings are a major determinant of nursing intervention.

Wellness

Wellness, as defined in the literature, is very similiar to the open ended, or eudaimonistic model of health, and, in this book, will be considered synonomous. Dunn (1977, p. 9) describes wellness as "an integrated method of functioning which is oriented toward maximizing the potential of which the individual is capable, within the environment where he is functioning." Others have characterized wellness as "an integrated state of optimum function" (Auger, 1976, p. 4), "a continually evolving and changing process" (Bruhn *et al.* Spring 1977, p. 209), and ability to "function at (his) perceived maximum capacity and satisfaction" (Bruhn and Cordova, November-December 1977, p. 248).

Wellness (health) is probably best conceptualized as an active process, continuing in time, that involves initiative, ability to assume responsibility for health, value

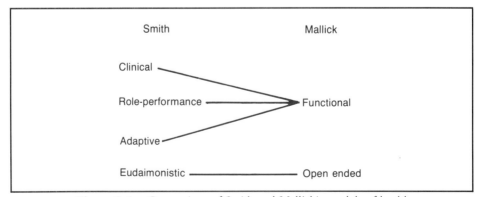

Figure 9–1. Comparison of Smith and Mallick's models of health.

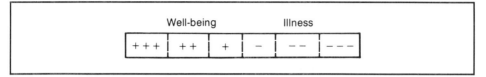

Figure 9–2. The well-being continuum. (Modified from Terris M: Approaches to an epidemiology of health. Am J Public Health 65:1039, 1975. Used with permission of the publisher)

judgements, and an integration of the total individual. It is a goal, a fluid process, rather than an actual state. Thus, wellness is difficult to quantify for objective evaluation. However, indications might include the capacity of the person to perform to the best of his ability, ability to adjust and adapt to varying situations, a reported feeling of well-being, and a feeling that "everything is together."

Possible Relationships

What is the relationship between health and illness? Are the concepts of health and illness at a comparable level as the literature implies, or might health be viewed as a much broader process (the eudaimonistic model), encompassing a definable illness status at any point in time? Four alternatives will be considered: health and illness as dichotomous opposites, health as a separate dimension from illness, health on a graduated scale with illness (Wu, 1973, p. 76), and holistic health as a concept encompassing illness.

Health as Dichotomous from Illness

In the "health as dichotomous from illness" approach, there are no degrees of health or illness. A person is either ill or healthy. For example, Wu defines illness as "an event . . . causing an impairment of capacity to meet minimum . . . requirements for appropriate functioning . . ." (Wu, 1973, p. 23). In her view, "health-wellness is . . . a capacity to perform to the best of one's ability" (Wu, 1973, p. 86). If the person is not able to perform at his best, his capacity is "impaired."

This approach, which defines the terms in relation to each other, is not consistent with observations of the real world. The view of health as a static state is not compatible with constantly changing open systems. Since there are no degrees of health, there is no room to acknowledge healthy behaviors in a person who is ill. This approach emphasizes illness and weaknesses, with intervention focused on curing the problem.

Well-being and Illness as Two Separate Dimensions

In order for well-being and illness to be considered two separate dimensions, they must be described independently, in observable terms. Hadley (1974, pp. 24–25), attempts to define physical and physiologic criteria as within or outside normal limits of size, composition, and function as determined by a physician. Examples of her social-psychologic criteria that demonstrate their linear relationship as bipolar opposites are as follows:

	Wellness	*Illness*
	Independence	Dependence
	Industry	Passive avoidance of obligations
	Initiative	Guilt
	Vigor	Impotence
	Capableness	Helplessness
	Confidence	Uncertainty

Jahoda (Wu, 1973, p. 82), views health and illness on two dimensions. She believes that every person has healthy and sick aspects simultaneously, with one or the other predominating. Since a person can only be viewed as a whole, the predominating behavior will determine whether he is considered ill or well by an observer. The predominant behavior will also affect the person's perception of his condition.

To engage in research, it is desirable to be able to describe health and illness in observable terms. However, critics argue that since health is subjective, culturally influenced, and relative, it is an abstraction that cannot totally be measured objectively (Siegel, 1973, pp. 282–283). At this point in time, only aspects of health can be measured. It is also questionable whether it is ordinarily useful or even possible to define a person's status at one point in time. Since the person is constantly changing, the most important consideration clinically would seem to be the ability of the observer to assess which behaviors are healthy (strengths), and which indicate possible need for assistance (weaknesses).

Continuum Approach

As soon as the need to measure health and illness in discrete terms is waived, the graduated scale or continuum approach appears more desirable. Well-being status can be conceptualized as constantly changing toward illness or well-being as various influences affect the balance of the individual. Dunn (1959) described a health (well-being) grid, made up of the health axis, the environmental axis, and the resulting health and wellness quadrants. The intent of his model is to suggest the possible effects of environmental interaction with a well-being–illness continuum. A person at the lower end of the well-being–illness continuum might be ill if placed in an unfavorable environment, but might not demonstrate symptoms if the environment was protective (Fig. 9–3).

In another approach, Twaddle proposes that "since no one attains perfect health and not everyone is defined as sick, there must be a range of less than perfect health that is defined as normal" (Twaddle, 1977, p. 103). In Twaddle's continuum (Fig. 9–4) there is considerable overlap among "normal" and "ill" behaviors, and there is provision for change in the person's relative position on the continuum over time. Healthy and ill behaviors can coexist.

Holistic Health

Holistic health is based on the theory that the whole is more than the sum of its parts. "Things and events cannot be analyzed by reducing them to component parts without destroying or distorting the integrity of the whole" (Flynn, 1980, p. 9). This theory is very different from other prevalent models that consider the person to be a composite of a variety of subsystems, such as physiologic, psychologic, social, and so forth. If a person demonstrates grief after a death in the family, other models would have the "problem" classified as psychologic, and the nurse would

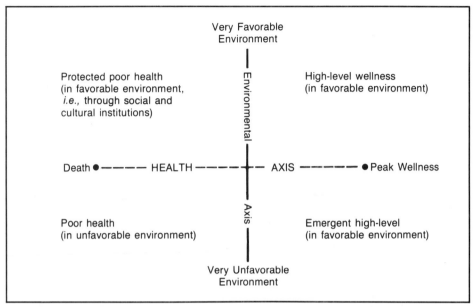

Figure 9-3. The health grid, its axes and quadrants. (Dunn HL: High-level wellness for man and society. Am J Public Health 49:788, 1959)

design psychologic interventions. In the holistic health model, the nurse would explore the impact of the loss on the whole person. The meaning of the death would be related to previous experiences of the person, and the influence on variables such as the person's mood, appetite, energy, well-being, and functioning, would be assessed. Intervention would be aimed at restoration of harmony, based on the individual's concept of direction and sense of meaning of his life.

Within the concept of holistic health, illness is viewed as a positive opportunity for growth of the individual. Illness indicates a degree of imbalance in the "harmonic integration of the body, mind, spirit and environment" (Flynn, 1980, p. 12). Illness offers the individual an opportunity to "further clarify values, affirm individual priorities and direction, and deepen a sense of the meaning and value of life" (Flynn, 1980, p. 28).

The holistic health model is compatible with systems theory. Emphasis is placed on the effect of the interaction between various variables on the individual. Since the individual is an open system, there is continuous interaction with the environment. Change in any one variable affects the entire system. The individual experiences ongoing change that can be a positive influence on development.

Health is a goal and a process. The ability to define a person's momentary posi-

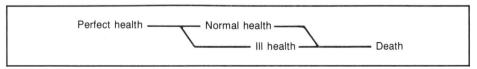

Figure 9-4. Health continuum. (Reprinted with permission from Twaddle AC: A Sociology of Health, p 103. St. Louis, CV Mosby, 1977)

tion on a continuum is less important than promoting positive change toward well-being and health. The nurse must be able to effectively assess a range of behaviors, and intervene to help the individual support and capitalize on his strengths as well as to help improve weaknesses. The next section discusses the multideterminants that can affect well-being, and thus should be considered during the nursing assessment of a client's well-being status.

MULTIDETERMINANTS OF WELL-BEING

Endogenous Factors (Factors Internal to the Individual)

Biologic Factors

Genetic Inheritance. Genetic inheritance has been related to susceptibility to specific diseases. For example, blood group A has been associated with gastric cancer and with pernicious anemia (Harrison, 1966, p. 295). A family history has been demonstrated in the incidence of breast cancer and diabetes (Bower, 1980, pp. 20–21). People with sickle cell anemia have an increased susceptibility to salmonella infection, and rheumatic fever is also believed to be under some genetic control (Sodeman and Sodeman, 1967, p. 54). In addition, resistance to certain diseases has been associated with genetic inheritance. For example, resistance to malaria appears to be related to carrying the sickle cell trait.

Gender. Gender influences the distribution of disease. For example, diseases found to be more prevalent among males include tuberculosis, parasitic diseases, arteriosclerotic heart disease, hemorrhoids, respiratory diseases, stomach ulcers, and abdominal hernias. Conditions more common among females include neoplasms, asthma, thyroid disease, diabetes mellitus, obesity, and gall bladder diseases (Mechanic, 1978, p. 210). In addition, a variety of biologically and socioculturally influenced behavior is related to gender. For example, males have been found to be more aggressive than females from infancy on, a phenomenon thought to be at least partially due to hormonal differences.

Age. Age has been related to distribution of disease. For example, for white males between 30 to 34, the greatest mortality risk factor is arteriosclerotic heart disease (Bower, 1980, p. 18). Age has also been associated with developmental needs or tasks that have a major impact on potential health behavior. For example, associated with the physical growth in puberty, the needs of the adolescent to determine an identity but also conform with peers (Bruhn and Cordova, January-February 1977, p. 17) has an impact on life-style, risk taking, and the practice of healthy behaviors.

Race. Race has also been associated with disease distribution. American Indians have a higher rate of diabetes, and blacks are more likely to develop sickle cell anemia or hypertension (Bower, 1980, p. 18).

Nutrition. Nutrition is another biologic variable with a major impact on health status. Obesity is prevalent in American society. The reasons for ingestion of food over and above nutritional needs are related to psychologic, socioeconomic, and cultural variables. However, being overweight has clearly been implicated in the incidence of heart disease (Haggerty, 1977, p. 277) and increases the risk of developing arteriosclerosis, diabetes, hypertension, and hernia, among other diseases.

Malnutrition is less publicized, but is a major health problem in many parts of the world (including pockets of American society). Poverty is the most frequently cited reason for eating fewer nutrients than needed, but cultural beliefs and crash diets also are associated with an unbalanced diet. Nutritional disorders due to physiologic causes may result in an inability to use ingested nutrients because of malabsorption or diarrhea. A third factor may be an increase in metabolic demands due to developmental changes (*e.g.,* pregnancy, infancy, or adolescence). Nutritional needs must be related to metabolic needs, cultural constraints, and coexistence of disease.

Cognitive Structures

There is a continuing controversy about the determination of intelligence. It appears clear that genetic inheritance affects potential. It is not clear however, if environmental influences can alter the potential or only affect the full realization of potential. In any case, intelligence has been found to be positively related to occupation, socioeconomic status, aptitudes, and performance variables (Auger, 1976, p. 119). Clearly, methods used for health education will be influenced by the ability of the person to understand. The nurse must modify her level of instruction to the client's ability to understand and accept the information.

Cognitive structure also influences learning style and the situations within which decisions about health are made. For example, some people need to have all the pertinent information about a situation and then analyze the various alternatives in a logical fashion to make a decision. Others may act more spontaneously, based on intuition, impulse, or wish. Thus, teaching methods must also be modified to meet the needs of the individual client.

Behavioral Patterning

An important factor influencing the degree of comfort with change is the person's *personality and temperament.* Individuals vary in the amount of change with which they are comfortable. In fact, a person varies in comfort with change from day to day or even from minute to minute. A person's emotional satisfaction and adaptability are partially the result of past experiences. Tolerance for stressors, inclination to take risks, and the value placed on short-term satisfaction are behaviors that have a major impact on health behavior. It is not clear if a person's behavior is consistent enough to be able to predict from previous experience how a person will behave in a specific situation. Thus, each specific situation should be assessed in relation to past history, but the possibility of novel responses should also be considered.

Another set of factors affecting behavior is a person's *life-style.* "One's lifestyle, including patterns of eating, exercise, drinking, coping with stress, and use of tobacco and drugs, together with environmental hazards, are the major known modifiable causes of illnesses in America today. Medical care, on which we spend so much has, in comparison, only a weak effect on health" (Haggerty, 1977, p. 276).

It has been shown that the length of life can be increased by modifying simple habits of life-style. Seven health habits have been associated with better health and increased life span: adequate sleep (7–8 hours), eating regular meals (not eating between meals), recreational activity (long walks, working in the garden, swimming), moderate to no drinking, never having smoked, near average weight, and usually eating breakfast, (Belloc and Breslow, 1972).

Life-style is influenced by cultural expectations. Certain values have been associated with the "American culture" (Parsons, 1958, pp. 178–179). Examples of these are the need to master the environment, in the name of ideals and goals, through hard work. Illness is a challenge to be met. Progress means moving in the "right" direction. Health is to be valued because it underlies the capacity for achievement. Because of these attitudes, a person who is sick is expected to work toward recovery. "Dependency is the primary threat to achievement capacity" (Parsons, 1958, p. 185).

Many specific diseases have been linked with life habits. Cigarette smoking has been associated with lung cancer, emphysema, and cardiovascular diseases. Presence of refined sugar in the mouth has been associated with the incidence of dental caries (Haggerty, 1977, p. 277).

Standard of Living

Standard of living and major familial and occupational *roles* are major determinants of food consumption, housing, and leisure patterns (Lerner, 1977, pp. 77–79). A large number of studies link *social class* with morbidity and mortality. In addition, *income, occupation,* and *education,* which are major components of social class, are each generally positively correlated with health status and negatively correlated with morbidity and mortality (Haggerty, 1977).

Socioeconomic class is also associated with certain values that affect health. For example, middle-class values stem from the original "Protestant ethic." Some of the characteristics of middle-class values are deferral of immediate gratification in the interest of long-term goals, placement of high value on rationality (*e.g.,* foresight, deliberate planning, and allocation of resources in an efficient way), assignment of a high premium on individual responsibility, resourcefulness, and self-reliance, and cleanliness, all of which are viewed as an index to the morals and virtue of the individual. In comparison, lower-class values have been described as immediate gratification, present time orientation, reciprocity, particularly within the family, and a more casual approach to cleanliness (Simmons, 1958, p. 111).

Financial status, especially poverty, affects a person's total life. Associated with poverty are high-risk characteristics such as lack of education, old age, physical disability, or racial discrimination. In addition, the poor tend to have a "present" orientation that may interfere with planning for future health needs. Emphasis may be on maintenance of essential earning ability rather than on prevention of illness, which may not seem as crucial.

Other characteristics that influence health include a person's *hygiene* habits and patterns that are usually learned early in life, *food preferences* and habits, and the *propensity to seek health* and follow health regimens. It has been said that "five dimensions constitute the framework for a wellness lifestyle. Self responsibility, nutritional awareness, physical fitness, stress management and environmental sensitivity" (Ardell, 1979, p. 19). The effect of health education on life-style is discussed later in this chapter.

Exogenous Factors (Factors External to the Individual)

Social Groups

People have a number of social support systems. These social networks are crucially important in shaping beliefs and behavior. The expectations of friends and influential others exert pressure on the individual. The school, church, peers, and the media have all been delegated responsibility for teaching health values. These social networks become a lay referral system that is consulted to help individuals interpret systems and decide if professional advice is needed.

A major support system is the family. "The family is a primary factor in the learning of wellness behavior" (Bruhn and Cordova, November–December 1977, p. 249). The family is the link between the person and the larger world. Since families share a common perspective derived from ethnic, religious, social class, and regional background influences, they help the individual to understand and define objects and events that impinge upon him. If a person is to learn healthy habits, the primary influence will be the parents. Even in adolescence, when approval by peers becomes an important consideration, modeling and parental influence continue to control values and attitudes (Bruhn and Cordova, 1978, p. 17).

Culture

All people are influenced by culture, a "way of life belonging to a designated group of people. Each cultural group has a special pattern of living and interacting together" (Leininger, 1967, p. 41), which results in distinctive, recurrent norms for behavior that are standardized throughout the group. "These cultural norms are the stable rules of behavior that prescribe the behavior to be followed, and they tend to consciously and unconsciously regulate our lives and help us solve many life problems" (Leininger, 1967, p. 42). How a person perceives, experiences, and copes with health and illness are based on his cultural beliefs.

Each culture is a systematic and integrated whole with closely interrelated and understood practices, values, and beliefs (Leininger, 1967, p. 41). For example, the Navajo Indian, who believes that man is an integral part of nature, includes little mention of clock time in his language, stressing instead types of activity, duration, or aspects of movement (Givens, 1977). Beliefs, values, and their associated patterns of living all influence the health status of a cultural group. In addition, "individuals from different cultures perceive and classify their health problems in specific ways and have certain expectations about the way they should be helped" (Leininger, 1967, p. 44). An understanding of the culture of an individual is just as important for effective health care as is knowledge of the physiologic and psychologic aspects. The nurse should also be aware of the possible effect of hospitalization on the individual. The sudden change into the hospital culture may create a kind of "culture shock" that will affect health status and response to nursing intervention.

Even similar reactions to symptoms by members of different ethnocultural groups do not necessarily reflect similiar attitudes. Zborowski (1958, pp. 261–263) studied pain responses of hospitalized Italians and Jews. He found that both groups were very sensitive to pain, emotional in response to pain, and tended to exaggerate pain. However, the two groups were very different in the meanings they attached to the symptom. The Italians were concerned with the immediacy of pain and the actual pain sensation. They expressed discomfort with pain, and were happy when the pain was relieved. They expressed confidence in the physician, and provoked sympathy from their friends toward their suffering. The Jews on the other hand, associated pain with meaning and significance for their health and welfare, and expressed worries and anxiety. They were reluctant to accept drugs because they only gave temporary relief, and even when the pain was relieved they remained depressed and worried about its recurrance. They were skeptical about the effectiveness of the physician, and they provoked worry and concern among their family and friends about their general health. This study demonstrates the need for the nurse to understand the meaning of the symptom for the patient. Misinterpretation can occur when the nurse intervenes on the basis of stereotyped assumptions.

Perception of being sick or being well is largely a cultural phenomenon that may vary significantly from "the 'scientific' health worker who may be defining health and disease in a special way and within a limited social and cultural frame of reference" (Leininger, 1967, p. 45). This influence on the health professional is known as the "provider culture." Each health professional is a member of a specific subculture that presupposes certain unconscious beliefs and patterns of behavior. In addition, providers of health care have been socialized into a professional culture that is characterized by specific beliefs, practices, habits, likes, dislikes, norms, and rituals (Spector, 1979, p. 78). Examples include specialized medical terminology, valuing of technology, and usually, an assumption that the provider knows what is best for the patient.

Consumers of health care represent a variety of cultural beliefs, different from each other and from the provider culture.

> Insight into what people believe causes illness will help the nurse understand client behaviors, such as at what point during an illness episode a client will seek Western health care, and with what treatments the client will or will not comply, and what influences whether or not the client will return for follow-up care, if needed. (Hautman, 1979, p. 23)

The nurse should also be aware of an unconscious belief in the superiority of her own cultural group or its beliefs and practices. This is known as ethnocentrism. In order to avoid imposing her own values on the client, or judging the client by her own values, the nurse must consciously try to understand health needs and the "why" of a person's behavior from his viewpoint, regardless of his specific cultural affiliation.

Kleinman *et al* (1978, p. 256) have suggested several questions that can help assess the "patient's model" of his cultural approach to illness:

1. What do you think has caused your problem?
2. Why do you think it started when it did?
3. What do you think your illness does to you? How does it work?
4. How severe is your sickness? Will it have a short or a long course?
5. What kind of treatment do you think you should receive?

Health and illness mean many different things to culturally different people. One client may be ill despite the absence of demonstrable organic pathology (*e.g.,* hysterical mental illness), while another may have a disease but not an illness (*e.g.,* controlled diabetes) (Hautman, 1979, p. 23). The nurse should try to understand health needs from the viewpoint of the members of different cultures. The nurse should try to avoid assuming that a person will hold certain beliefs *just* because he belongs to a certain cultural group. Each person expresses individual differences. However, the why of human behavior from a cultural viewpoint must be understood in order to deal with culturally conditioned behavior (Leininger, 1967, p. 46).

Physical and Ecologic Environment

The community provides a number of services that are necessary for group living. Some of these services include sanitation, sewage disposal, transportation, and health care services. Each of these factors can affect health.

Toffler (1970) describes rapidly accelerating changes in our ecosystem. Current research seeks to clarify the effects on health of nonnutritive chemical additives, airborne radioactive and chemical pollution, energy consumption, urban decay, population growth and crowding, and medically induced changes such as drug reactions and organism mutation.

An understanding of the various multideterminants of well-being status is necessary for the nurse. These factors must be assessed to identify the need for nursing intervention. In addition, the nurse needs an understanding of client behavior that might be associated with illness, sickness, or well-being. These behaviors are discussed in the next section.

ILLNESS, SICKNESS, AND WELL-BEING BEHAVIOR

Illness Behavior

Illness behavior is "any activity, undertaken by a person who feels ill, to define the state of his health and to discover a suitable remedy" (Igun, 1979, p. 445). Illness behavior depends on the way in which the person perceives illness, and is selectively affected by multiple determinants. For example, age, sex, occupation, socioeconomic status, religion, ethnicity, psychologic stability, personality, education, meaning attached to symptoms, modes of coping with anxiety, attitude toward self, prior health-illness experiences, availability of resources, and degree, type, and duration of concurrent stress situations are all factors that may be related to illness behavior (Wu, 1973; Kasl and Cobb, 1966; and Falek and Britten, 1974).

The meaning that the experience of illness has for the person may be a factor. For example, if illness is viewed as punishment for past sins, the person may be depressed because of fear of ostracism, or relieved at having been punished. Incapacity may be seen as an escape from a stressful situation, a solution for conflict, or an obstacle to achievement of goals (Martin and Prange, 1962, p. 168).

While illness behavior is an individually determined reaction, certain behaviors have been found to be associated with various stages of illness. Igun (1979, pp. 445–456) describes eleven stages of illness. These stages are composed of sequences of events that vary in duration. Some may occur simultaneously or very closely combined.

Stages of Illness

Symptoms Experience. The symptoms experience stage consists of four possible steps: the actual physical experience, an awareness that something could be wrong, the label and meaning that the person gives to the symptoms, and the associated response of fear or anxiety. While the symptoms are nonspecific, the person may unconsciously deny the symptoms to avoid anxiety. When the symptoms become specific, emotional acknowledgment is necessary, and at this point, anxiety usually becomes apparent (Martin and Prange, 1962, p. 169).

Factors that could influence a judgement of severity of symptoms include the extent to which the symptoms interfere with normal activities, the "obviousness" of the symptoms, the tolerance threshold and the meaning of illness for the person, the familiarity, seriousness, and speed of change of the symptoms, assumptions about cause and prognosis, and other concurrent crises in the person's life (Twaddle, 1977, pp. 125–127).

Self-treatment. If the person understands and can label the symptoms, and perceives the symptoms as not serious, he may choose to treat himself. Possible methods include staying home from work, drinking fluids, bedrest, and self-medication with over-the-counter drugs.

Communication to Significant Others. If sufficiently concerned, the person may communicate that concern to his immediate family, friends, or health care practitioners. The likelihood is that the person will consult a professional when the culture of the patient is similiar to that of the professional. People of lower social class are less likely to seek consultation with health professionals even in the presence of symptoms (Twaddle, 1977, p. 129).

Assessment of Symptoms. The assessment of symptoms stage determines the diagnosis and whether or not the person should legitimately assume the sick role. The diagnosis may be made by the person or significant others, but many people associate legitimacy with diagnosis by a health professional. Observable symptoms such as fever or vomiting help to reinforce legitimacy.

Assumption of the Sick Role. The person has accepted his illness, has been defined as sick, and has assumed the sick role. At this point, some patients regress in their behavior. They may become more typical and predictable, and may rely on others to make decisions for them. They try to delegate their worry and concern, but they are still anxious. Sick role behavior is discussed more fully in the next section.

Expression of Concern. Family, friends, and significant others offer sympathy, moral encouragement, and possible referral to others whom they believe may be able to help the patient. This stage occurs almost simultaneously with the following stage.

Assessment of Probable Efficacy of or Appropriateness of Sources of Treatment. A variety of possible treatments may be assessed. Previous experience, either positive or negative, may affect the perception of what treatment is desirable.

Selection of Treatment Plan. The patient, with possible consultation, assesses the costs and the benefits of the plans that he perceives as appropriate. Unfortunately, many people are not fully informed of possible treatment choices or the effects of the treatment chosen. They may defer to what the health provider says is "best."

Treatment. The selected treatment is implemented.

Evaluation of Effects of Treatment. When the patient enters the assessment of effects of treatment stage, there are several possible outcomes. If the treatment has been effective, the patient will recover and become well. Even if the initial treatment is not effective, eventual recovery is possible with alternate intervention. For some, recovery will leave partial disability, and some patients will not recover.

The patient may return to any of the earlier stages at this point. There is usually a lag between physical events and their psychologic significance. Intervention may be needed at this stage to help deal with lack of congruence between the perceptions of the patient and the caregiver. For example, the patient may insist on maintaining the sick role in the absence of validation by the health professional. In this case, it would be helpful to explore why the patient needs to maintain the sick role. Alternately, the professional may insist that the patient is sick, but the person may not accept that role. The person may need help to slow down and continue treatment even though he insists that he feels well. The professional may need to accept the person's right to reject treatment.

Recovery and Rehabilitation. The usual roles of the healthy person may be reassumed abruptly or gradually.

In the case of chronic disability (*e.g.,* diabetes, polio paralysis), the person is not usually considered to be sick. Such persons are incapacitated, and thus deviate from societal standards of what is normal, but the new capacity level must be considered as the new "normal" for the individual. Usually they are expected to engage in everyday activities as much as possible within the limits of the impairment (Twaddle, 1977, p. 131).

People with a chronic disability have to deal with a modified capacity and perception of well-being on a daily basis. How an individual deals with the perception of a stressor is called the coping process, which is discussed in the next section.

Stressing Life Events (Coping)

Many people consider stress "bad," a judgement reinforced by the extensive literature documenting an association between stressing life events and illness. The measurement of life events as stressors has been actively researched, especially since the Social Readjustment Rating Scale was developed by Holmes and Rahe in 1967. Since that time the scale has been modified several times, and a number of specific scales have been developed using the Holmes-Rahe scale as a model.

The amount of adjustment required by particularly stressing life events (*e.g.,* divorce, marital separation or death of a spouse, or personal illness or injury) has been found to be perceived similarly by a wide range of culturally diverse groups of people. For example, if marriage is given an arbitrary mean value on a scale of 0 to 100, death of a spouse would require twice as much adjustment (100 on the scale), while a change in living conditions or beginning or ending school would require half as much adjustment (25 on the scale) in the pattern of daily life. It has been assumed that "life-change events . . . lower bodily resistance and enhance the probability of disease occurrence" (Holmes and Masuda, 1974). However, the relationship between illness and the incidence of stressing life events has been found to involve a number of variables.

The way that an individual reacts to environmental events (copes) is highly variable. The parameters that must be considered include "the independence of life events from illness, the desirability of life events, the predictability and control of life events, the measurement of illness versus illness behavior, the past history of illness, possible threshold effects for life stress, and the individual impact of life events" (Bieliauskas, 1982, p. 63).

Ursin *et al* (1978) view coping as the mastery of something threatening. Lazarus *et al* (1980) have extended the definition of the coping process to include individual psychologic effectiveness that either increases or decreases the risk of maladaptive illness. In his view the essential mediator of the stress response is psychologic and the cognitive appraisal of threat is all important in initiating a response. The success or failure of the coping process will determine whether the stress response will be relaxed or maintained.

Falek and Britton (1974, pp. 2–4) describe a sequence of behavior that may be manifested in the process of coping with an overwhelming stressor. At first, the individual may appear stunned or dazed, as if he does not comprehend what he has been told. Unconsciously, these behaviors are related to shock and *denial.* This stage is usually short-lived, but at this stage the patient has no motivation for change. It is too early to give information or expect decision-making.

As awareness begins the patient may appear tired and nervous. He may be trying to deal with *anxiety* by dealing with the situation intellectually. He may seek information in order to understand or to identify ways to "undo" his diagnosis. Full impact is often associated with *anger.* The patient has not fully accepted the diagnosis, and may attempt to blame others for his situation.

Acceptance of the diagnosis is often associated with *depression,* at which point the patient can begin to deal with reality. However, these stages often recycle, with fluctuating behaviors. Each person will have a different pattern of behavior within these broad parameters. The family and health professionals should try to respond to the feelings beneath the patient's behavior. As a general rule it will be helpful to emphasize a person's abilities rather than disabilities, point to life accomplishments, and emphasize hope within the reality of the individual situation.

Sick Role Behavior

Sick role behavior "is the activity undertaken by those who consider themselves ill, for the purpose of getting well" (Igun, 1979, p. 445). The sick role was first sociologically described by Parsons in 1951. He views behavior during illness as a special kind of deviancy, which, in comparison with criminal behavior, is legitimized by society. Parsons describes four behavioral expectations of a patient who has assumed the sick role:

1. Exemption from moral responsibility for being ill.
2. Exemption from usual role tasks and responsibilities.
3. An obligation to seek and cooperate with technically competent helpers.
4. The obligation to want to get well. (Parsons, 1958, pp. 176–177)

The sick person is allowed to become dependent and temporarily give up some or all of his usual responsibilities without blame or guilt. But the patient is required to try to get well and give up the sick role.

This theoretical formulation has been criticized because the model does not include timing nor mechanism for change from one stage to another of illness. It also presents only one approach, although people react to illness in many different ways. The role performance, expectations, and perceptions of the person when he is healthy and cultural variables must be known. The sick role does not apply in all conditions (*e.g.,* pregnancy, trivial and incurable conditions). It is limited in its applicability to chronic disease. It is not valid during self-treatment or consultation with nonprofessionals unless they are considered to be experts by the client. In addition, it may not be applicable in non-western societies (Twaddle, 1977, p. 118).

Despite its limitations, the sick role theory does help us to understand some illness behavior. People who are labeled as ill by health professionals and who accept the sick role are allowed to give up their usual responsibilities and become dependent on others. In our society people who are seriously ill are usually hospitalized at least briefly. The nurse is often the one who assumes responsibility for daily activities until the patient is able to relinquish the sick role.

People are highly variable in their behavior when sick. Some people accept the sick role easily, are cooperative with treatment, and give up the sick role without problems at an appropriate time. Others have a great deal of difficulty accepting dependency, struggle against the loss of autonomy, and project their anger and anxiety on the nurse. Some people have difficulty giving up the sick role and refuse to reassume responsibility even though the health provider may perceive that the person should be "well enough" to resume usual activities of daily living.

Some health providers have a great deal of difficulty accepting such behavior, labeling the client as a "malingerer" and a "difficult" patient.

The nurse must assess each patient individually to determine his perceptions and motivations in illness. By developing a relationship with the patient and allowing the expression of anxiety (regardless of how it is expressed), the nurse can support the patient while collecting data that will form a basis for individualized therapeutic intervention.

Well-being Behavior

Igun (1979, pp. 445–456) defines well-being (health) behavior as "any activity undertaken by a person believing himself to be healthy, for the purpose of preventing disease or detecting it in an asymptomatic stage." In addition to this illness orientation, well-being behavior may be performed to promote well-being (*e.g.,* a person engaging in regular exercise to increase resiliance).

The health care system in the United States is disease-oriented. Approximately 90% of the national expenditure for medical care goes for the cure and control of illness, whereas only 3% is spent for prevention and 1% for health education (Dayani, 1979, p. 34). Even efforts toward prevention and health education are illness-oriented. For example, children are taught to brush their teeth to avoid cavities (not because the mouth will feel, look, taste, and smell better) and to dress warmly so they will not "catch cold," (rather than so that they will feel better).

Theories of Preventive Well-being Behavior

Motivation Theory. There are various theories to predict the liklihood that an individual will engage in a well-being—related behavior. One is motivation theory. Rosenstock (1966), in his Health Belief model, included (1) perceived susceptibility (patient's perception of his likelihood of experiencing a particular illness), (2) perceived severity (patient's perception of the severity of the illness and its potential impact on his life), (3) benefits of action (patient's assessment of the potential of the health action to reduce susceptibility and/or severity), and (4) costs of action (patient's estimate of financial costs, time and effort, inconvenience, and possible side-effects such as pain or discomfort). Rosenstock also included cues that trigger health-seeking behaviors in his model. Cues may be external information such as information in newspapers or on television, or internal signals such as symptoms. Patient compliance with a therapeutic regimen has been associated with knowledge and understanding of the regimen, complexity of the regimen, and interpersonal relationships with the health care provider and significant others (Loustau, 1979, p. 242).

The Health Belief model is a "rational" model for well-being behavior. The model assumes that well-being is a common objective for all. Individual differences are explained largely in terms of differing perceptions in interaction with motivation. Kasl and Cobb (1966) extended the basic model by specifying a relatively positive variable, the "perceived importance of health matters," in addition to perceived value and perceived threat. Becker (1975) expanded the model even further by including positive health motivation.

Pender (1975) believes that preventive well-being behavior manifests itself in two phases: decision-making and action. The three main determinants to the decision-making phase are personal, interpersonal, and situational factors.

Personal determinants include (1) the importance of well-being (*e.g.,* what is valued by the individual is made possible by well-being), (2) perceived vulnerability (*e.g.,* family history, part of a high risk group), (3) perceived value of early detection, (4) perceived seriousness (due to degree of threat, visibility, effect on roles, and communicability to others), (5) perceived efficacy of action (alternative with the highest chance of success with the lowest risk or inconvenience), (6) level of internal versus external control (belief of ability to influence the environment). Those who believe they can influence the course of their own health (internal control) will use preventive services to a greater extent than those who feel powerless (Pender, 1975, p. 387).

Interpersonal determinants include (1) concern of significant others (*e.g.,* family), (2) family patterns of use (early childhood patterns are important), (3) expectations of friends, and (4) information from professionals. A specific kind of interpersonal determinant is the individual's *support system,* first described by Cobb (1976). A support system has been defined as "a set of persons consisting of a focal or anchor person, all the family, all the friends and all the helping persons who stand ready to serve the anchor person, and the linkages or relationships among those people" (Hogue, 1977, p. 68). Support systems have their own patterning, made up of continuing and intermittent ties and high information exchange properties (Hogue, 1977, p. 68). The strengths of the individual are augmented through provision of emotional support and task-oriented assistance. Situational determinants include (1) cultural acceptance of health behaviors, (2) societal group norms and pressures, and (3) information from nonpersonal sources (*e.g.,* mass communication).

Once an individual has decided to engage in preventive behavior, the action phase begins. A cue from the outside or an internal signal will trigger action. The intensity of the cue needed depends on the readiness to act. If the cue is too strong, overwhelming anxiety may inhibit rather than encourage action.

Well-being related behaviors are likely to be performed by people who are concerned about their health, perceive a value to reducing the threat of disease, believe that health action will reduce the threat, and possess a set of demographic, structural, and enabling factors that promote such behavior (Harris and Guten, 1979, p. 19).

Social Learning Theory. Why do individuals behave in certain ways in certain situations? What kinds of nursing intervention would be most effective in modifying behavior? One approach to these questions is social learning theory that is concerned with "the analysis of why individuals behave in certain ways under given conditions and the effects of certain reinforcement patterns on their behavior" (Lowery, 1981, p. 294). Rotter, a leading social learning theorist, developed the concept of locus of control to differentiate people who have a general expectancy that rewards are based on internal resources such as effort from those who expect that rewards are externally related to things like luck, chance, or powerful others (Rotter, 1954).

It has been suggested that locus of control is associated with mastery of health information, motivation, effective problem-solving, sense of responsibility, desire for active participation in health care, and the ability to defer gratification (Arakelian, 1980). It is a stable personality factor that exists on a continuum but can be modified through new experiences. However, there are numerous questions about measurement of the concept. The scales used to measure locus of control have been found to have items related to control ideology (the extent to which people generally have control) including beliefs in how modifiable, just, predictable, difficult, or politically responsive the world is as well as personal control beliefs (Arakelian, 1980, p. 28). In addition, it appears that locus of control is a mediating rather than a causal factor in determining behavior, and that it is only one of a number of significant variables. For example, Weiner suggests that the *amount* of control the person has over the cause and how *stable* (*i.e.,* variable or enduring) the control is as well as the *locus* of the control should be considered (Weiner, 1979).

It appears that locus of control may be one factor that interacts with multiple others to affect behavior. An understanding of this concept might help to indicate desirable intervention strategies to promote preventive health behavior. However, it would be inappropriate to predict certain kinds of responses on the basis of the client's locus of control, or to assume that this is the only or even the dominant determinant of behavior.

In addition to motivational and social learning theories for preventive well-being behavior, investigators have focused on the influence of environmental factors (such as the social milieu), the influence of feedback and reinforcement in promoting individual surveillance and autonomy, and finally, the philosophy of enabling self-care, which maintains that it is the individual's responsibility to determine his own health and health care practices. The individual must evaluate possible risk factors in relation to life-style and make his own decisions (Ruffing, 1979).

Practically everyone performs some regular and routine "health protective behavior." This has been defined as "any behavior performed by a person, regardless of his or her perceived or actual health status, in order to protect, promote, or maintain his or her health, whether or not such behavior is objectively effective toward that end" (Harris and Guten, 1979, p. 18). In a study of health protective behaviors, almost three fourths of the sample considered nutritional and/or eating habits to be health protective behavior (71.3%), but less than one tenth of the sample considered weight (9.7%), smoking (8.8%), medications (7.8%), or alcohol consumption (6.8%) in that way. It is interesting that only 18.8% of the sample thought of contact with the health care system in terms of health protective behavior! (Harris and Guten, 1979, p. 28).

Prevention of Illness

Prevention has been classified as primary, secondary (AMA, 1951), or tertiary. Secondary prevention is the early diagnosis and prompt treatment of disease, while "tertiary prevention is concerned with conditions that cannot be cured or reversed, but which can be alleviated or improved by rehabilitative measures" (Fielding *et al,* 1978, p. 569).

Primary prevention may be accomplished in the period before pathology occurs "by measures designed to promote general optimum health or by the specific protection of man against disease agents or the establishment of barriers against agents in the environment" (Leavell and Clark, 1965, p. 20). One technique that has been used to identify possible susceptibility to disease is a health risk appraisal, first designed by Robbins and Hall in 1970. Health risk appraisal instruments estimate the odds that a person with a given set of characteristics will become ill or die from selected diseases in a given time span. It is hoped that persons learning about their odds will act to improve them.

There are three steps. First, an estimate is made of present and future risk through a computer analysis of the 10-year chance of survival considering such factors as the personal and family history of certain diseases; life-style factors such as smoking, drinking, exercise, driving practices, stress on the job; physical measures such as blood pressure, weight and blood analysis; and presence in or absence from a high risk group as revealed by recent screening (*e.g.,* breast or cervical cancer). Next, the person and the appraiser consider possible preventive measures to reduce the identified risks, and design a health management program. The object is to try to prevent "premature death."

Health risk appraisals provide *probabilities* of an individual developing a specific disease or of dying within a defined period of time. These are not diagnoses, and are determined solely on the basis of statistical probabilities. There are criticisms of this approach based on concerns about the variability of the instruments being used for assessment, lack of adequate follow-up after the client has been assessed, and abuses by inadequately prepared appraisers. On the other hand, health risk appraisal can benefit the consumer by providing reinforcement for behaviors in risk situations where there are no symptoms (*e.g.,* seat belt use, elevated blood pressure), and provides a document that can be used to track progress toward defined goals. There are also benefits to the community as an additional statistic to gauge the risk of various preventable diseases.

The nurse must be aware of the factors that prompt or inhibit preventive health behavior. The client must be given information to promote his realistic perception of vulnerability to specific problems, as well as the consequences of the illness for which he may be at risk. Information about various measures that can be taken to decrease vulnerability may help to reduce anxiety to manageable levels and promote cooperation. The nurse may also be able to facilitate use of preventive services by suggesting appropriate resources and expressing approval of the client's intent to change his behavior.

Promotion of Well-being

Health promotion has frequently been combined with health maintenance and disease prevention. Brubaker, however, defines health promotion as "health care directed toward high-level wellness through processes that encourage alteration of personal habits or the environment in which people live. It occurs after health stability is present and assumes disease prevention and health maintenance as pre-requisites or by-products" (Brubaker, 1983, p. 12). This definition assumes maintenance and prevention as the "bottom line," and focuses on the growth potential of promotion.

Until fairly recently, limited attention had been paid to positive efforts to promote individual responsibility for well-being and health. Probably a person's first awareness of "wellness" comes from role models in the immediate environment, the family. Bruhn and Cordova (November–December 1977) have suggested that at each stage along a developmental continuum there are minimal levels or thresholds for well-being that must be completed to the satisfaction of each individual. At each stage the individual should be given reinforcement for practicing positive behavior. The family, school, peers, and mass media have a major impact on the development of a value system. The individual is viewed as an active participant in shaping the direction of his life.

For example, health teaching in late childhood must build on the trust and sense of autonomy that were developed in infancy. A positive self-concept and a view that health is important were initiated in early childhood, but need reinforcement. At this stage the person is also ready for intellectual knowledge of techniques and rationale related to positive health habits. The emphasis is on building positive health behavior into the value structure (Bruhn and Cordova, November–December 1977). By early adulthood however, the person has usually adopted the work ethic. Efforts to promote self-control in the person's life-style should receive the major attention.

Promotion of well-being efforts have often relied on health education programs, with controversial results. Most health education programs have focused on acquisition of knowledge, relying on knowledge transfer to achieve change in behavior. Strong motivation on the part of the client seems to be the stimulus that is lacking in many programs. Since beliefs usually precede motivation, knowledge of the person's values and attitudes is needed before attempting to persuade a person to change well-being behavior. The nurse may be able to stimulate motivation for health promotion in the absence of any immediate threat to the client's health. Use of the client's desire to conform to social norms may be helpful (*e.g.,* "I saw your friend at the immunization clinic with her children"). Unfortunately, it appears that even with the most successful techniques, only modest behavior change is probable unless strong motivation is reinforced by the social group (Haggerty, 1977, p. 280). For this reason a group (social network) is often used to facilitate behavior change (*e.g.,* groups to lose weight or stop smoking).

Yet there are strong indications that the public has become more aware of the relative importance of various factors to health, and may be more willing to adapt life-styles to promote well-being. For example, "over the last fifteen years, the United States has experienced marked improvements in the control of high blood pressure. The proportion of smokers in the adult population has declined by more than 20%. The aggregate consumption of foods high in total fat, saturated fat, and cholesterol has decreased by 10% to 15% or more between 1968 and 1978. The proportion of the population reporting regular exercise has increased by as much as 100%" (McGinnis, 1982, pp. 296–297). Promotion activities and advertising are making a difference in well-being and health.

SUMMARY

In our society, responsibility for illness has been delegated to "health" professionals who have been prepared and rewarded for delivery of care for the sick. Short-term incentives and rewards to maintain health do not exist for the recipient. The health care system is not organized to reward the provider for keeping the client well. Individuals must be encouraged to assume an increased concern and responsibility for their own health potential.

"Health professionals need to stop dictating and exhorting. Teachers of health care need to be expert in techniques or strategies for motivating, exploring, experiential learning, placing responsibility, facilitating, negotiating health care goals, practices or regimens, and for persuading and rewarding successes" (Norris, 1979, p. 489). By using the nursing process applied through the leadership role, nurses can support, facilitate and encourage those positive skills, qualities and plans that will promote the process of health and foster well-being potential. Intervention can then be worked out collaboratively by the patient and the nurse, based on goals and a timetable determined by the patient. The nursing process and the leadership role of the nurse are discussed in later chapters.

REFERENCES

American Medical Association, Commission on Chronic Illness. Proceedings of the Conference on Preventive Aspects of Chronic Disease, Chicago, March 12–14, 1951

Arakelian M: An assessment and nursing application of the concept of locus of control. Adv Nurs Sci 3:25–42, October 1980

Ardell DB: The nature and implications of high level wellness, or why 'normal health' is a rather sorry state of existence. Health Values 3:17–24, January–February 1979

Auger JR: Behavioral Systems and Nursing. Englewood Cliffs, Prentice-Hall, 1976

Becker MH, Maiman LA: Sociobehavioral determinants of compliance with health and medical care recommendations. Med Care 13:10–24, 1975

Belloc NB, Breslow L: Relationship of physical health status and health practices. Prev Med 1:409–21, August 1972

Bieliauskas LA: Stress and its Relationship to Health and Illness. Boulder, Westview Press, 1982

Bower FL (ed): Health Maintenance. New York, John Wiley & Sons, 1980

Brubaker BH: Health promotion: A linguistic analysis. Adv Nurs Sci 6:1–14, April 1983

Bruhn JG, Cordova FD, Williams JA et al: The Wellness Process. J Comm Health 2:209–221, Spring 1977

Bruhn JG, Cordova FD: A Developmental Approach to Learning Wellness Behavior. I. Infancy to Early Adolescence. Health Values 1:246–254, November–December 1977

Bruhn JG, Cordova FD: A Developmental Approach to Learning Wellness Behavior. II: Adolescence to Maturity. Health Values 2:16–21, January–February 1978

Cobb S: Social support as a moderator of life stress. Psychosom Med 38:300–314, September–October 1976

Dayani E: Concepts of Wellness. Nurs Prac:31–34, January–February 1979

Dubos R: Health and creative adaptation. Human Nature 1:74–82, January 1978

Dunn HL: What high-level wellness means. Health Values 1:9–16, January February 1977

Dunn HL: High-level wellness for man and society. Am J Pub H 49:786–792, 1959

Falek A, Britton S: Phases in coping: The hypothesis and its implications. Soc Biol 21:1–7, Spring 1974

Fielding JE, Hyde J Jr, Russo PK: A program for prevention in Massachusetts. Prev Med 7:564–640, December 1978

Flynn PAR: Holistic Health. Bowie, Robert J. Brady, 1980

Givens D: An Analysis of Navajo Temporality. Washington, University Press of America, 1977

Greifinger RB, Grossman RL: Toward a language of health. Health Values 1:297–299, September–October 1977

Hadley BJ: Current concepts of wellness and illness: Their relevances for nursing. Image 6:21–27, 1974

Haggerty RJ: Changing lifestyles to improve health. Prev Med:276–289, 1977

Harris DM, Guten S: Health-protective behavior: An exploratory study. J Health Soc Behav 20:17–29, March 1979

Harrison TR: Principles of Internal Medicine. New York, McGraw-Hill 1966

Hautman MA: Folk health and illness beliefs. Nurs Prac:23–27, 31, 34, July–August 1979

Hogue CC: Support systems for health promotion. In Hall JE, Weaver BR (eds): Distributive Nursing Practice, pp 65–80. Philadelphia, JB Lippincott, 1977

Hollen P: A holistic model of individual and family health based on a continuum of choice. Adv Nurs Sci 3:27–42, July 1981

Holmes TH, Masuda M: Life Change and Illness Susceptibility. In Dohrenwend BS,

Dohrenwend BP (eds.): Stressful Life Events: Their Nature and Effects. New York, John Wiley & Sons, 1974

Holmes TH, Rahe RH: The Social Readjustment Rating Scale. J Psychosom Res 11:213–218, 1967

Igun UA: Stages in health-seeking: A descriptive model. Soc Sci Med 13A:445–456, 1979

Kasl S, Cobb S: Health behavior, illness behavior and sick role behavior. Arch Environ Health 12:246–266, 1966

Keller MJ: Toward a definition of health. Adv Nurs Sci:43–82, October 1981

Kleinman A, Eisenberg L, Good B: Culture, illness and care. Ann Int Med 88:251–258, February 1978

Lazarus RS, Cohen JB, Folkman S et al: Psychological stress and adaptation: Some unresolved issues. *In* Selye H (ed): Selye's Guide to Stress Research, vol 1. New York, Van Nostrand, 1980

Leavell HR, Clark EG (eds.): Preventive Medicine for the Doctor in His Community, ed 3. New York, McGraw-Hill, 1965

Leininger M: The Culture Concept and Its Relevance to Nursing. J Nurs Ed 6:27–37, April 1967

Lerner M: The Non-Health Services' determinants of health levels: Conceptualization and public policy recommendations. Med Care 15:74–83 Suppl, May 1977

Loustau A: Using the health belief model to predict patient compliance. Health Values 3:241–245, September–October 1979

Lowery BJ: Misconceptions and limitations of locus of control and the I-E scale. Nurs Res 30:294–98, September–October 1981

McGinnis JM: Targeting progress in health. Public Health Rep 97:295–307, July–August 1982

Mallick MJ: Defining Health: The Step "Before" The Nursing Assessment. J Geront Nurs 5:30–33, May–June 1979

Martin HW, Prange AJ Jr: The stages of illness-psychosocial approach. Nurs Outlook 10:168–171, March 1962

Mechanic D: Sex, Illness, Illness Behavior, and the Use of Health Services. Soc Sci Med 12:207–214, July 1978

Murray RB, Zentner JP: Nursing Concepts for Health Promotion. Englewood Cliffs, Prentice-Hall, 1979

Norris CM: Self care. Am J Nurs 79:486–489, March 1979

Offer D, Sabshin M: Normality. New York, Basic Books, 1966

Parsons T: Definitions of health and illness in the light of american values and social structure. In Jaco EG (ed): Patients, Physicians and Illness, pp 165–187. Illinois, The Free Press, 1958

Pender NJ: A conceptual model for preventive health behavior. Nurs Outlook 23:385–390, June 1975

Robbins L, Hall J: How to Practice Prospective Medicine. Indianapolis, Methodist Hospital of Indiana, 1970

Rosenstock IM: Why People Use Health Services. Milbank Mem Fund Quart 44:94–127, July 1966

Rotter JB: Social Learning and Clinical Psychology. Englewood Cliffs, Prentice-Hall, 1954

Ruffing MA: Preventive health behavior: A theoretical review and synthesis. Health Values 3:235–240, September-October 1979

Siegel H: To Your Health-Whatever That May Mean. Nurs Forum 12:280–89, 1973

Simmons O: Implications of social class for public health. *In* Jaco EG (ed): Patients, Physicians and Illness, p 111. Illinois, The Free Press, 1958

Smith JA: The idea of health: A philosophical inquiry. Adv Nurs Sci: 43–50, April 1981

Sodeman WA, Sodeman WA Jr: Pathologic Physiology. Mechanisms of Disease. Philadelphia, WB Saunders, 1967

Spector RE: Cultural Diversity in Health and Illness. New York, Appleton-Century-Crofts, 1979

Toffler A: Future Shock. New York, Random House, 1970

Twaddle AC: A Sociology of Health. St Louis, CV Mosby, 1977

Ursin H, Baade E, Levine S: Psychobiology of Stress-A Study of Coping Men. New York, Academic Press, 1978

Weiner B: Theory of motivation for some classroom experiences. J Educ Psych 71:3–25, February 1979

Wu R: Behavior and Illness. Englewood Cliffs, Prentice-Hall, 1973

Wylie CM: The definition and measurement of health and disease. Public Health Rep 85:100–104, February 1970

Zborowski M: Cultural components in responses to pain. *In* Jaco EG (ed): Patients, Physicians and Illness, pp 256–268. Illinois, The Free Press, 1958

From an understanding of what produces good health and from a given viewpoint of what is socially desirable, it is then possible to deduce what is required of society in the way of institutions, relationships, sciences, and individual participation to improve health. (Blum, 1983, p. xiii)

Chapter 10

Professional Nursing Within the Health Care Delivery System

Marie G. Finamore and Eleanor Rudick

THOUGHT QUESTIONS

1. Why is it suggested that health care delivery is really not a system in the United States today?

2. What is the role of government in the delivery of health care in the United States today?

3. What are the different kinds of health care delivery institutions and how does organizational power differ among them?

4. What are some of the things nurses must do to gain control of nursing practice in health care delivery systems?

5. Compare the characteristics of collaboration, cooperation, and competition among health care disciplines in the health care delivery system.

6. What are some of the factors to be considered in reducing the costs of health care in the United States today?

7. What are some of the changes suggested that should enable nurses to become more effective members of the interdisciplinary health care delivery team?

We desire to prepare a visionary leader who is more concerned about recasting health care institutions for the benefit of humankind than with ruling the institutions. It is believed that the manner in which health care is defined directs the manner in which the Health Care Delivery System (HCDS) is organized. If health care continues to be equated with medical care the present system for the delivery of health care will continue unchanged. If, however, the focus is placed on well-being rather than illness, and health care rather than medical or nursing care, the process used to deliver health care will be vastly different as will the use made of the various health care professionals.

In this chapter the HCDS as it presently exists is discussed. Then ways to change the HCDS to achieve improved health care are examined. Initially, the focus will be on the organizational structure of the HCDS. Next, the mission of the HCDS, the appropriate responsibility and accountability of professional nursing in a variety of health care delivery settings, and the use of planned change theory to facilitate effective delivery of health care services are discussed.

THE ORGANIZATIONAL STRUCTURE OF THE HEALTH CARE DELIVERY SYSTEM

The HCDS in the United States is described as highly pluralistic—a complex mix of multiple types of public and private organizations with multiple sources of funding, many points of decision-making, and numerous unskilled personnel. This system has been undergoing continuous and often rapid change. Wilson and Neuhauser categorize its components into *institutional care* rendered to persons who stay for short- or long-term periods in hospitals, nursing homes, and other institutions, and *ambulatory care* for clients in the community. They state that society's values and priorities are manifested by regulation, financing, consumerism, and technology interacting with the health care system. They suggest that the complex educational and research system, the collection of manufacturers and suppliers of equipment, drugs, and numerous other items, and the many providers of services also support and interact with the basic components (Wilson and Neuhauser, 1982, p. 1).

The word *system* implies that in the United States the delivery of health services is organized, and has a boundary, component parts, and relationships. Others would argue that it is a nonsystem implying that it is chaotic and in need of reorganization along more rational lines. Multiple causes have been given for the present state of the HCDS. Some of these causes include escalating costs, maldistribution of personnel and services, limitations and loopholes in insurance coverage, and confusing and fragmented organization of hospital services. There appears to be common agreement that Americans are convinced that there is a health care crisis in the United States. The crisis in public health is, of course, only part of the larger crisis in American life. Health is linked to all aspects of life. Fundamental progress in health depends on solving the major issues that challenge our entire national life.

The Role of Government

In principle, the responsibility for the general health, safety, and welfare of the people resides with the states that enact and implement appropriate laws under the inherent police powers of the sovereign states. Despite the steadily rising influence of the federal government in recent years, these basic powers and responsibilities have remained with the states, which have a major and expanding role in many aspects of health care, including extensive regulation of health facilities and manpower. Certain powers and functions are delegated to the local governments of counties, cities, and towns either directly or through state charters, which permit many cities and towns to function with considerable autonomy (Wilson and Neuhauser, 1982, p. 229).

Even though the federal government does not have a constitutionally defined role in health, over the years there has been a gradual development of the federal presence in the field of health. Wilson and Neuhauser identify the sources of this still expanding role as:

1. The special responsibility for certain population groups, such as merchant seaman, members of the armed forces, veterans, and American Indians.
2. The Constitutional power to regulate interstate commerce; much of the regulatory power of the federal government in health as in other areas derives from this power. An example is the regulation of food and drugs.
3. Grants-in-aid to states, institutions, and individuals for a wide variety of activities.
4. Most recently, sponsorship and financial participation in the health insurance program for the elderly (Medicare). (Wilson and Neuhauser, 1982, p. 137)

The federal government, through the Health Planning and Resources Development Act (Public Law 93-641) signed in January 1975, has also exerted leadership in establishing four new structures that assist in the setting of national priorities and provide opportunities for nurse and consumer participation. These structures are the National Council on Health Planning and Development (NCHPD), a state health planning and development (SHPDA) agency in each state, statewide health coordinating councils (SHCCs), and health systems agencies (HSAs) in each state (Chopoorian and Craig, 1976, p. 1988). Most federal health-related functions are consolidated in the various units of the Department of Health and Human Services. Many functions, however, are among the responsibilities of a variety of other departments, agencies, and bureaus, where they represent only a part of or are incidental to the main activities of the unit (Wilson and Neuhauser, 1983, p. 139).

As a basis for understanding the present HCDS, the power structure within the HCDS is examined. Both formal and informal power are defined and described and their relationship to responsibility and accountability is discussed.

Formal Power, Responsibility, and Accountability

Power, as defined by MacKenzie, means the capability to affect people, to change the paths of their lives. He further states that for power to be effective it must be made legitimate by responsibility within a system (MacKenzie, 1979, pp. 6–7).

The types of power have been identified by French and Raven as reward, coercive, referent, legitimate, expert, and informational. Their theory of social influence and power is limited to the influence on the person produced by a social agent that can be either another person, a role, a group, or a part of a group. Reward power is based on the person's perception that the agent has the ability to mediate rewards for him while coercive power is based on the perception that the agent has the ability to mediate punishments. Legitimate power is based on the person's perception that the agent has a right to prescribe behavior for him. Referent power is based on the person's identification with the agent, and expert power is based on the perception that the agent has some special knowledge or expertise (French and Raven, 1959, pp. 155, 156).

Other categorizations of power are identified by Stevens as positional and functional or personal power. She states that positional power that is combined with the authority existing in an organization inherently has legitimate and reward power. The legitimate power exists as authority and the reward power may include the right to hire, fire, promote, recognize, and grant raises. This combination is referred to as formal or positional power. Functional or personal power may be independent of formal power and may exist with or without it. Functional power may be used to convince others to grant more formal power to one's position (Stevens, 1983, p. 12).

Chaney and Knebel view power in health care agencies as both unique and in certain respects similar to power in other organizations. Power in health care agencies is supported not only by expert and reward power, but also by legitimate or positional power. Legitimate or positional power, which may or may not be earned, is merely the result of an individual holding a specific position. Positional power, unlike authority, need not be legitimized by subordinates to be exercised. Legitimate or positional power is generally prescribed by organizational design and organizations are designed with varying degrees of complexity, depending on the classification and size of the agency. Diversity and complexity are reflected in the classification of health care institutions. The classification of the institution structures its responsibility and accountability to the public.

More than 7,000 hospitals provide most of the medical care to the acutely ill. There are also about 4,000 extended care facilities and approximately 23,000 nursing homes that provide other than acute care. Hospitals are classified in a variety of ways. The classification may be done according to size (number of beds, exclusive of bassinets for newborns); type (general, mental, tuberculosis, or other specialty, such as maternity, orthopedic, eye and ear, rehabilitation, chronic disease, alcoholism, or narcotic addiction); length of stay (short term, average stay less than 30 days or long term, 30 days or more; or ownership (public or private, including the for-profit investor-owned proprietary hospital or not-for-profit voluntary hospital, which may be owned by religious, fraternity, or community groups) (Kelly, 1981, p. 118). Because of this variety in organizational classification it is difficult to draw one picture of the formal power structure within hospitals.

In voluntary hospitals power formally rests in the board of trustees, a governing board generally made up of individuals representing various business and professional groups interested in the community. Most of these unsalaried and volunteer board members are influential citizens who are able to assist in helping to raise money needed to support the hospital. Presently, because of the complaints of some consumer groups that the boards are not representative of consumers in general, some boards are gradually acquiring broader representation. Other changes in the degree of trustee power are possible if hospitals adopt a corporate model, integrating the board of trustees and the administrators of the hospital, with the board having full-time and salaried presidents and vice presidents. There is also an increase in the growth of mergers, consortia, and holding companies that are creating new business oriented hospital systems. These changes will also contribute to changes in the role of trustees (Kelly, 1981, pp. 120–121).

The flow of organizational power differs in public hospitals. Hospital administrators are directly responsible to their administrative supervisors in the governmental hierarchy, which may be a state board of health, a commissioner, a department (as the Veteran's Administration) or some public corporation with appointed officials. The hospital administrator, the direct agent of a governing board, implements its policies, advises on new policies, and is responsible for the day-to-day operations of the hospital. Usually the hospital administrator is a lay person with management education and experience, although in the past physicians and nurses frequently filled these positions (Kelly, 1981, p. 121).

The medical staff, through their exclusive control over the admission of patients to hospitals and reimbursement for services, establish and maintain a monopoly over the services they wish to deliver, and are an impressive power in the hospital (DeSantis, 1982, p. 17). Expert power is seen as the base from which physicians practice medicine. Usually the medical staff organization is parallel to and not subordinate to that of hospital administration, although some changes are occurring in this area. For example, nurses and representatives from other disciplines are joining the hospital committees concerned with patient care and are engaged in the decision-making process. Physicians also control through their committees, including the Credentials Committee, not only medical practice, but all patient care in the hospital (Kelly, 1981, p. 121).

Because medical staff members have such responsibility for patient care they are held accountable for the quality of this care. (See Chapter 11 for a discussion of accountability.) Outside pressures have been applied to achieve this end. Increasingly the public is resorting to the law, through malpractice suits, to obtain their rights as consumers of health care. This pressure has resulted in the establishment of utilization review boards within the hospital that are required under Medicare law to review records to determine whether the patient's admission is valid, the treatment is appropriate, and discharge occurs within a reasonable time. The Professional Services Review Organization (PSRO) looks at these and other factors. It is important that nurses participate on these committees and they do, in some instances, even on a full time basis (Kelly, 1981, p. 122).

Nursing has not enjoyed a power base broad enough to enable the nurse to influence policy decisions that could dramatically improve the delivery of health care although the nurse is in an excellent position to do so. Since health care is a system wherein a great deal of politics and power are used to control or create change, it is argued that the development of nursing power, which would allow nurses to increase their impact on the HCDS, has been delayed by the characteristics of the profession and by the bureaucratic setting in which nurses practice. Nurses are unfamiliar with the game and rules of corporate politics and they accept their traditional role of low status in a low-risk situation with little accountability (Stevens, 1983, pp. 4–7,20). In addition, nurses employed in hospitals encounter another problem because they are seen to have dual responsibility to the administration that employs them and to the physicians who are seen to have overall responsibility for patient care. When these two groups differ the nurse is caught in the middle. How the nurse reacts to these situations is changing in some instances where nurses are beginning to recognize their responsibility to both themselves and to their clients. The legal responsibility of the nurse to the client is receiving new attention and nurses are seeking more autonomy (Kelly, 1981, p. 122). Nurses are beginning to recognize their importance in the delivery of health care and are beginning to develop power. However, developing power is just the first step in making changes. A critical step remains. That step is to learn the rules by which the game of organizational politics is played (Stevens, 1983, p. 13). Learning these rules help nurses gain control over their practice.

Cleland identifies a control problem for nursing. That problem is the fact that nursing charges are incorporated into the per diem hospital charge. Outcomes of this are that (1) nursing does not have clear control over its budget, which results in lack of control in personnel decisions, and (2) the professional contribution of nursing to well-being cannot be separated from the technical services of the institution. Cleland states that the nursing profession cannot be held accountable for the cost and effectiveness of nursing care until nurses have more control over the appropriate use of nursing resources, and adds that only with appropriate use of nurses by level of education and experience can nursing have a significant impact on the availability, continuity, quality, and cost of health services. Health systems goals cannot be achieved without active participation by nurses in the documentation and quantification of their contributions (Cleland, 1983, p. 19). Nurses who are trying to achieve the goal of separating nursing costs from the total institutional cost are given significant opportunities to participate in the game of organizational politics.

Nurses must use power in order to realize their full professional potential and maximize their contributions to health care and society at large (Stevens, 1983, p. 3). Formal power has been discussed. However, it is agreed that informal power exists within every system. This source of power must also be understood by nurses if they are to use it effectively.

Informal Power, Authority, and Responsibility

"There is no doubt that within organizations there are individuals who possess power despite the fact that they do not hold a formal source of power such as a significant position or degree of expertise" (Chaney and Knebel, 1983, p. 134). Informal power is referred to as functional authority by Claus and Bailey who state that the source of this power is derived from professional-technical knowledge, expertise and experience, and the knowledge of management techniques and human relations. Within any organizational structure there is generally much unused functional authority. Three reasons are given for this: organizations do not see that they can positively encourage the acquisition of functional authority, rather they rely heavily on the formal authority vested in position, roles, or offices that are perceived as legitimate; because nurses are generally not risk takers, they tend to be fearful of using functional personal power; and finally, traditional line organizational concepts support the underlying feeling that it is dangerous to permit power to be distributed informally throughout an organization. In the case of the HCDS this concern is focused on legal liability problems (Claus and Bailey, 1977, pp. 56,58). Hospital administrators are having to relinquish control over the HCDS because of civil rights acts, the women's movement, the Nurse Practice Act, expanded roles for nurses, the rise of consumerism, a more humanistic approach to management, the complexities of organizational structures, and the increased level of preparation of nurses. Nurses must learn to use the untapped power of functional authority. It should be remembered, however, that the acquisition of authority is not an end in itself. The person who acquires authority or power must be willing to be held responsible for the actions taken based on that authority (Claus and Bailey, 1977, pp. 58–63).

Professional Disciplines Within the System–Their Intradisciplinary and Interdisciplinary Relationships

Nursing is a segment of the system in which health care is provided through the services of many professions, including nursing, medicine, pharmacy, social work, and dentistry, among others. The term health care refers to a composite of planned care provided by interdependent professions whose members collaborate with individuals and groups being served (ANA, 1980, p. 13). The following sections examine the concepts of collaboration, cooperation, and competition; the processes that occur between members of the interdisciplinary health team.

Collaboration

The most desirable relationship, both intradisciplinary and interdisciplinary, is that of collaboration. Collaboration is defined as the mutual responsibility for the adjustment of behavior to perceived needs in order to work together toward achievement of goals and is achieved through interpersonal communication. Collaboration means shared responsibility for planning, problem-solving, and evaluating with clients and others in the HCDS. Collaboration represents "real" sensitivity to others, whereby individuals clearly adjust behavior to the perceived needs of others. Thus collaboration promotes growth. Collaborative team effort is characterized by a high degree of information exchange, clarity of communication, and mutual trust and respect, and is inherent in order to accomplish goals of the group or organization.

Nursing, as is true of all other professions, is viewed as dynamic rather than static and change is observed in the scope of practice. One characteristic used by the ANA to define the scope of nursing practice—the content of the nursing segment of health care—is intersections. *Intersections* are defined as the meeting points at which nursing extends its practice into the domains of other professions and are not viewed as hard and fast lines. In situations where collaborative joint practice exists, the relations between nursing and medicine are especially fluid and unproblematic. All of the health care professions interact, share the same overall mission, have access to the same published scientific literature, and in some degree overlap in their activities (ANA, 1980, p. 16). Collaboration is characterized by mutuality in decision-making and planning affecting all and respecting the authority and responsibility of the experts at given times. It may also be viewed as equal sharing in the planning and implementation of mutually determined goals.

Cooperation

Next in degree of effectiveness in the interpersonal processes that occur between members of the HCD team is cooperation. Cooperation implies two or more persons or entities acting jointly for their mutual profit or common benefit. However, the mutuality exhibited through all the steps of the collaborative process is missing. There are not, for example, mutually derived goals. In the delivery of health care there is minimally a provider and a consumer. On a larger scale, there can be a group of several disciplines who might cooperate in providing health care to an entire community. The major goals for all would be achieving the highest level of well-being for the consumers of care. The providers of care would experience rewards from those health outcomes as a result of their participation and activities—the satisfaction of a job well done (MacElveen-Hoehn, 1983, p. 516).

Cooperation and Collaboration with the Consumer

Due to the shift in the politics of health care the issue of patient power must be considered. In the past the patient was expected to follow the doctor's orders. Now, however, with a population better educated and more knowledgeable about health, the old model is becoming obsolete. There is a move to a more democratic model where the client, family members, and the care providers work together and the emphasis is on the setting of goals and the identification of the means to achieve these goals. The hope is that with greater client involvement and agreement on goals, health behaviors will change.

Most care providers desire a specific level of health for their clients. However, clients frequently differ in their perception of what is achievable by them, or what price they are willing to pay to achieve a specific level of wellness. As an alternative to the problem of what to do when the only option to care is viewed by the client as that of treatment or no treatment, MacElveen-Hoehn suggests a negotiated level of health. She views this as better than no care. Care providers need to consider whether they believe that the individual has the right to make an informed choice, and whether they are willing to negotiate with the client the level of health they will agree to work on together (MacElveen-Hoehn, 1983, p. 522). To the extent that collaboration is present the consumer and the provider share mutual decision-making.

In order to participate effectively in planning and decision-making, health care consumers usually require information, knowledge, and skills. When the care provider makes these available to the client, the client is empowered, whereas the traditional medical approach exchanged power for care. The inclusion of the family, through a cooperative triad model, allows for its participation along with the client and the care giver. When the client is unable to be actively involved, an alliance of care provider and family is then formed. This model of providing services is seen to alter the role of the care provider; not, however, by diminishing that role but rather by expanding it. The expanded role of the care provider allows greater emphasis to be placed on teaching the client and the family necessary skills. The relationships established are viewed as interdependent, with power and status differences deemphasized and the consumer, the family, and the care provider feeling more satisfied (MacElveen-Hoehn, 1983, p. 524).

An example of just such a cooperative model is the innovative program, which combines patient education and family participation in health care while substantially reducing costs, established in 1979 at New York University (NYU) Medical Center. This Cooperative Care unit admits only those clients who do not require constant nursing supervision. The "care partner" must accompany the client, stays without charge in the client's room, and is taught to perform many tasks traditionally handled by the nursing staff. Some clients and their partners find the emotional responsibility or the physical demands of a co-op care setting overwhelming. Nevertheless, the concept is growing in popularity for two important reasons. The first reason is the economic one. The average bill in the co-op care unit is 40% to 45% less than it would be for the same number of days in a traditional hospital. The second reason is that it encourages clients to become active participants in their own health care and dramatically alters the traditional delivery of health care in this country (Berg, 1983, pp. 90,91). The concept of each individual being responsible for his own health status is an important one. When all members of the professional disciplines within the HCDS recognize this and collaborate with clients and their families, then major changes in the HCDS will take place. This point has not yet been fully appreciated although there is movement in this direction.

Competition

Competition is defined as the act of striving to outdo another for supremacy. It is viewed as the least effective way for professional disciplines to conduct their intradisciplinary and interdiscipilinary relationships within the HCDS. The ability to compete implies the presence of an equal relationship but nurses and doctors, for example, do not presently have an equal relationship. Therefore they cannot compete on an equal basis. The previously described collaborative relationship stresses the importance of working together. The competitive relationship implies just the opposite. In competition all members strive to attain the same goal(s) but only one may attain the goal(s) to the exclusion of others. Most goals are oriented to superior positions or power to control others and individual and private efforts are used to pursue the goals. Therefore, interdependency is low. The sharing of information and resources is limited and selected. When resources are limited the competition for these resources becomes more intense. Chaska writes of a phenomenon that is coming to light in the evolution of the professionalization of nursing. She states that the lack of support, compassion, and empathy for one another as professionals shows itself in intense competition and dissension within the profession. It is suggested that the lack of what is referred to as professional bonding may be the most significant source of conflicts within the profession and might be the result of the absence of opportunities for women to be socialized as team members through participation in team sports. This serves to hinder their progress through the developmental stages to cooperation and collaboration (Chaska, 1983, pp. 873, 874).

At no time in our society, Chaska states, has collaboration been more essential between and among professionals. No one health professional or health profession can effectively begin to meet all the needs of clients. With the knowledge explosion and rapid obsolescence, technology, economics, and costs of health care it is demanded that every health professional be more accountable. No single health profession can afford to stand alone or predominate (Chaska, 1983, p. 873).

Competition has been discussed in a negative sense, however, competition can also be viewed in a positive sense when discussed within an economic framework. Fagin identifies a new approach to containing the high cost of health and medical care as the injection of competition into the health insurance and health delivery systems. She states that competition, with minimal regulation and no addition to federal health financing will be palliative for health care inflation. When examining the so-called consumer choice pro-competition bills, Fagin found several important components of choice and competition to be lacking. The consumer, she states, is barely visible in any proposal, and competition, where it exists, is competition among the already-present conglomerate of providers who cannot be assumed to be any more competitive under the proposed organizations than under previous efforts (Fagin, 1982. pp. 56, 57). Two conditions must be present for competition to operate in a system. These are identified as the active involvement of the consumer in choosing alternatives, and the free entry of qualified providers into the system (Griffith, 1983, p. 263).

Both Fagin and Griffith argue for the inclusion of nursing into these competitive models. Fagin documents her argument with multiple examples of studies demonstrating over the past 20 years the importance of nursing and nursing care in affecting patient outcomes in and out of hospitals and showing that nursing services can contribute to the goals of a competitive delivery system. She further comments on the suitability of alternative nursing services for higher-cost hospital services and states that it has been shown that a variety of predominately nursing interventions have low-cost/high benefit results. The examples she gives include use of home care, skilled nursing facility care, nurse-aided family care, and rehabilitative care with or without prior hospitalization. Fagin urges that the present push toward competition in health delivery should be seized as an opportunity to lobby for legitimizing nursing's roles and realizing its potential. Whatever constrains nursing from its potential—be it legal interpretations, third-party payments, insurance policies, or public image—should be fought (Fagin, 1982, pp. 57, 60).

Griffith identifies strategies for advancing nursing's interest in developing competition as increasing legislative visibility, achieving direct third-party reimbursement and interpreting the nurse's role in preventive care, geriatric care, and consumer education (Griffith, 1983, p. 265). Many of these strategies have now been adopted by the American Nurses' Association (ANA) and included in their national agenda for health policy. This agenda will be advanced by a new political education and action project called "Nurses: Visible in Politics." This collaborative effort between the ANA and the state associations is aimed at encouraging nurses to become knowledgeable about candidates for national office and issues of importance—especially those related to health care; help elect delegates or become a delegate to the Democratic or Republican national convention; contribute to the Nurses' Coalition for Action in Politics (N-CAP), ANAs political action arm, and to the political action committees (PACs) operated by some state nurses associations; and support candidates who support nursing's national agenda for health policy (The American Nurse, 1983, p. 1).

The agenda lists seven categories and examples of legislative actions that the ANA advocates in each category. Of particular interest are the sections on access to health care and financing of health care. The aims are to assure access to quality health care services, especially to vulnerable populations such as children, the disadvantaged, and the aged; and to assure access to nursing care services with emphasis on the role of nurses as qualified providers of health care services. Under the category of financing health care, the ANA seeks to assure that the federal government maintains an appropriate role in determining the nature of basic health care services and the quality of those services. The ANA also wishes to assure that the federal government continues to work with state and local governments to provide a stable source of funding to meet health care needs, including recognition and remuneration for services rendered by nurses. ANA supports legislation to remove barriers to the financing of nursing services and provides a rational mechanism of payment for nursing services (The American Nurse, 1983, p. 5). The realization of these identified goals would have a major impact on the national health policy and therefore on the HCDS.

Leadership as a responsible use of infuence is discussed in Chapter 14. However, it should be noted that an organizational structure impacts on the style of leadership possible in that institution. Conversely, the leadership style that is practiced will impact on the existing organizational structure. Historically, the leadership roles that existed were developed over time to maintain the status quo—that is, the physician in charge, the nurse, the employee of the institution and the assistant to the physician, and the patient, the receiver. A changing order will produce a nurse whose responsibility is to herself and her clients. Changes are already beginning to be evident in some systems where nurses are appearing on governing boards with voice and vote. The role of all professionals is changing. When man is viewed holistically, the requirements for care change and leadership on the multiprofessional team can no longer be the role of one but is determined by the demonstrable needs of the client. Administration therefore, has to be responsive to input in policy-making from the representatives of all the people involved, including all givers and receivers of care.

THE MISSION OF THE HEALTH CARE
DELIVERY SYSTEM

A mission, when accepted by a group or assigned to a group, implies that there is agreement on purpose and in the case of the HCDS, agreement as well on who shall be served and how they shall be served. There is agreement that health care providers will offer the finest health care that is possible given the knowledges and skills available. But there is little agreement on a definition of health and so little agreement on what constitutes health care. There is also little agreement on where and how health care shall be offered. And finally little agreement about who shall offer it and to whom it shall be offered. As an example, the primary objective of Medicaid is to provide people of low income equal access to health care. Yet in a study of Medicaid participation by pediatricians, reported in *Pediatrics*, the following statement was made: "A pediatrician makes several decisions regarding Medicaid participation. One is simply whether or not to treat Medicaid patients. This decision is of importance because nonparticipation of pediatricians has a pronounced effect on the access of low-income children to health care in private physicians' offices" (Davidson, 1983, p. 553).

The concept of health is changing from mere absence of disease to one that encompasses various states of being and we accept that the health status of the individual results to a greater extent from his interaction with his environment than it does from medical care. The system is still heavily invested in illness care rather than in the improvement of health through the correction of factors detrimental to good health. There is much agitation for change—the nature of which is ill-defined (except by vested interests) primarily because we have not evolved a national policy with relation to health (policy defined as a course of action adopted and pursued by a government at any level). Policy is formed by many social forces and special interest groups within and without a system. "Nonetheless," says Banta, "the broad outlines of a national health policy are beginning to emerge. There is general agreement on certain critical needs concerning the organization of medical and health care: the need to assure access to primary health care services; to plan and organize health services in a region; to foster group practice and team medicine; to train health manpower to carry out the tasks of the future; and to establish a national health insurance system" (Banta, 1981, p. 353).

There is increasing dissatisfaction with the system(s) of delivery of health care, with the fragmentation, impersonality, and above all—the cost. We, as a nation, pride ourselves on the mixture of the public and the private controls in other areas of resource—as in higher education—where the combination is viewed as a national strength. The history of the HCDS is other than that of higher education in which the government was involved quite early. Entrance of the government into the delivery of health care is a comparatively recent phenomenon. Its role still needs to be defined so that the combined public-private contributions result in effective services.

There have been a variety of proposals for National Health Insurance (NHI) offered during the Carter administration and several in the Reagan administration—each in its way anomalous either because it represents the wishes of a particular group or it tries to be satisfying to all and succeeds in satisfying none. Most crucial to our assessment of any plan is the understanding that change in the method of payment—NHI alone—without change in the way the health care is delivered is not responsive to human needs. Testimony to this is available in the results of Medicare and Medicaid—that provided a change of payment for care but no change in delivery of that care with subsequent abuses.

Although, as Banta has written, the broad outlines of a national health policy are beginning to appear, the government, concerned about excessive costs of Medicare and the inconsistencies of charges among institutions has embarked on a new payment system for hospitals. Heretofore, Medicare paid the hospital whatever it claimed as the cost of care, and claims varied from institution to institution. In order to remedy the inconsistencies and to cut costs, on October 1, 1983 another form of reimbursement, diagnosis related group (DRG), began a 3-year phasing in period. "By late 1986 every hospital will receive a flat fee for each Medicare patient based on the DRG that describes his condition" (Hunt, 1983, p. 262). As stated in the introduction to Title VI (Social Security Amendment P.L. 98-21), "The bill is intended to improve the medicare program's ability to act as a prudent purchaser of services, and to provide predictability payment amounts for both the Government and hospitals. More important, it is intended to reform the financial incentives hospitals face, promoting efficiency in the provision of services by rewarding cost/effective hospital practices." Some of the changes provided in the amendment are: (1) Rates are prospectively determined. (2) Capital related costs (depreciation, interest, rent) are excluded from the prospective payment system—but covered on a "reasonable cost basis" pro tem. There is a phase-out of return of equity to proprietary hospitals. (3) Direct and indirect expenses for medical education are excluded from payment determinations. Such expenses (including nursing education programs) will be paid on the basis of "reasonable cost." There will, however, continue to be consideration for the special needs of teaching hospitals. (4) Psychiatric, long-term care, rehabilitation, and children's hospitals are exempted. The DRG system was developed for short-term acute care hospitals. There are provisions for admissions and quality review. (5) The Secretary is authorized to approve a state cost control system meeting specific criteria. Health maintenance organizations (HMOs) require special treatment since use of hospital services by their members vary from that of individuals covered by health insurance plans. (6) The Secretary will begin to collect data and study the feasibility and appropriateness of including physicians payments under the DRG system as soon as possible.

Speculating on the meaning of the DRG system for nursing it might be the time to reaffirm the cost-effectiveness of professional nursing, and to present once more the nursing alternative to high-cost care-prevention. "Nursing should be actively involved in the design of programs of health promotion and disease prevention that will ultimately reduce reliance on higher-cost technological interventions" (Fagin, 1982, p. 59). Theoretically, at least, DRG offers an opportunity to free nursing service costs from lump per diem hospital rates and to calculate nursing costs for patients in different classifications. That it will affect all of us—consumers and caregivers—is certain. Not so certain is the nature of the effects. Systems theory teaches that change in one part of a system affects the other parts of the system. A possible system change in the delivery of health care that has been proposed is a national health service (NHS), designed to provide comprehensive services for the entire population and entirely supported by tax monies. There is no evidence of legislative moves in such a direction at this time.

The heart of the matter at this time is health planning which, since the delivery system affects every American, should be done by representation from the broad spectrum of consumers and the various groups of providers. All voices need to be heard and all concerns and priorities identified. The process of planning itself then becomes a means of education for narrowing the existing HCDS gaps and preventing the institution of two levels of care. At this point in time there seem to be at least two divergent views of the future of health care—the one that of movement toward a NHS, the other as Starr states toward corporate management. "Medical care in America now appears to be in the early stages of a major transformation in its institutional structure. Corporations have begun to integrate a hitherto decentralized hospital system." With the entry of a variety of other health care businesses and the consolidation of ownership and control, the health care delivery system may eventually become an industry dominated by huge health care conglomerates (Starr, 1982, p. 428). Starr notes that the change to a corporate philosophy has already given rise to a "marketing mentality" in health care; medical care organizations are headed by business school graduates; the professional ideal no longer dominates. The new health care conglomerates will exercise powerful political force opposed to a national health program and resistive to public participation and accountability. The for-profit institution is more likely to limit care to those who are privately insured. Voluntarism is not a characteristic of the corporate ethic.

THE RIGHTFUL RESPONSIBILITY AND ACCOUNTABILITY OF PROFESSIONAL NURSING IN A VARIETY OF HEALTH CARE DELIVERY SETTINGS

Regardless of the structure of the HCDS, the profession of nursing has rights and responsibilities in the delivery of nursing care. The basic right of any profession is the control of its practice. The basic responsibility of any profession is that it is accountable for the service it purports to offer.

Control of Professional Nursing Decisions: The Administration and Practice of Nursing

The ANA as the professional society for nursing in the United States, is responsible for defining and establishing the scope of nursing practice. The document *Nursing: A Social Policy Statement* was published in 1980 to address this responsibility. Burge writes that the social policy statement gives very specific and clear interpretations of the practice of nursing while it also identifies nursing's responsibility to the public and other health professionals (Burge, 1983, p. 65). Two other documents produced by the ANA contribute to the standards of nursing care that will assure consumer protection. These two documents are the *Standards of Practice* written in 1975, and the *Policy Guide for State Nursing Practice Acts* written in 1980. The standards identify assumptions and beliefs basic to the area of practice, descriptions of types of practitioners, qualifications related to educational preparation, and scope of practice. The ANA policy guide reinforces the premise that the public's health and welfare should be protected with a minimum of governmental regulation and that there are checks and balances between governmental and professional regulation of the practice of nursing (Burge, 1983, p. 64). These standards are discussed in Chapter 12, "The Nursing Process."

Control of nursing must be in the hands of nurses. For nursing to be accorded true professional status, it must function autonomously in the formation of policy and in the control of its activity. To be an autonomous body implies that an occupational group has been granted authority to define its scope of practice, delineate its specific functions and roles, and determine its goals and responsibilities in delivery of its services. The degree of professional autonomy accorded an occupational group depends on the effectiveness of the group's efforts at governance. Without governance, there is no autonomy. Without autonomy, full professional status is unattainable (Aydelotte, 1983, p. 832). Therefore, in order to gain control of nursing, nurses must be involved with governance planning.

The term governance refers to the establishment and maintenance of social, political, and economic arrangements by which practitioners maintain control over their practice, their self-discipline, their working conditions, and their professional affairs. Until recently, nursing has been unable to implement effective arrangements for governance because of several obstacles. Aydelotte identifies the foremost obstacle in nursing's drive for governance as the bureaucratic organization of hospitals that prevents nurses from assuming autonomous roles in the delivery of nursing services. In addition, she states that the insufficient number of well-prepared nursing leaders in nursing, and the recent push by labor unions to add nurses to their membership ranks are also obstacles (Aydelotte, 1983, pp. 835–837).

To assist nursing in gaining control through governance, the ANAs 1981 Commission on Nursing Services offered some ways of achieving the desired control. According to testimony presented to the National Commission on Nursing in February 1981, nursing needs to assume autonomy and budgetary control in order to be responsible and accountable for the quality of nursing practice. Institutional policies with mechanisms for shared governance, continuing education for practitioners, joint practice committees, and incentives for promotion and scholarship need to be in place.

Implementation of these suggestions could assist nurses to overcome obstacles caused by the bureaucratic organization of hospitals and assume more control over their practice. Also, further development of well-prepared nursing leaders is essential to the advancement of an autonomous profession. The professional association is responsible for representing the professional interests and concerns of nurses. To be accorded true professional status, Aydelotte believes that nurses at all employment levels and in all patient care settings must participate in determining the terms and conditions of their employment and must share in decision-making that affects the quality of nursing care they provide, whether as employees or as self-employed individuals (Aydelotte, 1983, p. 837).

The issue of membership on the interdisciplinary health care delivery team is essential to any discussion of the rightful responsibility and accountability of professional nursing. Therefore, that issue will be explored and the problems for nurses participating as full members will be identified.

Participation on the Interdisciplinary Health Care Delivery Team

It is desirable for nurses to participate as full contributing members on interdisciplinary health care delivery teams (IHCDT). There is common agreement that all members are needed by the client and the goal of helping the client is mutually agreed upon. However, problems exist with the full participation of nurses. Participation implies equality of status and for reasons of identity, educational preparation, and role-relations, nurses are not yet equal partners. Because the theory base from which nursing practices is uneven and not fully developed and the basic credential for entry into nursing practice has not been agreed upon, an unequal participation results. Therefore, more work is needed in theory development and nurses must agree on the baccalaureate in nursing (BSN) degree as the minimum requirement for entry into professional practice. When progress in these areas is achieved participation by nurses as full members of the IHCDT will be more likely.

Several authors have looked past the present level of participation on IHCDT and envisioned a much larger role for nurses. La Monica writes that with the emphasis on prevention first and cure second the control of health care by the American Medical Association (AMA) is threatened and it is placed in a defensive fight for survival because of consumer dissatisfaction with health care. La Monica suggests that nurses can grasp the personal power being lost by the physicians to carve its unique place in tomorrow's picture of health care. If nurses do seize this power La Monica believes that tomorrow's professional nurse will be primarily an independent primary health care practitioner or "helper" to clients as clients seek to maintain and optimize their individual healthy states. These nurses who will practice collaboratively with all health care providers, will call in the physician as a consultant, for example, when cure of disease is necessary or the social worker, as another example, when that expertise is warranted. This nurse is seen to coordinate all health services for the client and be *the* primary health care provider in either private practice or as the leader in a multidisciplinary health care team such as seen at the present time in health maintenance organizations and clinics. These professional nurses will admit and follow clients in hospitals and plan the comprehensive, individualized nursing care that follows the nursing process together with technical nurses, who will be employed by the hospital, and other health care personnel. La Monica further differentiates the practice of the professional nurse and states that when health maintenance is the principal focus for the client, the professional nurse will function independently; when cure or rehabilitation is the priority, the professional nurse will be interdependent with the physician and others; and when life sustenance is predominant, the nurse may be independent or interdependent (La Monica, 1983, pp. 490–491).

However, Rogers points out a problem. She states that as nursing moves rapidly toward scientific identity and independent actions there is increased conflict with power and profit interests. This conflict will be overcome because the public is demanding freedom of choice, informed consent, and alternatives in health providers and health services. Therefore, in the world of tomorrow Rogers (1983, p. 799) envisions autonomous nursing centers augmenting the independent professional practice of nursing.

Another view of the future of nursing tied into the interdisciplinary health care delivery team is expressed by Christman who states that there will be a growth of operational alliances between the disciplines and the professions manifested by a sharp decrease in territoriality and an equally sharp increase in cooperative enterprises. To achieve this state all the health professions, including the nursing profession, will have doctoral preparation as the entry level to practice and all will take their preparation from the same clinical base. This, Christman believes, will reduce communication difficulties, and achieve the full democratization of the professions. Especially in nursing the overwhelming white female makeup will yield to societal pressures and all health professions will contain equal sex ratios, and minority groups will reach appropriate representation. He further states that the intense need to rely on scientific training will alter the organization of care into new patterns. "One may see primary multidisciplinary teams replacing primary nursing because this matrix form may be the basic requirement for effective management of patient care" (Christman, 1983, pp. 803, 804).

These views of nursing in the future are exciting for nurses currently practicing. It must be remembered, however, that as we change there is a vast unevenness in our rate of progress and in the points from which we start. In the variety of settings in which nursing is practiced one sees major differences manifested in how nursing is practiced. Starting from such unequal points presents a major challenge. Whether nursing is able to accept this challenge and work collaboratively is a major question.

Planned change theory is discussed in Chapter 15. Planned change theory must be used to facilitate the effective delivery of health care services and maintain the integrity of the delivery system. However, change must begin first with the individual nurse and her vision of nursing, then proceed to change within the profession, and finally change should be reflected within the HCDS. If we believe that change begins with the individual this must be reflected in the educational programs that should seek to develop within each practitioner an understanding of one's selfhood and its relationship to practice. Leaders prepared in this way will be able to assist their colleagues to effect change within the nursing profession. Nursing professionals who are convinced of their worth develop credibility as change agents and therefore, will be effective in making changes within the larger HCDS.

REFERENCES

ANA starts project to advance national health policy agenda. Am Nurs 15: 1,20, 1983

Aydelotte ML: Professional nursing: The drive for governance. *In* Chaska N (ed): The Nursing Profession: A Time to Speak. New York, McGraw-Hill, 1983

Banta D: The federal legislative process and health care. *In* Jonas S (ed): Health Care Delivery in the United States. New York, Springer, 1981

Berg B: A touch of home in hospital care. NY Times Magazine, 90–98, Nov 27, 1983

Blum HL: Expanding Health Care Horizons, ed 2. Oakland, Third Party, 1983

Burge JM: The power of organizations. *In* Stevens K (ed): Power and Influence: A Source Book for Nurses. New York, John Wiley & Sons, 1983

Chaney HS, Knebel EA: Health care agencies and power. *In* Stevens K (ed): Power and Influence: A Source Book for Nurses. New York, John Wiley & Sons, 1983

Chaska NL (ed): The Nursing Profession: A Time to Speak. New York, McGraw-Hill, 1983

Chaska NL: Winter of discontent and invincible springs. *In* Chaska N (ed): The Nursing Profession: A Time to Speak. New York, McGraw-Hill, 1983

Chopoorian T, Craig MM: Nursing and health care delivery. Am J Nurs, 76: 1988–1991, 1976

Christman L: The future of nursing is predicated by the state of science and technology. *In* Chaska N (ed): The Nursing Profession: A Time to Speak. New York, McGraw-Hill, 1983

Claus KE, Bailey JT: Power and Influence in Health Care: A New Approach to Leadership. St Louis, CV Mosby, 1977

Cleland VS: Reimbursement for nursing practice. *In* Chaska N (ed): The Nursing Profession: A Time to Speak. New York, McGraw-Hill, 1983

Davidson SM: Full and limited Medicaid participation among pediatricians. Pediatr 72: 552–559, 1983

DeSantis G: Power, tactics, and the professionalization process. Nurs Health Care 3: 14–17,24, 1982

Fagin CM: Nursing as an alternative to high-cost care. Am J Nurs 82: 56–60, 1982

French JRP Jr, Raven B: The bases of social power. *In* Cartwright D (ed): Studies in Social Power. Ann Arbor, University of Michigan, 1959

Griffith H: Competition in health care. Nurs Outlook 31: 262–265, 1983

Hunt K: DRG-what it is, how it works, and why it will hurt, Med Eco: 262–272, 1983

Kelly LY: Dimensions of Professional Care, ed 4. New York, Macmillan, 1981

La Monica EL: The nurse as helper: Today and tomorrow. *In* Chaska N (ed): The Nursing Profession: A Time to Speak. New York, McGraw-Hill, 1983

MacElveen-Hoehn P: The cooperation model for care in health and illness. *In* Chaska N (ed): The Nursing Profession: A Time to Speak. New York, McGraw-Hill, 1983

MacKenzie WJM: Power and Responsibility in Health Care. Oxford, England, Oxford University, 1979

Nursing: A social policy statement. Kansas City, Mo, American Nurses' Association, 1980

Rogers ME: Beyond the horizon. *In* Chaska N (ed): The Nursing Profession: A Time to Speak. New York, McGraw-Hill, 1983

Starr P: The Social Transformation of American Medicine. New York, Basic Books, 1982

Stevens KR (ed): Power and Influence: A Source Book for Nurses. New York, John Wiley & Sons, 1983

Stevens KR: Power as a positive force. *In* Stevens KR (ed): Power and Influence: A Source Book for Nurses. New York, John Wiley & Sons, 1983

Wilson FA, Neuhauser D: Health Services in the United States, ed 2. Cambridge, Ballinger, 1982

Chapter 11

Accountability to the Public, the Profession, the Employer, and the Self

Susan E. Gordon

THOUGHT QUESTIONS

1. What differentiates accountability from autonomy and authority?
2. What are the essential questions the professional nurse must answer in order to be accountable to the client/public?
3. What is the relationship between the educational level of the practitioner of nursing and accountability in practice?
4. What are some of the positive outcomes of the nurse becoming accountable to clients, profession, self, and employing institution?
5. Using the checklist provided, how do you evaluate yourself on accountability?

Accountability is a concept that has been present in nursing for a very long time, although the use of the word itself is relatively recent. In its simplest sense, accountability is synonomous with responsibility and, in this regard, permeates the writing of Florence Nightingale. When she discusses the nurse's responsibility for the state of the sick-room (Nightingale, 1859, p. 45) or the need for careful observation on the part of the nurse in order to avoid patient accidents (Nightingale, 1859, p. 66), or the fact that "I have often seen really good nurses distressed, because they could not impress the doctor with the real danger of their patients" (Nightingale, 1859, p. 68), she is expressing the responsibility or accountability of that nurse to her patient.

Perhaps the epitome of the accountable nurse is the private duty nurse of old, who took a "case" and remained with it until the patient had no further need of nursing care. The patient was very much this nurse's responsiblity and, in turn, the nurse was very much in charge of and accountable for the nursing care, life, and space of that patient.

However, after the Great Depression of the 1930s the percentage of nurses choosing private duty nursing decreased and more turned to staff nursing (Dachelet, 1979, p. 15) with its highly functional orientation at that time. Accountability became harder to pinpoint and remained that way, with the care of the individual patient split over several different nurses and nurses' aides. Accountability became limited to the provision of isolated treatments, any of which, if overlooked or performed improperly, might prove to be the downfall of the nurse. The notion of accountability, therefore, became tied to negative situations and picked up a punative connotation. Nurses were legally liable for their actions or the omission of necessary actions, but often were unaware of this. The belief of many was that the ultimate liability remained with the institution, which would "cover" them in the event of a lawsuit. Accountability, in a professional sense, was not functioning and the entire concept certainly had no positive attributes as far as the individual nurse was concerned. This has remained the situation up to the current time (Clifford, 1981, p. 20).

Now, in the 1980s, accountability has come to the forefront and assumed an importance and visibility it never before possessed. Why is accountability the byword of the future for the nursing profession? Why is it a newly created subject heading in the *Cumulative Index of Nursing and Allied Health Literature?* Why is it the subject of countless articles and workshops and why is it so inextricably caught up with the emerging professional status of nursing?

DEFINITION OF ACCOUNTABILITY AND RELATED CONCEPTS

Before embarking on the answers to the above and other questions it is necessary to define the word accountability. It is a term that is increasingly confused with and used in place of autonomy and authority, although it is synonomous with neither, but related to both (Batey, 1982, p. 13). The meaning of this trio of terms must be clarified.

Accountability continues to retain its original meaning of responsibility but has an added dimension, that of answerability, the necessity of offering answers and explanations to certain others. That answerability can be to the public, to the other members of one's profession and allied professions, to the agency in which one is employed, and to oneself. As the American Nurses' Association (ANA) Code for Nurses states, this accountability

> refers to being answerable to someone for something one has done. It means providing an explanation to self, to the client, to the employing agency, and to the nursing profession. (American Nurses' Association, 1976, p. 10)

Yet, an additional dimension to accountability is the reporting aspect of it, which is embodied in the following definition:

> (accountability is) . . . the fulfillment of a formal obligation to disclose to referent others the purposes, principles, procedures, relationships, results, income and expenditures for which one has authority. This disclosure is systematic, periodic, and carried out in consistent form . . . Initiating the disclosure is the responsibility of the one accountable and not of others. (Batey, 1982, p. 10)

Accountability, then, is the state of being responsible and answerable for those behaviors and their outcomes that are included in one's professional role, as it is reflected in the periodic written reporting of those behaviors and their outcomes.

In distinction to this, autonomy refers to independence of functioning. Autonomy means that one can perform one's total professional function on the basis of one's own knowledge and judgement and, further, that one is recognized by others as having the right to do so. Obviously, this concept is related to accountability, as one who functions autonomously must be accountable for his behavior.

The last of the trio is authority. Authority can be defined as being in a position to make decisions and to influence others to act in a manner determined by those decisions. Again, this term is certainly related to accountability, in that one in authority is accountable for the decisions she makes and for the actions of herself and others who act on the basis of her decisions. Further, authority is related to autonomy because those in authority often act autonomously in performing all or part of their respective roles.

One can see these relationships further developed in the nursing literature. According to Batey:

> Responsibility, authority, autonomy, and accountability are inextricably related. Responsibility and authority are necessary conditions for both autonomy and accountability. It is illogical and inappropriate for an organization to hold a department or an individual accountable for those activities over which the department or individual has no authority. . . . Autonomy within the areas in which nursing service has responsibility is also a necessary condition for accountability. . . . Accountability is an exercise in futility and an experience in failure unless it is linked to nursing service's autonomy. The process of fulfilling nursing's formal obligation to disclose requires that nursing services have the formal and legitimate power to carry out relevant actions. Without the opportunity to make binding decisions, accountability is a hollow concept. (Batey, 1982, p. 13)

Bergman sees this relationship somewhat differently by considering responsibility and authority (along with ability) as preconditions leading to accountability. As she states:

> The basic precondition is to have the ability . . . to decide and act on a specific issue. One must be given or take, the responsibility to carry out that action. Next, one needs the authority, i.e. formal backing, legal right to carry the responsibility. Then, with the preconditions, one can be accountable for the action one takes. (Bergman, 1981, pp. 54–55)

What can be seen developing here, then, is a grouping of concepts, all related but not synonomous, projecting an image of a responsible, independent individual, who is able to make decisions and influence others to act on them, and who is answerable for her behavior and the behavior of her associates. This image is clearly that toward which the profession of nursing is striving for its members and provides the reason for the current upsurge in interest and relevance of the concept of accountability. As the selected watchword for the International Council of Nurses for the quadrennium 1977 to 1981, "accountability" is an inherent part of the image of the professional nurse of the 1980s and beyond (Bergman, 1981, p. 54). In fact, it is part of the image of any professional person. Accountability is a necessary attribute in all those who wish to exercise authority and act autonomously—and this characterizes nurses today.

ACCOUNTABILITY OF A PROFESSION _____

As nursing has come closer to being a true profession, it is to be expected that its concern with accountability has been increasing. Accountability has always been acknowledged as one of the hallmarks of a profession. This view is supported in Flexner's work characterizing a profession, in which he indicates that a profession is likely to be more responsive to public interest than are unorganized and isolated individuals (Flexner, 1915). In terms of nursing's involvement with its own professionalization in the 1950s and 1960s, it is evident in the Bixlers' (1959, p. 1142) conviction that a profession functions autonomously in the formulation of professional policy and in the control of professional activity. McGlothlin explains that a profession undertakes tasks that require exercise of judgement in applying knowledge to the solutions of problems and accepts responsibility for the results (McGlothlin, 1961, p. 214).

However, in order to be accountable, a profession must know that for which it is accountable. To do this, the profession must establish professional standards and attempt to enforce them. The ANA, nursing's major professional organization has, in fact, done this, with its Standards of Nursing Practice, Service, and Education. In doing so it has complied with one of the functions of a professional organization, according to Merton (1958, p. 50), that is, of providing the means by which members of the profession can judge the competency of its members. Through the Standards the ANA has contributed greatly to the ability of the nursing profession to be accountable.

By using the Standards of Nursing Practice (American Nurses' Association Congress for Nursing Practice, 1973, pp. 1–6) as a guide, the individual nurse can see, clearly laid out, the scope and the limits of practice. She can internalize that for which she is accountable. Through the use of the Standards of Nursing Service, a nursing service organization can monitor its collective accountability.

Additionally, the nurse has another document to guide her in practice, the Code for Nurses, also developed by the ANA. More in the nature of an ethical code, this provides a clear framework within which the nurse can seek to uphold the standards of care. Should there be any further doubt about accountability of the nursing profession, the Code lays this to rest by confronting the issue head on. As stated in item #4 of the Code, "The nurse assumes responsibility and accountability for individual nursing judgments and actions" (American Nurses' Association, 1976, p. 10).

Other items in the Code do not address the area of accountability directly but, by discussing various factors that are necessary underpinnings for accountability, indirectly support the concept. These factors include the presumed competence of the nurse, her use of informed judgement, and her participation in nursing research.

It should be highly evident by this point that nursing is accountable as a profession and that its individual practitioners are accountable, as well. It has been implied throughout the foregoing discussion that nurses are accountable to the public and to the profession itself. Additionally, with most nurses remaining employed by health agencies, rather than being independently employed, one must also consider the area of accountability to the institution. In light of current emphases on self-actualization and growth, it is important to add that the professional nurse must be accountable to herself as well.

Accountability to the Client/Public

A profession exists to provide service to the public. While it may be intellectually stimulating, gratifying, and exciting to the professional to perform her role, ultimately the reason for that role lies in its relationship with the public. Therefore, almost by definition, a profession must be accountable to that public. The consumer has the right to receive the best possible quality care, care grounded in a firm knowledge base and performed by those who can make use of that knowlege base through the application of sound judgement and a clear and appropriate value system.

As the consumer is becoming more knowledgeable through formal education and access to informal education as provided by a vast array of mixed media, he is able to know more about what the professions are supposed to be doing. He is able to demand more and to make those demands more effectively and more visibly. Nursing must be aware of this increased knowledge and sophistication on the part of the consumer and must be prepared to respond to it in an equally knowledgeable and sophisticated manner. The nurse must be able to demonstrate clearly those principles and concepts on which practice is based. The nurse must be able to demonstrate the ability to call into play a problem-solving method in order to properly use those principles and concepts. The nurse must know the importance of documenting her work and the processes used in accomplishing her goals, and the place served in the demonstration of her abilities by this documentation. The nurse must be able to formulate and present to others the bases for the judgement exercised in the performance of her role by indicating the depth and breadth of nursing science and of her educational preparation. The nurse must be able to formulate and present to others the ethical code or value system to which she refers when making her judgements and using her knowledge base. In other words, she must be able to answer the questions, from the consumer and others of "why did you do that?," and "how did you come to that decision?," and "what makes you believe this is the most effective course of action?" Furthermore, she must be able to answer these questions without becoming defensive about them or about the questioner, for the consumer has the right to know and, if the nurse is truly a professional, it's her responsibility to give the answers. She is accountable to the public.

Accountability to the Profession

The profession of nursing is exercising its accountability toward itself in the performance of its duty to formulate its own policy and control its activities. Its standards for licensure and certification, as well as those that exist for entry into a variety of professional groups and associations (such as the Association of Operating Room Nursing, the Association of Critical Care Nurses, and the American Academy of Nursing) all attest to nursing's attempts to set policy for its organization and performance. Further, the committees on professional conduct and discipline that exist on the state level, and are heavily staffed by nurses, are testimony to the profession's work in terms of controlling its activities and the work-related activities of its practitioners.

In connection with this aspect of accountability, the individual nurse must understand the necessity of being aware of and accountable for not only her own actions but those of her colleagues. Often the professional nurse is the only one who is present to observe the behaviors of her co-nurse, or the only one competent to evaluate her co-workers's care. While sharing apparent evidences of poor practice with the appropriate authorities (within the agency or without) may not be an attractive course of action, it is the only possible one if nursing is to strive toward ensuring quality care to all its recipients, and toward functioning in a truly professional manner. Approaching the capable individual first with the evidence of her failure would serve to emphasize the observing nurse's empathy for and concern about her, while eliminating the secrecy or spying aspect so detestable in our society.

Accountability to Self

While the professional person is perhaps more committed to her career as a source of satisfaction and as a lifelong pursuit than is one who is following an occupation or who is working only in order to earn a living, it is now accepted that her professional life is but one aspect of her life. The nurse is no longer expected to live on the premises in which she works, she is no longer expected to work most of her waking hours without time away from her duties, and she is no longer considered a piece of property belonging to the agency in which she works. She is seen as a free and independent person with other aspects and facets to her life besides the professional side. However, the exigencies of the job situation often cause her and others to overlook these basic facts. Additionally, the nurse's activities in her other life roles often have bearing on her professional performance in some way. Thus, the nurse must be the one accountable to herself for her own actions both on the job and off, because of the ways in which these actions will affect her and others.

The nurse who appears on the job still suffering the effects of too much celebrating over her days off is not prepared to function in the manner expected of her. Fatique, jet lag, minor illness, or the effects of alcohol or drugs make the nurse a liability rather than an asset in the work situation. Conversely, the nurse who puts in too much overtime, who allows herself to be placed in a position far beyond her ability and knowledge and is always functioning in a highly stressed state because of it, the nurse who constantly fills in for those in the next tour who fail to show up, is not prepared to function in her social and personal life in the way expected of her. Significant others cannot always be expected to take second place to one's work, while one's work cannot always be expected to play second fiddle to one's social and personal relationships. A certain balance is needed. Overdoing the amount of time and energy expected on the job will often lead to the burnout of which we hear, with the nurse no longer able or willing to do adequate work. This burnout, however, can extend into one's personal and social life as well, with one's relationships in that sphere suffering (Chaska, 1983, pp. 874–875).

The nurse's accountability to herself comes across here very clearly. She must be the one responsible for her own mental and physical health, for assuring that she keeps all aspects of her life in a balanced perspective. She must decide when to give more energy to her work and when to give more energy to other areas, but never sabotaging her wholeness as a person by allowing one aspect of her life to swallow her completely. She must be at her fullest capacity when on the job and yet pace herself to avoid the staleness and despair that come when the throttle is constantly on full speed ahead.

The nurse's accountability to herself includes refusing to work in situations that she considers unsafe. This may be by virtue of her own lack of knowledge or experience of the area or because of insufficient staffing or some other problem inherent in the situation itself. She must be able to see this as ultimately of service to the consumer and the profession, although she must also be aware of the sanctions that may be applied to her.

It further involves her acknowledging her limitations and knowing when she is in need of further education in order to more fully and safely perform her role. The decisions of others (perhaps to promote to head nurse only those with the B.S. degree) should not be the controlling factor in this; the nurse's personal accountability is on the line here.

Accountability to the Employing Agency

The final domain of the nurse's accountability is the agency in which that nurse is employed. This has been left for last in this discussion of those to whom the nurse is accountable because it is not the primary area of the nurse's accountability. While not unimportant, accountability to the agency has received too much emphasis in the past. It more rightfully takes a back seat to the client/public, the profession, and the nurse herself—but it *does* have a place.

The agency is accountable to the public for the care provided under its auspices. Therefore, in turn, it has the right to expect the nurse to be accountable to that agency.

The quality of the nurse's work is one aspect in which she must be accountable to the agency. This includes her own preparation for the job, as well as her fitness each time she appears on the job. The agency has contracted with the nurse for a specific job to be done at a specific time and place, for a specific wage. The nurse, then, must uphold her end of the bargain in all of these areas. She is accountable, as well, for the nature of her peers' performance and, should this be found lacking, should proceed as indicated earlier. Further, she is accountable for those over whom she has authority in the work setting, and must be aware of what they are doing and how they are doing it, in order to exercise that accountability.

The nurse must refuse to work in areas and situations that she considers to be unsafe. This further fulfills her accountability to the agency (as well as herself) because she is saying, in effect, "I will not put the agency in the position of giving unsafe care."

An additional aspect of the nurse's accountability to the agency involves the attitude toward that agency that she projects to the client. It should be one of objectivity and honesty. It is appropriate to promote the strengths of the agency to the extent that it has them, in a realistic manner. It is also necessary that its shortcomings not be exaggerated. Sometimes, in the heat of the moment, when particularly taxed, or following a disagreement, the nurse may denigrate an agency to a far greater extent than is deserved. She has not, then, acted maturely or accountably for she is probably unaware of the impact of her statement on the client and on the agency.

Nurses have, for too long, maintained their accountability to the agency above their accountability to all others. This has not enhanced the desirable image of nurses as working primarily in the public interest. It has, instead fostered the impression of the nurse as being subservient to and totally under the control of the employing institution. It is time to fully recognize and implement nursing's accountability towards its primary foci: the client/public, the profession, and the self. However, one must not lose sight of the nurse's accountability toward the employing agency. To do so, is to remain with an incomplete notion of the nurse's true answerability.

THE GROUNDWORK FOR ACCOUNTABILITY

From the foregoing description of accountability, it should be evident that this quality cannot appear overnight and without adequate preparation in either a profession or its practitioners. It is necessary to provide a substantive service about which to be accountable as well as to possess a variety of skills and attributes that enable one to exercise that accountability. A definite foundation or groundwork must be laid.

Research and the Establishment of a Theoretical Base for Nursing

One of the major factors in the accelerating pace of nursing's movement toward professional status is the growth of its theoretical and conceptual base for practice. It is this growth that allows the nurse to be truly accountable in this technologic and scientific era. This is what is now available, in some instances, and will be available increasingly in others, as the result of nursing research.

However, it is also not sufficient for the research to be done and the reasons to be available if they are ignored by nurses themselves in their practice. While those involved in doing research and nurses enrolled in nursing educational programs are highly cognizant of the amount, quality, and distribution of nursing research, this is not universal among nurses. The percolation of the results of nursing research to those in the front lines, to those from whom accountability in practice is most commonly demanded, has not occurred. It is the rare nurse who introduces a new component into her practice because of research findings. It is the rare nurse who justifies, or accounts for, her actions or judgements on the basis of research findings. It is the rare supervisor or administrator who calls on those under her authority to institute change based on the findings of nursing research.

Among the reasons for this problem is the inability of many of these individuals to comprehend and evaluate the research studies they may read. This leads to a general "uncomfortableness" around nursing research and causes these nurses to bypass the research literature altogether when planning change or implementing practice. Urgently needed are programs to help the practicing nurse to understand the available research reports, and to apply the findings to work situations. These can be provided under the auspices of staff development departments, nursing associations, continuing education departments, or degree programs, but they are a necessity.

Competence in Practice

If there is one attribute that has always been expected of the professional nurse, it is that she be competent in her practice. Just what that practice encompasses has been a matter of discussion and dissension at various times, and just what the "professional" before the word nurse really means has also been hotly contended. However, everyone, on all sides of these issues has always agreed that whatever it is that any type of nurse does, it must be done well. Currently, with many levels of nurse being reflected in the makeup of the health care team, it is imperative that each level have a clear idea of the scope of practice at that level and responsibly perform to the maximum limit of that level. The nurse's accountability may be called into question if she is functioning beyond the limits of her particular level. It is no more appropriate for the nurse who has been educated at the baccalaureate level to restrict her professional activities to those she may have exercised at the associate degree level than it is for her to assume the role of the masters prepared nurse practitioner.

The key to expertise in practice lies both in the knowledge and the skills area, a somewhat artificial distinction, which, nevertheless, allows for more clarity in this discussion. Nursing has always had a strong manual skills component and, to the extent that the nurse is in a role that contains this kind of activity, gentleness, quickness, and accuracy remain hallmarks of excellence. Where the skills required are in the areas of communication, teaching, leadership, and research (the so-called hands-off skills), the matter of expertise is no less pressing. Underlying all skills is an excellence in terms of one's command of "nursing knowledge." Nurses can never expect to contribute significantly to health care in its planning, implementation, and evaluation aspects if they do whatever they do in a mediocre manner. Competence is an absolute prerequisite for accountability.

Leadership Skills

Leadership development frequently brings questions and puzzlement when first introduced to nursing students. A frequent response is, "Not everyone can be a head nurse or a supervisor, or wants to be an instructor. I don't want to be a leader; I just want to be a nurse." The fact is, that inherent in that "nurse" role the elements of leadership are deeply inbedded. Leadership ability is one of the most important areas in laying the ground-work for accountability. The nurse's accountability extends into the areas of health maintenance and promotion, as well as the area of promoting the self care of the ill, as long as they are able to accomplish it. She is a constant catalyst in the process of change, at this highly individual level at the very least, especially if she is "just" a nurse. To satisfactorily fulfill this portion of her role, she must be well versed in the theory and practice of change, which is practically synonymous with saying she must be able to exercise leadership. She is a leader in working with her patients, their families, and significant others. She is a leader in regard to health care in her contacts with friends and acquaintances in her community. She is a leader in performing and making certain that she is permitted to perform her role as a professional involved in health promotion, maintenance and restoration of the public. The accountable nurse cannot function without leadership skills.

Ethical Framework

The nurse is accountable within an ethical framework. She cannot be accountable in a moral vacuum. She must have as her guide standards and values in which she believes, and to which she refers. To some extent these are determined by the collective values of the profession—and these in turn are partly determined by what the public expects of that profession and partly by what the profession demands of itself. In nursing, these professional values are formalized by the Code for Nursing referred to earlier. However, in large measure, this ethical code is a personal one, developed in the course and the context of the individual's total life experience. It includes those values learned in the home, in the schools, from social groups, during religious training, in the work setting and from the activities and contacts of daily life. It is influenced by one's ethnic and religious background, the area of the country in which one lives, and one's own personality. It is highly individual.

One's ethical code is also often something of which one is relatively unaware. It is unconsciously used in making decisions and running one's life, but is rarely if ever pulled out and scrutinized or even acknowledged as existing. It is this that is so essential in the professional nurse. She must be aware of her own ethical code, of how it affects her decisions and actions, and of where it is congruent with or departs from the more standard codes of the profession. These conflicts, then, must be worked through and compromise must be sought so that the nurse can feel comfortable with and confident in the ethical basis in which her practice is rooted.

Education to the Baccalaureate and/or Beyond

It is obvious from the discussion thus far on laying the groundwork for accountability that this is neither a simple nor a short-term task. It is not one that can be accomplished in a weekend and, for most individuals, it is not one which can be accomplished on one's own. Rather, it is a task that continues over a long period of time, during which various ideas are explored, analyzed, tested, and absorbed into the individual's makeup. It is a task that is partially contributed to by others, guided at times by others, and discussed and shared with others. It is a task most ideally accomplished within the context of a higher education.

This educational experience should provide opportunities for the student to take responsibility and to exercise accountability. It should be an education toward the ability to make decisions and be accountable for them (Lanara, 1982, p. 10). In reviewing the areas requiring attention in the preparation for accountability, this desirability for addressing them within a baccalaureate or higher degree program in nursing becomes evident.

While most educational programs in nursing are based on a conceptual framework, it is at the baccalaureate level that significant time is devoted to understanding some of the outstanding conceptual/theoretical frameworks for nursing practice. It is also at this level that the relationship between these conceptual/theoretical frameworks and the research process is explored. The research course often included in a baccalaureate program provides the opportunity for learning how to read research, adequately evaluate it, and judge its potential applicability within a work setting. It is only after the nurse can knowledgeably read and interpret research findings, that she can use them to improve her practice. It is at the point of usage of and referral to research findings that this area of nursing activity adds immeasurably to the nurse's accountability.

Expertise in practice is not confined to those with a higher education in nursing. The associate degree and diploma programs of the present day, along with the individual's work experience, continuing education courses, and orientation and inservice programs, create input to this area. However, as a vitally important area in the preparation for accountability, it can be enhanced by the years and the liberalizing influence offered in the baccalaureate or higher degree program.

The area of leadership truly comes into its own in the baccalaureate and higher degree program. It is here that styles of leadership behavior, health care delivery systems, characteristics of bureaucracies, and change theory are explored. It is here where the nurse who in practice may already be in a leadership position, learns how to function more effectively and more accountably in her role, why some of her programs have succeeded and others have not, and how to inculcate greater levels of accountability in her staff. It is here where she learns the extent to which she is accountable for the actions of others and it is here where she begins to learn something of the institution's accountability (or lack of it) in regard to the care she and others are providing. It is here where she will both work with and analyze the professional behavior of leaders in nursing, role models from whom she can learn accountability—for it is a learned behavior (Clifford, 1981, p. 20).

Finally, in the area of ethics and values, it is at the university level that the nurse can and is encouraged to contemplate her own value system, to uncover it and see its relationship to her practice and to the other aspects of her life. This is where she can learn of the different value systems of others and of how they have sought to make their own ethical codes complementary to those of the profession.

In summary, it takes all of what the nurse is and does as a person to prepare her for functioning in an accountable manner (Lanara, 1982, p. 10). It is a lifelong process engaged in along with others in both structured and unstructured ways and it is interwoven with the nurse's preparation as a professional person.

THE POSITIVE ASPECT OF ACCOUNTABILITY

The image conjured up in the mind of the average nurse when accountability is mentioned is often a negative one, permeated with punishments, negative sanctions, reprisals, and "being called on the carpet" for tasks undone or done incorrectly (Clifford, 1981, p. 20). This is indeed an unfortunate state of affairs. Quite the contrary, accountability should be looked at as a highly positive concept, permeated with visions of respect, reward, effectiveness, control, and action. In addition, concepts such as power, leadership, accomplishment, choice, and yes, even professionalism, are associated with it.

Nursing is striving for a voice in setting policy for health care delivery at every level, from that of the individual and institution, to those national in scope. Nursing is increasingly seeking to define the extent of its own practice and then to practice to the limits of that definition. Nurses are seeking to be vice presidents of hospitals, to influence legislators in Washington, to determine what kind of teaching their patients should receive, and to decide when beds must be closed because of inadequate staffing. But to have the autonomy, the authority, and the power to make these kinds of decisions and perform these kinds of activities, the nurse must be ready to be accountable. She must be willing to allow the buck to stop with her. She must stop blaming others for the leaks and problems in health care (Schorr, 1981, p. 9). She must be willing to take the risks of her accountability. However, and this is what is often overlooked, she will also reap the rewards. She will be the one responsible for and commended for maintaining safe standards for patients. She will be the one responsible for and acknowledged as the vehicle for the patient's increased level of knowledge and understanding of his health situation. She will be responsible for more progressive health care legislation and recognized as such, and she will be responsible for and respected for determining what nursing is and what it does in a particular institution. She will reap many benefits and rewards. She will gain self-respect. She will finally have control over her practice and that practice will truly be professional in nature.

A CHECKLIST FOR ACCOUNTABILITY

In attempting to prepare oneself to act in an accountable manner, and to evaluate one's actions, the following questions may serve as guides to the nurse. The list is not all inclusive but serves merely as a beginning tool for working the concept of accountability into one's life and work.

Accountability to the Client

Am I providing the best care of which I am capable?

Is that care sufficient to meet the needs of the client in this situation?

Is this client entitled to more than I can offer and am I turning elsewhere to obtain that additional dimension?

Am I incorporating what I know of nursing theory and research into my practice in this situation?

Am I using my leadership skills to encourage others to function at their optimal ability levels in the care of this patient?

Am I acting in accordance with my own ethical code and that of the profession?

If by meeting the needs of this patient I am in conflict with my ethical code, am I seeking some alternative method or person to satisfy those needs?

Have I given the patient information that he wants and/or needs to know about his health status, while considering the effect on him of that knowledge?

Accountability to the Public

Am I seeking to improve health and nursing care?

Am I speaking out against abuses I see in health and nursing care?

Am I acting as a community resource in the areas of health and nursing?

Am I remaining an active and contributing member of the profession after using public funds to finance my education?

Am I attempting to increase the knowledge of the public to enable it to make more knowledgeable choices about health and nursing care?

Accountability to the Profession

Am I fulfilling my professional role in accordance with the requirements of the profession?

Are other nurses in my setting doing the same?

If I or others are not performing satisfactorily am I taking steps to remedy that situation?

Am I a participant in professional meetings, organizations, seminars, conferences, and so forth, so that I may express my views on nursing to those in nursing?

Am I working within the profession to improve practice, education, and/or research?

Am I complying with the ethical code of the profession?

Accountability to the Self

Am I satisfied with my chosen profession?

Am I prepared in the best possible way for the professional role I am assuming?

Should I seek further preparation for that role?

Should I withdraw from that role until I receive further preparation?

In those areas where I am dissatisfied, am I seeking alternative modes of action and/or thought?

Am I comfortable, ethically, with the way in which I am performing my professional role?

Am I shortchanging my patients, my significant others, or myself in the way I am performing my professional role?

Am I satisfied with the position this role assumes within my total life-style?

Accountability to the Agency

Am I performing in accordance with the job description for the position for which I was employed?

If I am not satisfied with that job description, am I seeking appropriate ways to change it?

Am I seeking to ensure that I am practicing under safe, if not optimal, conditions?

Am I giving the institution its money's worth in terms of my work?

Am I working in accordance with the policies and procedures of the institution?

If I am not satisfied with those policies and procedures, am I seeking to change them using principles of leadership and change, and with the total mission of the institution in mind?

It would be quite the superperson, indeed, who could look through this checklist and confidently say she currently is carrying out all of the above activities. Some of them are more appropriate than others for nurses in different settings and at different times. However, these and other questions must be considered by the nurse who is to act in an accountable manner and/or increase the accountability of her decisions and actions. They must be considered by the person who wishes to call herself a professional nurse.

SUMMARY _____

After a brief discussion of the history of accountability in nursing, definitions are given of accountability and the related concepts of autonomy and authority. The idea of accountability as a characteristic of a profession is then presented. The accountability of the nurse to the client/public, the profession, the self, and the employing agency is discussed at some length. Following this, the necessity is expressed for a groundwork to be laid in order for the nurse to act in an accountable manner, along with specific areas to be covered during this educational process. The positive aspects of being accountable are presented, and, finally, a check list appears, which can be used by the nurse in determining if she is, in fact, acting as or developing into an accountable professional.

REFERENCES

American Nurses' Association Congress for Nursing Practice: Standards for Nursing Practice. Kansas City, American Nurses' Association, 1973

Batey MV, Lewis FM: Clarifying autonomy and accountability in nursing service: 2. J Nurs Adm 12:10–15, 1982

Bergman R: Accountability—definition and dimensions. Int Nurs Rev 28:53–59, 1981

Bixler GK, Bixler RW: The professional status of nursing. Am J Nurs 59:1142, 1959

Chaska NL: The Nursing Profession: A Time to Speak. New York, McGraw Hill, 1983

Clifford JC: Managerial control vs. professional autonomy: A paradox. J Nurs Adm 11:19–21, 1981

Code for Nurses with Interpretive Statements. Kansas City, American Nurses' Association, 1976

Dachelet CZ, Sullivan JA: Autonomy in practice. Nurse Prac 4:15, 1979

Flexner A: Is social work a profession? Proceedings of the National Conference of Charities and Correction, pp 576–590. Chicago, Heldman, 1915

Lanara VA: Responsibility in nursing. Int Nurs Rev 29:7–10, 1982

McGlothlin WJ: The place of nursing among the professions. Nurs Outlook 9:214, 1961

Merton RK: The functions of the professional association. Am J Nurs 58:50, 1958

Nightingale F: Notes on Nursing: What It Is and What It Is Not. Philadelphia, JB Lippincott, 1946 (facsimile of 1st ed, London, Harrison & Sons, 1859)

Schorr T: Unity, authority, accountability—nursing's imperatives for the 80's. Washington State J Nurs 53:7–10, 1981

Section 4

Professional Practice

Chapter 12

The Nursing Process

THOUGHT QUESTIONS

1. Why is it desirable to use the nursing process when giving care?
2. How do nursing diagnoses differ from medical diagnoses?
3. How does the choice of a nursing model affect the nursing process?
4. What are the standards for nursing care? How are standards related to nursing process?

The integrated use of cognitive, interpersonal, and psychomotor skills in client care is basic to the practice of professional nursing. The nursing process provides a logical and rational way for the nurse to organize information so that the care she gives is appropriate, efficient, and effective.

A number of books have been written on the nursing process. Invariably the process is presented as a series of four or five phases, with a number of steps within each phase. The net effect is a procedure that appears linear (or at best overlapping or circular) and cumbersome. Unfortunately, in many practice settings, there is a perception that the nursing process is desirable but too time consuming to be practical. If it is not valued, it is not used, and many nurses continue to intervene using standardized procedures based on medical diagnoses, rather than a rationale based on assessment, planning, and evaluation feedback.

The emphasis in this chapter is on the relationship of the nursing process to the practice of professional nursing, the "why for" rather than the "how to." It is hoped that the student will grow to value the process and thus apply it as an integral part of her practice.

RELATIONSHIP OF PROCESS TO PHILOSOPHY OF NURSING

Consider the nature of nursing when it is based on a model of dependence on medical practice. Much nursing as taught and practiced is standardized according to medical diagnoses and supports medical intervention. The physician does the assess-

211

ment needed for the medical diagnosis and this planning is the basis for the medical orders. The focus of nursing is the support of the medical regimen in order to cure the patient's disease. "Nursing knowledge" includes detailed knowledge of pathophysiology, symptoms of disease, and standard medical intervention, and the "best way" to perform procedures and treatments.

In contrast, consider the nature of nursing when it is based on a model of autonomous professional practice. The focus has become support of the client in order to improve well-being status and potential. Needed knowledge includes information about the client's well-being status including strengths as well as weaknesses, support systems, knowledge, beliefs, and values about health, life-style, and health-related goals. If the client has a disease, knowledge is also needed about that process and its medical treatment. The rationale for nursing intervention is knowledge based on assessment, planning, and feedback from evaluation.

The model of nursing accepted by the practitioner can have a major impact on the knowledge needed and the nature of practice. Acceptance of the professional model mandates the acceptance of responsibility for nursing knowledge based on a rationale for practice. The nursing process provides a systematic approach to nursing practice. The process remains the same regardless of which framework or model is used to integrate theoretical formulations. Examples from the six nursing models that were discussed in Chapter 8, "Models of Nursing," are used in this chapter.

The nursing process is defined as "a set of actions leading to a particular goal" (Wolff *et al*, 1979, p. 54). All parts of the process are interrelated and influence the whole. The parts, or phases of the nursing process occur sequentially but they are not linear. Planning may lead to intervention, or evaluation during the process of planning may result in more assessment. Figure 12–1 attempts to depict the nursing process when viewed from an interactional perspective.

The American Nurses' Association (ANA) has developed eight Standards of Nursing Practice (ANA, 1973) that are related to application of the nursing process as shown in Table 12–1. "Nursing practice in all settings must possess the characteristics identified by these Standards if clients/patients are to receive a high quality of nursing care" (ANA, 1973). These standards are used to organize the following discussion of the nursing process.

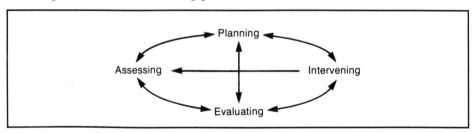

Figure 12–1. An interactional approach to the nursing process.

STANDARDS OF NURSING PRACTICE

Standard I

The collection of data about the health status of the client/patient is systematic and continuous. The data are accessible, communicated, and recorded.
Before the nurse can begin collecting data about the client, a degree of trust

TABLE 12-1. Correspondance Between Phases of the Nursing Process and Nursing Practice Standards

Phases of the Nursing Process	Nursing Practice Standards
Assessing	Standard I
Planning	Standards II–IV
Intervening	Standards V–VI
Evaluating	Standards VII–VIII

must be established between the nurse and the client. The nurse should initiate a relationship with the client, and begin the definition of the roles each will play in the client's care. This contact provides an opportunity for the client to "voice initial fears, raise pressing questions, and begin to feel a degree of comfort in the client role" (Yura and Walsh, 1983, p. 131). In this way a positive environment for mutuality in the process can be established.

In establishing the nurse-client relationship, "the nurse needs to identify specific actions that communicate trust (consistency, honesty), empathy (touch, sincerity), caring (genuineness, eye contact), autonomy (nonjudgemental, nonthreatening), and mutuality (inclusion of client in decision-making) (Griffith and Christensen, 1982, p. 30). (For a full discussion of communication in the nursing process, see Chapter 13, "Communication and Helping Relationships.")

The collection of data should be an organized process. The nurse has to decide which data are desirable to collect in the particular situation, and determine what sources and methods are appropriate to obtain the desired data. The nature of the nurse-client contact influences the data collection process. For example, the data needed for an outpatient admission for minor surgery are far different than those appropriate in lengthy hospitalization for a life-threatening disease. The data collected in each situation should be appropriate and necessary for planning nursing intervention. The data should supplement rather than duplicate those data collected by other health professionals (*e.g.,* history), and should focus on information needed for nursing care. As data are collected they are reviewed to determine additional needed data, and to begin the process of organization of the data for planning purposes.

Data will be needed about who is the client, why is the client being considered for care, and what factors are influencing his present health status? Data the nurse needs to collect include the client's name, age, sex, marital status, occupation, education, economic status, knowledge about his health/illness status, attitudes of the family and significant others toward health care and the client's status, personal habits and communication styles, cultural influences, growth and development status, learning capacity, supports and resources, previous experience with the health care system, medical diagnosis and regimen, coping patterns, and direction of change desired by the client. Other needed data are related to the conceptual model being used to organize care, as suggested in Table 12–2. The elements have many similarities, but the emphasis varies among the models.

Yura and Walsh (1983, p. 141) have summarized assumptions about behavior that reinforce the need to understand the client from his frame of reference when collecting data.

TABLE 12–2.	Implications for Data Collection of Selected Nursing Models
Nursing Model	**Indications for Data Collection**
Peplau	Physiologic and personality needs, illness symptoms, significant others, influences on establishment and maintenance of the nurse-client relationship
Johnson	Functioning of the behavioral subsystems, symptoms of disturbed equilibrium
Orem	Therapeutic self-care demand, presence of self-care deficits, ability of client to meet self-care requisites
Roy	Adaptation level (related to three classes of stimuli), coping in relation to modes of adaptation, position on the health-illness continuum
Neuman	Stressors, indications of disruption of the lines of defense, resistance factors
Rogers	Characteristics of patterning, health potential, environmental influences

1. A person's behavior is governed by available energy.
2. Behavior has a purpose, although it is not always obvious.
3. A person's response to a particular situation is the best he is capable of at that time.
4. A person's perception of what is happening has a greater influence than what is actually happening or how it is interpreted by someone else.
5. Each person has a potential for striving forward.

As data are collected they must be validated with the client and other sources. If discrepancies are noted they should be clarified, and those data should not be used as the basis for inferences or judgements. Evaluation of the data should consider accuracy and whether all relevant factors have been included. As data collection continues the organization and analysis of patterns within the data proceeds concurrently, which may indicate additional data collection needs.

Standard II

Nursing diagnoses are derived from health status data. "Client data are evaluated by categorizing, identifying data gaps, determining patterns, applying standards (comparing), establishing relationships, and identifying strengths and health concerns" (Griffith and Christensen, 1982, p. 89). The analysis and synthesis of data require objectivity, deliberation, judgement, and discrimination. It is important for the nurse to identify strengths as well as obvious and potential problems, but problems should not be created if they do not exist.

Brill (1980, p. 154) defines a nursing diagnosis as a "statement of probable relationship between an identified negative health behavior and the factor(s) most likely contributing to its occurrence." Others would suggest that a nursing diagnosis may also relate to a potential health problem (Gordon, 1976; Price, 1980). Nursing actions may support the strengths or address the weaknesses of the client in order to address the underlying cause of the health problem. In contrast to medical diagnoses that identify precise pathologic diseases, nursing diagnoses identify problems "that nurses are qualified and licensed to treat" (Price, 1980, p. 668).

Yura and Walsh (1983, pp. 152–154) have developed a classification for possible nursing diagnoses:

1. No problem exists and the client's state of wellness is affirmed. A plan to maintain wellness is developed with the client that the client then implements. Periodic reassessment of wellness will be made, and the client will be present for these at given intervals. The client will seek reassessment sooner if a problem is suspected.

2. No problem exists, but there is a potential problem that may be offset by giving the client information on prevention and planning for a future interview. It may be necessary to refer the client to another health care member.

3. A problem exists but is being handled successfully by the client or the family or both. Plans for periodic reassessment will be formulated, but the client will return for these at nonscheduled times if the client thinks it is necessary.

4. A problem exists that the client needs help in handling. Providing this assistance . . . will either resolve the problem or make it easier for the client, family, neighbors, or some combination to handle it. . . . Implementation continues until evaluation indicates that the problem has been resolved or has decreased or reassessment deems a change in plans is necessary.

5. A problem exists that the client cannot handle at this time and its nature prevents family and neighbors from helping to resolve it. Health care intervention is needed. Specific members of the health care team, such as the physician, nurse, dentist . . . may be assigned to help the client. With health care intervention, the problem can be specifically diagnosed, treated, and resolved (*e.g.,* dental caries).

6. A problem exists that must be studied further and diagnosed to resolve it or keep it within manageable proportions. Ambulatory or inpatient health and nursing services may be needed (*e.g.,* elevated blood sugar, obstruction).

7. A problem exists that is not incapacitating to the client at present, but its resolution requires intervention that would render the client dependent for a specific period or indefinitely. Inpatient care is generally necessary (*e.g.,* surgery).

8. A problem exists that places heavy demands on the client's ability to cope with it and that the family cannot resolve. Immediate and continued intervention by members of the health care team, on an inpatient basis, is required (*e.g.,* myocardial infarction, bleeding peptic ulcer).

9. A problem is imposed unexpectedly on the client or the family because of an accident, injury, or natural disaster, or is self-imposed (attempted suicide). The problem may or may not be a threat to life.

10. Problems exist that are long term and permanent. The client is able to cope with some but not all problems, and other persons may have to intervene to cope with the problem and provide care on a continuing basis (*e.g.,* congenital disability).

There are three components of a nursing diagnosis: (1) the client's actual or potential health problem, combined with, (2) the etiologic factor(s), and supported by (3) the signs and symptoms (Gordon, 1976; Price, 1980). The National Conference Group for Classification of Nursing Diagnoses has accepted a list of diagnoses for clinical testing (Kim and Moritz, 1982). These diagnoses, organized by functional health pattern areas, appear in Table 12–3.

The diagnostic categories provide an approach to terminology for expressing the client's existing or potential health problem that is currently being tested. The other part of the diagnosis, the etiologic factor(s) "identifies the probable factors causing or maintaining the client's health problem" (Gordon, 1982, p. 8). The etiology

---

TABLE 12–3.   Grouping of Currently Accepted Diagnoses Under Functional Health Pattern Areas

---

Health-perception–health-management pattern

Noncompliance (specify)
Injury, potential for
Poisoning, potential for
Suffocation, potential for
Trauma, potential for
Nutritional–metabolic pattern

Skin integrity, impairment of: actual
Skin integrity, impairment of: potential
Nutrition, alterations in: less than body requirements
Nutrition, alterations in: more than body requirements
Nutrition, alterations in: potential for more than body requirements
Fluid volume deficit: actual
Fluid volume deficit: potential
Elimination pattern

Urinary elimination, alterations in patterns of
Bowel elimination, alterations in: constipation
Bowel elimination, alterations in: diarrhea
Bowel elimination, alterations in: incontinence
Activity–exercise pattern

Home maintenance management, impaired
Mobility, impaired physical
Self-care deficit (specify level): total
Self-care deficit (specify level): feeding
Self-care deficit (specify level): bathing/hygiene
Self-care deficit (specify level): dressing/grooming

(Continues)

TABLE 12–3.   Grouping of Currently Accepted Diagnoses
                Under Functional Health Pattern Areas
                (*Continued*)

Self-care deficit (specify level): toileting
Airway clearance, ineffective
Gas exchange, impaired
Breathing pattern, ineffective
Diversional activity, deficit
Tissue perfusion, alteration in (cerebral, cardiopulmonary, renal,
    gastrointestinal, peripheral)
Cardiac output, alterations in: decreased
Sleep–rest pattern

Sleep pattern disturbance
Cognitive–perceptual pattern

Knowledge deficit (specify)
Sensory perceptual alterations (visual, auditory, kinesthetic, gus-
    tatory, tactile, olfactory)
Comfort, alterations in: pain
Thought processes: alterations in
Self-perception–self-concept pattern

Fear (specify)
Self–concept, disturbance in (body image, self-esteem, role per-
    formance, personal identity)
Role-relationship pattern

Grieving, anticipatory
Grieving, dysfunctional
Parenting, alterations in: actual
Parenting, alterations in: potential
Communication, impaired verbal
Violence, potential for
Sexuality–reproductive pattern

Sexual dysfunction
Rape-trauma syndrome
Rape-trauma: compound reaction
Rape-trauma: silent reaction
Coping–stress-tolerance pattern

Coping, ineffective individual
Coping, ineffective family: compromised
Coping, ineffective family: disabling
Coping, family: potential for growth
Value–belief pattern

Spiritual distress (distress of the human spirit)

(Gordon M: Nursing Diagnosis: Process and Application, pp 327–
328. New York, McGraw-Hill, 1982. Used by permission of the
publisher.)

makes the diagnosis specific to the client, and provides the rationale for potential nursing intervention strategies.

All diagnostic categories are associated with a cluster of signs and symptoms that permit discriminations between health problems. A goal is the standardization and publication of nursing diagnostic clusters of signs and symptoms. These are the cues or indications that a particular health problem exists. The signs and symptoms determine the diagnosis and, as changes occur, can be used to monitor progress and evaluate the effectiveness of the nursing care plan.

Figure 12–2 indicates several possible etiologic factors associated with a diagnostic category. A diagnostic category may be related to one or to multiple etiologic factors. Examples of specific diagnoses from Figure 12–2 include potential for injury to the surgical incision related to noncompliance with bedrest, or potential for injury related to alteration in thought processes from medication.

Nursing diagnoses are developed by the nurse. However, they are based on data that have been validated with the client. The nurse and client then need to review the diagnoses to identify the goals (objectives) that will determine what outcomes are to be expected as the result of implementation of planned care.

Standard III

The plan of nursing care includes goals derived from the nursing diagnoses.

"Goals state the criteria for what observable behavior will occur as a result of the change and the time frame within which it will occur" (Brill, 1980, p. 157). The conceptual model being used to organize care can influence broad goals of care as suggested in Table 12–4. All of the models except Rogers' stress the maintenance or restoration of balance as the goal of care. Rogers alone conceptualizes the goal of care as facilitation of more complex patterning, a kind of "becoming" of the person.

The overall goal must be agreed on by the nurse and client from within the categories of health restoration, maintenance, or promotion. Specific objectives then can be broken down by time frame into long-range, intermediate-range, and short-term behaviors that are going to be expected. It is important that the objectives be as realistic as possible and clearly stated, because they will be the basis for evaluation of the effectiveness of the plan of care. The objectives are determined by the client, in consultation with the nurse, with consideration given to his capabilities, limitations, and desired life-style. The client's preferences may be very difficult for the nurse to accept, particularly if they differ from what would be her own choices or what she "thinks is best for the client." However, the nurse cannot plan objectives in isolation from the client nor can she impose her will on him. Using change

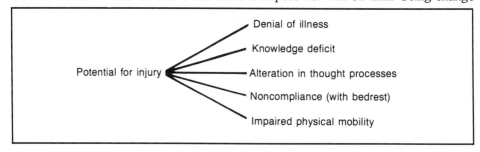

Figure 12–2.   Diagnostic category with multiple etiologic subcategories.

TABLE 12–4.   Broad Guidelines for Goal Setting of Selected Nursing Models

Nursing Model	Broad Guidelines for Goal Setting
Peplau	Physiologic or psychologic equilibrium, met needs, capabilities demonstrated
Johnson	Maintainance or restoration of balance
Orem	Restoration of internal and external constancy
Roy	Promotion of adaptation from successful coping
Neuman	Maintenance or restoration of dynamic equilibrium of the normal line of defense
Rogers	Increasing complexity and innovativeness of patterning

strategies (see Chapter 15, "The Professional Nurse As A Change Agent"), she can attempt to influence goal setting. However, once the objectives have been identified, the nurses' role must be to support their accomplishment.

Standard IV

The plan of nursing care includes priorities and the prescribed nursing approaches or measures to achieve the goals derived from the nursing diagnoses.
The purposes of the nursing care plan are to:

1. Give direction, guidance, and meaning to nursing care.
2. Provide a means of communicating, synchronizing, and organizing activities of the nursing team.
3. Provide for continuity of care (Griffith and Christensen, 1982).

"The nursing care plan includes precise data about a specific client. These data are organized in a systematic, concise manner that facilitates overall nursing and health goals. It clearly communicates the nature of the client's problems. It contains all information about the client, the obvious and potential nursing diagnoses and the priorities assigned to each, problems and complications to be prevented, and expected outcomes with prescribed nursing actions" (Yura and Walsh, 1983, p. 177).

After the objectives for care have been selected, priorities must be set among them. When survival is threatened, physical needs must take precedence. Cost, available personnel and resources, and time factors may also influence priorities. For example, for a student with a broken leg, weight loss may be considered an important goal, but, because of the time needed to accomplish substantial weight loss, it may be assigned a lower priority than learning how to use crutches needed for mobility. The theories or model being used to organize care can also influence determination of priorities. For example, use of Maslow's theory would assign the highest priorities to physiologic, safety, and security needs, and a lesser priority to love, self-esteem, and self-actualization needs. In addition, as always, the client must be closely involved in the decisions.

Once the priorities among objectives have been determined, alternative options for care can be generated, and their probability for success predicted. The possible "solutions" or approaches are heavily influenced by availability of resources and by factors in the client's life-style and cultural background. For example, weight loss could be achieved by 2 weeks' residence at a clinic, adherence to a diet requiring weighing portions of food, an exercise program, and so forth. However, financial constraints may make the clinic nonfeasible, and time and life-style constraints may influence the desirability of the exercise and/or food weighing approaches.

This process of choosing approaches from among a number of alternatives is frequently neglected in the rush to "do." As a result the first "solution" thought of may be the one implemented, with limited assessment of its likelihood of success or its appropriateness in the particular situation. This tendency to avoid brainstorming is also fostered by the belief of some that there is "one best way" to accomplish a particular goal. A conscious effort may need to be made to avoid the "cookbook recipe," and for the nurse and client together to select the alternative that has the best likelihood of success. This approach can then be translated into specific actions, their desired frequency, who will be assigned to carry them out (*e.g.,* nurse, client, other health team members), and the timetable for expected achievement.

The writing of the nursing care plan by students is often a rigorous exercise in complexity and volume, which results in avoidance and dread of the procedure. However, once the intellectual process has been completed, the actual writing of the plan can be accomplished fairly quickly. The care plan should include (1) the nursing diagnosis, (2) the objectives associated with the diagnosis in order of priority, and (3) the "blueprint" to accomplish the objectives, including actions, assigned resources, and timetable.

The nursing activities involved in meeting standards I through IV include those often categorized into the assessing and planning phases of the nursing process. "Both the assessment and the planning phases draw heavily on intellectual skills—critical thinking, decision-making, judgement, observation—and interpersonal skills. The latter are used to establish rapport through verbal and nonverbal communication, including active attentive listening. Technical skills are used mainly in the assessment phase to obtain data but to a lesser extent than are intellectual and interpersonal skills. Intellectual and interpersonal skills are paramount in the planning phase" (Yura and Walsh, p. 176). The next two standards correspond to the intervention phase of the nursing process, and may involve psychomotor as well as cognitive and interpersonal skills.

Standard V

Nursing actions provide for client/patient participation in health promotion, maintenance, and restoration.

Standard VI

Nursing actions assist the client/patient to maximize his health capabilities.

The actions performed by the nurse are those previously determined to have the highest likelihood of success in meeting the objectives sought by the client. In addition, nursing actions support the medical regimen of care. The accomplishment of the actions will require diverse skills, possibly including teaching-learning, leadership, management, group process, psychomotor ability, and in all cases, communication. All interactions with the client should be goal-directed and purposeful. As the actions are carried out, the nurse continues her collaboration with the client and significant others, and continues to involve the client in his care. Interventions are carried out with sensitivity to the client's feelings and are based on the individuality of the client.

The conceptual model being used to organize care has possible implications for intervention strategies, as suggested in Table 12–5. A number of the models emphasize the dominant role of the nurse in manipulating the client and/or the environment. Peplau and Rogers stress the active role of the client in the process of change.

The results of actions and the client's reactions to them should be recorded so that the progress can be shared by all involved in the client's care. It is necessary for the nurse to remain flexible, so that modifications of actions can be made as needed. As data are accumulated, they are evaluated in relation to the behaviors sought and the previously set timetable. This assessment may indicate continuation of the plan, modification of the actions or timetable, or possibly the need to reconsider the importance of the previously defined objective. Thus, the process of intervention is integrally involved with concurrent evaluation of its effectiveness. The final two standards correspond to the evaluation phase of the nursing process.

TABLE 12–5.	Implications for Nursing Intervention of Selected Nursing Models
Nursing Model	**Indications for Intervention Strategies**
Peplau	Emphasis on the therapeutic relationship between the client and the nurse.
Johnson	Emphasis is on imposition of external controls on behavior, facilitating structural change through teaching, or providing resources to fulfill functional requirements of the subsystems
Orem	Emphasis is on self-care actions for or with the client that he is unable to perform for himself
Roy	Emphasis is on increasing, decreasing, or maintaining focal, contextual, and/or residual stimuli
Neuman	Emphasis is on primary, secondary, or tertiary prevention to reduce stressors or strengthen the lines of defense
Rogers	Emphasis is on mobilization of the clients' resources and repatterning of the man-environment interaction

Standard VII

The client's/patient's progress or lack of progress toward goal achievement is determined by the client/patient and the nurse.

Standard VIII

The client's/patient's progress or lack of progress toward goal achievement directs reassessment, reordering of priorities, new goal setting, and revision of the plan of nursing care.

Evaluation should be continuous and ongoing throughout the nursing process. At this phase however, the purpose of the evaluation is to compare changes in client behavior or health status with the desired behaviors or indicators defined in the objectives. "The outcome of the evaluation may indicate that the care planned must be reassessed, replanned, modified, and the revised plan implemented and evaluated" (Yura and Walsh, 1983, p. 194). The evaluation also may demonstrate that the plan is working, or that it might be improved with minor modifications.

Yura and Walsh (1983, pp. 194–195) have suggested that the outcome of evaluation may be any one or a combination of the following:

1. The client responded as expected and the problem is resolved. No further nursing action is needed. A plan to maintain the client's state of optimal wellness is formulated jointly by the nurse and the client. . . . A future appointment may be made to reaffirm the client's problem-free status.
2. Behavioral manifestations of the client's situation indicate that the problem has not been resolved; evidence demonstrates that short-term results, but not intermediate and long-range expectations have been achieved. . . . Reevaluation is to continue.
3. Behavioral manifestations of the client are similar to those evidenced during the assessment phase. Little or no evidence is available that the problem has been resolved. . . . Reassessment with replanning is needed.
4. Behavioral manifestations indicate new problems resulting from unmet or poorly met human needs. Assessing, planning, and implementing a plan of action to resolve these problems (nursing diagnoses) are in order. Planning action to resolve the new problem must be coordinated with the planning for the previously diagnosed problems. Evaluation will follow implementation.

Evaluation may be difficult because of the difficulty in developing valid and reliable tools to objectively measure progress toward some goals. It may be helpful to consider whether there are appropriate tools to measure progress toward goals when the goals are established. For example, weight loss and blood pressure reduction are easily validated. However, it is very difficult to objectively assess improved self-concept or valuing of a more healthful life-style. Assumptions must be made about the meaning of observed behavior and whether it contributes to the specified goal.

Because the nursing process is systematic, logical, and goal-directed, it is assumed that adherence to the process will result in accomplishment of the desired goals. When evaluation of progress indicates that the problem(s) is not resolved, it is necessary to consider possible reasons, which may involve the client, the nurse, significant others (to the client), or members of the health care team. Yura and Walsh (1983, pp. 201–202) suggest a number of possible reasons, including:

1. *Client*—Unrealistic expectations, lack of expected ability to cope, insufficient or inaccurate communication with nurse, or lack of acceptance of planned goals or strategies.
2. *Nurse*—Lack of knowledge, insufficient data, inappropriate delegation to team members, assigning priorities inappropriately, inadequate sharing with client and/or significant others, failure to consider client strengths, failure to set realistic goals, or ineffective or inadequate communication.
3. *Team members*—Insufficient information about the client, failure to communicate with nurse who is responsible for the care plan, poor nursing (*e.g.,* alienating the client, being insensitive, failure to record data), lack of valuing of the care plan, or having conflicting goals for the client.
4. *Significant others*—Lack of understanding or acceptance of the planned goals, failure to see that a problem exists, or limitation of resources (*e.g.,* transportation, emotional support, own fear).

Griffith and Christensen (1982, pp. 168–169) have suggested some questions to assist the nurse in evaluation of the process:

1. Was the assessment complete and appropriate?
2. Was the planning complete and sufficient?
3. Were the nursing diagnoses complete and appropriate?
4. Were the objectives appropriately stated?
5. Were the objectives met? Were all participants satisfied?
6. Was the intervention effective and efficient?
7. What changes were desirable in planning and intervention?
8. Were all steps communicated effectively?
9. What changes have occurred in the client's needs, health status, or coping ability? Are additional changes desirable?
10. How does the client feel about the outcomes?
11. What could have been done differently?

Depending on the outcome of the evaluation, the nurse and client may need to modify the goals and/or interventions, continue the planned strategies with a modified timetable, or, if the goals have been met and no new ones have emerged, terminate the relationship. Both the client and the nurse may have difficulty terminating the relationship. The client may be unsure of his ability to maintain the changes in health behavior or well-being status on his own. The nurse may be ambivalent about "not being needed any longer." However, awareness and an open sharing of these feelings can lead to satisfaction in having accomplished the desired goals, and acceptance of the need to end the relationship.

SUMMARY

The nursing process provides a systematic procedure for the nurse and client to accomplish mutually agreed on goals. The use of this process provides a cognitive base for autonomous practice based on a professional nursing model.

SAMPLE CARE PLAN USING THE NEUMAN MODEL*

Mrs. Jones

Nursing History

Mildred Jones is a 75-year-old widow. She came to Goodwill Clinic complaining of the inability to walk the 10 blocks to the grocery store without experiencing shortness of breath. The only other time this happened was shortly after her husband's death when she had a "heart attack." This time the problem is different and she would like to learn to take care of herself. Mrs. Jones reports that she's afraid that if it continues, she'll be dependent on her daughter for all her care, which she doesn't want.

Mrs. Jones noticed that she became less short of breath after the doctor prescribed her heart pill (Digoxin). She thinks her problem started slowly after she gained some weight (about 20 pounds). She reports that she really likes candy and has some that she shares with neighborhood children. She says that "nurses have helped her to lose weight in the past and hopes we can help her now." See Figure 12–3 for her care plan.

Intrapersonal Factors–Physiologic

75-year-old Caucasian female; 5'2"; *180 pounds; BP 160/94* T 98.6F P 84 *irregular* R 22; Gray hair, arcus senilicus around eyes; reports some difficulty hearing grandson when records are playing; no difficulty swallowing, no sore throat or swollen areas of neck; *reports SOB* when climbing stairs or walking 10 blocks against an incline to the store; lung sounds clear; pulses in all extremities 3–4+; *protuberant abdomen*; bowel sounds in all quadrants; reports *pain in ankles, hips, and knees* that doesn't interfere with ambulation; full ROM all joints except decreased flexion at knee; alert; CN 2–12 grossly intact; coordinated smooth movements; sensory pathways intact; equal strength, mass and tone in muscular system. Urine *2+ glucose*. Takes *Digoxin .25* mgm po q.d.

Intrapersonal Factors–Psychologic

Friendly woman. Has lived with daughter, son-in-law, and two teenaged grandchildren for 1 year.

Intrapersonal Factors–Sociocultural

Moved 1 year ago from home of 30 years (200 miles away). Contributes to household by doing light housekeeping duties. Widow of 2 years. Second daughter lives nearby.

Intrapersonal Factors–Developmental

Retired as a dressmaker 6 years ago. Enjoys grandchildren, whom she sees daily. Attends senior citizen functions 1–2 times a week.

Interpersonal Factors

See above. Receives health care at a local clinic.

Extrapersonal Factors

Income from combined social security and widow benefits from railroad pension totals $625 per month. Has medicare.

---

*Modified from sample care plan, School of Nursing, University of Wyoming, 1983

ASSESSMENT	PLAN	IMPLEMENTATION	EVALUATION
Stressors	**Nursing Diagnosis**		
1. Overweight for height and build. Recognizes her difficulty maintaining calorie intake and avoiding sweets.	Alteration in nutrition: More than body requirements—due to increased calorie intake and "sweet tooth"	*Primary prevention* 1. Record weekly weight taken at same time and on the same scale	Did she lose weight?
	Goals (in priority)	2. Describe diet regimen of 1500 calories intake	Can Mrs. J. and daughter describe foods that are appropriate to diet?
	1. Mrs. J. will have a 1-pound weight loss for each of the next 4 weeks (short term)	3. Assist Mrs. J. to read labels	
	2. Mrs J. will lose 10 pounds in the next 3 months (intermediate)	4. Give Mrs. J. a list of low calorie, low salt foods	Can Mrs. J. describe plan of 1500 calorie intake?
	3. Mrs. J. will maintain her weight loss for 1 year (long term)	*Secondary prevention* 1. Develop a maintenance diet for use after weight loss is complete	
	Nursing Diagnosis		
2. Exertion causes SOB	Ineffective breathing pattern—due to mildly enlarged heart and increased body weight	*Primary prevention* 1. Discuss the importance of a written record of episodes of SOB with Mrs. J. and her daughter	Review the record
	Goals		
	1. Mrs. J. will describe a schedule that will allow for rest periods before leaving clinic (short term)	*Secondary prevention* 1. Discuss a schedule that will alternate rest and activity periods	Can Mrs. J. report her activity periods?
	2. Mrs. J. will walk to the market without SOB within 6 months (long term)	2. Plan a gradual increase in activity to improve tolerance	How far can Mrs. J. walk without SOB?
	Nursing Diagnosis		
3. Pain. Mrs. J. reports pain in the morning and increased discomfort if "she sits too long"	Alteration in comfort—due to pain in joints	*Primary prevention* 1. Discuss importance of continuing to walk	
	Goals		
	1. Mrs. J. will describe side effects of medications before leaving clinic and again in 1 week (short term)	*Secondary prevention* 1. Discuss side effects of medications with Mrs. J. and her daughter	Does Mrs. J. know the side effects?
	2. Mrs. J. will report decreased pain on rising within 2 weeks (short term)	2. Teach Mrs. J. the best way to take the medication	
		3. Reinforce importance of following diet	Is Mrs. J. more comfortable?

Figure 12–3. Care plan for Mrs. Jones.

REFERENCES

ANA Standards for Practice. Kansas City, American Nurses Association, 1973

Brill EL: Foundations for Nursing, pp 108–170. New York, Appleton-Century-Crofts, 1980

Gordon M: Nursing Diagnosis and the Diagnostic Process. Am J Nurs 76:1298–1300, August 1976

Gordon M: Manual of Nursing Diagnosis. New York, McGraw-Hill, 1982

Griffith JW, Christensen PJ: Nursing Process: Application of Theories, Frameworks, and Models, pp 29–164. St Louis, CV Mosby, 1982

Kim MJ, Moritz DA (eds): Classification of Nursing Diagnoses: Proceedings of the Third and Fourth National Conferences (April 1978 and 1980). New York, McGraw-Hill, 1982

Price MR: Nursing diagnosis: Making a concept come alive. Am J Nurs 80:668–671, April 1980

Wolff L, Weitzel MH, Fuerst EV: Fundamentals of Nursing, ed 6, pp 54–81. Philadelphia, JB Lippincott, 1979

Yura H, Walsh MB: The Nursing Process. Norwalk, Appleton-Century-Crofts, 1983

Chapter 13

Communication and Helping Relationships

THOUGHT QUESTIONS

1. Why is communication considered to be an essential element of nursing?
2. What are the major purposes of communication? Cite the significance of each purpose for nursing.
3. Explain the significance of space in the nursing process. Cite an example of how the nurse can manipulate space to be helpful to the client.
4. What are three principles in the nurse-client relationship that ensure helpfulness in communication? Define each and describe its significance to the nursing process.
5. How does the client's role as a petitioner affect the nurse-client interaction? Relate the client's role as petitioner to the need for the nurse to act as an advocate.
6. What are the outcomes of mutuality in the helping relationships?
7. How does anxiety affect the relationship between the nurse and the client?
8. Using the lists of therapeutic and nontherapeutic communication techniques in this chapter, write your own example of each.

The axiom, long supported in the helping professions, that behavioral change occurs by way of emotional experience serves as the basis for placing great emphasis on communication in nursing practice. The human need for relatedness binds people together and communication serves as the exchange medium in these relationships. The verbal and nonverbal messages exchanged in human relationships determine, to a large extent, the structure and function of feelings in people. Indeed the whole existence and health status of humans are dependent on communication since the affective component of life cannot be separated from the biologic component.

COMMUNICATION AS INTERACTION _____

The client and the nurse in the nursing process both undergo emotional experiences as a function of the communication process that exists between them. Since the ultimate goals of the professional nurse are to maximize the potentials for health in the client and to actualize the best professional abilities of the self, the professional nurse must clearly understand the power of communication in shaping relationships. The quality of the communication process between the nurse and the client is, therefore, an essential determinant of the success of the professional relationship. Mutual goals cannot be defined or achieved in the relationship without effective communications that positively influence the emotions of both the client and the professional nurse. This chapter focuses on communication as the interpersonal component of the nursing process and the essential component of helping relationships.

The Interpersonal Component of the Nursing Process

Assuming that humans possess all the characteristics of an open system, the nurse concludes that people are influenced by and influence all human systems with whom they are associated. Indeed, this reciprocal process suggests that man's most important attribute is not only openness to interpersonal experiences but also power to influence self and others. Sullivan (1953, p. 32) assumes that "everyone is more simply human than otherwise."

Humans influence others primarily by communication. Communication is described as the "matrix for all thought and relationships between persons" (Murray and Zentner, 1979, p. 62). Through communication in the nursing process with clients, the professional nurse hopes to create new situations with the client that will influence the client to behave in a healthier manner. This goal can only be achieved if the nurse is knowledgeable about the content and process of the nurse-client relationship. To understand content in the nursing process, the nurse must have knowledge of the person as a human system interacting with the environment, health, and specific factors that promote positive change in human systems. To understand process in the nurse-client relationship, the nurse must have knowledge of communication and experience in developing "helping" relationships. Therefore, to participate effectively in nurse-client relationships, intradisciplinary or interdisciplinary relationships and personal relationships, the nurse must understand both the structure and functions of communication.

Nursing as an organized body has not always been successful in portraying an image of an autonomous professional discipline. Disagreement among theorists, practitioners, and educators in nursing about the meaning of the "diagnosis and treatment of *human responses* to actual or potential health problems" (Nurse Practice Act, New York State, 1972) has led to multiple and sometimes conflicting images of nursing. Now there is general agreement among all parties that nursing's unique business is dealing with the human responses in health and illness. These human responses are the substance of communication. Thus, professional nursing's business is communication and the purposeful use of communication in nurse-client relationships.

The Structure of Communication

Human communication has been defined as "the generation and transmission of meaning" (Pluckham, 1978, p. 6). It is dynamic interaction between two or more people in which ideas, goals, beliefs and values, feelings, and "feelings about feelings" are exchanged. Experiencing even a minute exchange results in change in both communicants in the process. It should be noted that communication is defined only in the context of "process." Since humans are continually and irrevocably exchanging energy with the environment and life is continually being repatterned, it can be assumed that the individual human reflects only dynamic actions. One is always affected by others and is always affecting others. One always communicates, thus, generates change in others and experiences change in self.

Although communcation is a dynamic process, it is possible to identify components and to analyze the interrelationships between the components. Berlo (1960), a noted authority on communications, traces the various models of communication from Aristotle to the 1960s. Aristotle identified the related components as the speaker, the speech, and the audience. After analyzing the several points of view and behavioral science research, Berlo (1960, pp. 30–32) has postulated a communication model generally accepted today:

1. A source—defined interpersonally as some person(s) with ideas, needs, intentions, information, and a reason for communicating.
2. A message—a coded, systematic set of symbols representing ideas, purposes, intentions, and feelings.
3. An encoder—the mechanism for expressing or translating the purpose of the communication into the message (in humans, the motor mechanisms (*e.g.,* the vocal mechanism for oral messages, the muscles of the hands for written messages, the muscle systems elsewhere in the body for production of gestures).
4. A channel—the medium for carrying the message.
5. A decoder—the mechanism for translating the message into a form that the recipient can use (in humans, the sensory mechanisms).
6. A receiver—the target or recipient of the message.

In this model, the transmission of meaning occurs by way of a dynamic process in which there is an intention or purpose (the communication source); that purpose is translated into communicable form by the person's set of motor mechanisms and skills (encoder); the message is transmitted through a channel; the message is translated into receivable form by the other person's sensory mechanisms and skills (decoder); the other person receives the message (the communication receiver).

Since this model was postulated, systems theorists have further explained the reciprocal relationship between the participants in the communication process. The individual person at any given time is both an active initiator and recipient of meanings in an interpersonal situation. Thus, it is important for the nurse to understand that she is simultaneously acting and reacting in the nursing process and that the client's meanings have an equal effect on the outcome of the purposeful relationship. The process just described has been labeled "transactional." The dynamic nature of the communication process dictates the need for professionals to evaluate their own actions and reactions throughout the nursing process with clients. Without such awareness and evaluation, the professional will be less likely to experience successful communication by the feeling of satisfaction associated with the transmission of clear meanings and the validation that the message intended was indeed the message received. Validation of meanings is essential to the achievement of any therapeutic goals in helping relationships.

Functions and Types of Communication

Synthesizing from several communication models, Cecchio proposes four major purposes of communication: to inquire, to inform, to persuade, and to entertain (Cecchio and Cecchio, 1982). Professional nurses may attempt to achieve any of these purposes with clients, the health care delivery system, peers, other personnel, and even the self. In attempting to achieve these purposes, the nurse transmits messages in the process. Messages are transmitted verbally and nonverbally as well as through meta-communication.

Implicit in all models of communication is the concept that communication has two interacting components: the content value of the message and the interactional or perceptual value of the message and its participants. The content value is the informational aspect of the message and is expressed in verbal and/or nonverbal forms. The interactional or perceptual value of the message (referred to as meta-communication) identifies how the content is to be interpreted as well as how the relationship is perceived between the participants. Meta-communication may also be expressed in both verbal and nonverbal forms.

Verbal Communication

Verbal communication in nursing is primarily associated with the spoken word. It requires functional physiologic and cognitive mechanisms that potentiate speech production and reception. Although the greatest influence on communication is not words (it is the nonverbal message), words are an essential tool of personal and cultural communication. Language is constituted by an entire system of symbols. Words are symbolic of actual objects or concepts. Lack of congruence between the nurse and the client in language usually interferes with initiation of relationships and creates obstacles to validation of meanings, the essential characteristic of an effective message.

Following are the primary influences on verbal communications:

1. Developmental age—Verbal abilities reflect the physiologic ability to change sounds into words and the cognitive ability to symbolize.
2. Cultural heritage—By the process of acculturation, the human develops variations from others in defining words. Although denotative meanings are equal (*i.e.,* the concrete representations or words are the same between and among people), the connotative meanings often vary between people because individuals vary in culture and the accompanying acculturation.

Associated with the fact that words are the symbols of communication are three types of problems with which the nurse needs to be concerned (Cecchio and Cecchio, 1982):

1. The technical problem—How accurately can one transmit the symbols of communication?

2. The semantic problem—How precise are the symbols in transmitting the intended message?

3. The influential problem—How effectively does the received meaning affect conduct?

The verbal content of communication can be used to evaluate the content theme of the communication process. If one evaluates the seemingly varied topics of discussion, the words that underlie or link together several ideas will reflect the what of the communication.

Nonverbal Communication

The nonverbal component of the message is the greatest influence on communication. Nonverbal communication consists of all forms of communication that do not involve the spoken or written word. Perception of nonverbal communication involves all the senses including hearing, which is used for the perception of verbal messages. Signs (gestures), actions or kinesics (all body movements that are not specific signs), objects (all intentional and nonintentional display of material things), and proxemics (the use of space) are all powerful nonverbal messages that are perceived by the senses.

The tactile senses represent the most primitive sensory process developed by humans. Important to infant development, bonding between the infant and parent figure occurs largely through nonverbal communication that results from touch. Touch remains a powerful communication tool throughout life. It is commonly accepted today that deprivation of tactile stimulation in infancy may impair the achievement of some developmental tasks. The young child orients himself to space through touch. As the child develops into the adult, touch as nonverbal communication takes on very specific cultural meanings. Taboos concerning touch and distance must be understood by the nurse if the nurse desires to be purposeful in nonverbal as well as verbal communication. For example, to one person a touch on the knee might mean concern, while, to another, it is interpreted as seduction. Used sensitively at the proper time and within the context of the client's culture, touch is a powerful nonverbal tool for the professional nurse.

All the sensory processes become powerful components of the communication process as humans exchange nonverbal as well as verbal messages with others throughout life. For example, the olfactory (smell) and gustatory (taste) senses make it possible for a person to learn which odors and tastes are pleasant and which are not. Once that physiologic capacity is present, odor and taste are significant nonverbal messages in the communication process. The nurse needs to manipulate the environment in the health care delivery system in such a way that nonverbal messages such as odor are controlled. Finally, in relation to the sensory aspects of nonverbal communication, the sense of hearing the spoken word has a nonverbal component: that of interpreting the qualities of the voice. Hunsaker and Alessandra (1980) state that the following voice qualities are strong determinants of effectiveness in communication: resonance (the intensity with which the voice fills the space), rhythm (the flow, pace, and movement of the voice), speed (how fast the voice is used), pitch (the highness or lowness of the voice related to the tightening of the vocal cords), volume (loudness), inflection (change in pitch or volume of voice), and clarity (articulation and enunciation capacity of the voice).

Motor or kinesic actions are perhaps most often performed with little or no awareness on the part of the communicant. Body movements are nonverbal communications that are largely determined through socialization. Developed in a particular psychosocial and cultural setting, motor actions vary according to sex, social class, age, and ethnic background. It is generally accepted that misinterpretations of kinesic behaviors that are culturally variable produce barriers to effective communication. For example, eye motions involved with eye contact communicate culturally specific messages. If the professional nurse does not assign the same meaning to this nonverbal communication, the effectiveness of the nurse-client relationship may be limited. Hunsaker and Alessandra (1980) suggest that 90% of meaning comes from nonverbal communication. Thus, nonverbal behavior has a significant impact on the recipient of the message communicated. Nonverbal behavior is therefore very significant in leaders. It conveys the greatest meaning to the persons involved in the leadership process. For example, the following motor actions (which are commonly observed) may be highly influential in the communication process (Hunsaker and Alessandra, 1980):

1. Gently rubbing behind the ear with the index finger—interpreted as doubt.
2. Casually rubbing the eyes with one finger—the recipient in the communication process does not understand what is being communicated.
3. Cupping hands over the mouth—participant in the interaction trying to hide something.
4. Leaning back with both hands supporting the head—interpreted as confidence or superiority.
5. Pinching the bridge of the nose with eyes closed—interpreted as thoughtful evaluation.
6. Moving eyeglasses to the lower bridge of the nose and peering over them —interpreted as a powerful negative evaluation.

Kinesics must be carefully examined in the nursing process. The nurse must be able to understand the specific meaning of the motor actions used by the client and to purposefully strive for congruence between her own nonverbal behaviors and the verbal communications she intends to convey.

Proxemics, or the function of space in nonverbal communication, play an important role in all aspects of life. Space is a constant. It either surrounds people or exists between them. Professional nurses must be concerned with the human's personal and environmental space. Hall (1966) studied the effect of culture on communication in terms of proxemics. Clearly, the Germans, English, and Americans vary in the interpretation of what constitutes intrusion into personal space and the valid use of personal and environmental space. In order to be effective, the nurse needs to consider the way body parts (such as the eyes) move within space, the position of bodies in space (e.g., are the nurse and client body parts oriented in the same or different directions), and the distance between bodies in space. The following properties of space are useful to the nurse's purposeful use of space:

1. Point behaviors occur in space—body parts move within space and orient themselves in some direction (e.g., the direction of the eyes' gaze gives a specific message).
2. Positional behaviors occur in space—four regions of the body (head-neck, upper torso, pelvis-thighs, and lower legs-feet) are oriented in space, either in the same or different directions, dependent on the message to be conveyed.

3. The position of the participants in the communication space represent the degree of affiliation between them. Persons use point and positional behaviors to show they are "with" someone, affiliated and sharing space, or "not with" someone, unaffiliated with one another and sharing *different* spaces.

4. Orientation and position between bodies in space represent patterns of commitment between the parties. Some configurations represent involvement and commitment between the parties in the spatial relationship. Other configurations represent lack of involvement and commitment between the parties. (Pasquali *et al,* 1981, pp. 183–184)

With an awareness of what a client perceives as acceptable use of space and how body position and direction affect the meaning of the relationship, the professional nurse can use manipulation of personal and environmental space for the benefit of the client in the nursing process. For example, the nurse who is attempting to teach a client how to give himself insulin cannot see the full picture of the client's nonverbal behavior if the nurse sits side-by-side with the client. In that position, the nurse's torso is not directed toward the client's, the head must be turned awkwardly to see facial expressions, and so forth. This position gives the client a message of the nurse not being with the client.

Meta-Communication

Meta-communication occurs on both the verbal and nonverbal levels, and represents an integrative level that defines the "what," the "who," and the relationship between the "what" and "who" of the communication process. Since this level of communication is influential in determining the effectiveness of relationships, the professional nurse must evaluate communication both in terms of its context and the relationships between the parts. Understanding themes of the relationship helps the nurse evaluate the meta-communication occurring in the nursing process. The nurse must search for the content theme (the central underlying idea or links), the mood theme (the emotion communicated—the how of the message), and the interaction theme (the dynamics between the communicating participants). Knowing that change occurs more readily and more effectively if there is congruence between the verbal and nonverbal components of communication, the nurse must be alert to indicators of the degree of agreement on meaning of the content and process of the relationship. When there is a discrepancy between verbal and nonverbal components, the nonverbal is usually the more accurate indicator. However, nonverbal behavior is more open to subjective meaning and variations, thus, it must be verbally validated. That validation process plays an important part in effectively using meta-communication in the nursing process.

Perception

Communication is possible between humans because they have the capacity for interpretation. Interpretation involves perception, symbolization, memory, and thinking. Perhaps the most important of these is perception, the basic component after which the others follow. Taylor (1977) defines perception as the selection and organization of sensations so that they are meaningful. She takes the position that perceptions are learned and that what is learned is dependent on experience during socialization. Perceptual expectations are influenced by emotions, language, and attitudes, and vary widely from one individual to another. One's interpretation ability therefore is highly dependent on perceptual abilities.

Factors affecting perception in the nurse-client relationship are the capacity for attention (reception of sensations) by nurse and client, the perspective each brings to the relationship, and the physical condition of the receptors. The presence of anxiety (the actual or anticipated negative appraisal by the other) in the nurse or the client limits the ability to be attentive in the communication process, interferes with the validation of individual perspectives, and decreases physical capacities. Thus, it is essential for anxiety to be controlled in nurse-client relationships. Validated perceptions between nurse and client are essential to goal setting and achievement.

The evolutionary nature and significance of perception can be seen in the following statement of relationship: How we perceive and feel about the world is a force for and a result of our pattern of organization as a living system. This pattern affects our perception and feelings at any point in time. Perceptions and feelings about them affect how we communicate. The nurse must constantly be aware of the power and influence of perception on the outcomes of verbal, nonverbal, and meta-communications.

Self-Concept

Another important factor affecting communication in the nursing process is the relationship between the participants in the process. The self-concept of each participant is a major determinant of that relationship. Self-awareness and awareness of others is dependent on self-concept. See Chapter 4, "Development of Professional Self-Concept" for an elaboration on the significance of the personal self-concept in developing professional abilities. In addition to self-awareness, other factors involved in the self-concept that are essential to effective communication are the ability to share with individuals (a function of achievement of interpersonal developmental tasks), the ability to establish, maintain, and terminate the kind of relationship in which one is comfortable (a function of the human's need to perpetuate his self-concept), and the ability to share power (a reflection of the person's view of self and others).

If the major reason for nurses' communicating with clients is to influence them in the direction of better health, it is essential for nurses to develop concepts of self that are most effective in actualizing the potential of the client for growth. Those concepts include awareness of one's own perceptions of and feelings about self, the ability to derive satisfaction by sharing responsibility for the nurse-client relationship, the ability to view the self as the therapeutic tool for implementing the nursing process, and the appreciation of the value of shared power in activities directed toward change.

Principles of Communication in Collaborative Relationships Between Nurse and Client

Vital characteristics possessed by effective communicators are the abilities to empathize, to demonstrate respect, and to respond genuinely. The process for achieving each of these characteristics represents a principle on which communications in the nursing process can be based. Collaborative relationships mandate that the nurse and the client mutually and equally share the responsibility and authority for the planning, implementation, and evaluation of the helping process. Such collaboration cannot occur without high levels of empathy, respect, and genuineness.

Empathy

For effective change to occur in any helping relationship, the principle of empathy must be observed: In order to be helpful, the nurse must demonstrate the ability to participate in the client's feelings or ideas by sensing, sharing, and accepting the client's feelings. Empathy is defined as (1) "the imaginative projection of a subjective state into an object so that an object appears to be infused with it"; and (2) "the capacity for participation in another's feelings or ideas" (Webster, 1949, p. 269). Hammond *et al* (1977) replicated and modified the research on empathy originally conducted by Carkhuff (1969). They view the empathic process as the creation of the world as we perceive it rather than simply responding to it. They suggest that the process is developmental, moving sequentially from:

1. The experience of the biologic state in which one experiences his own bodily actions.
2. A state in which his feelings become more differentiated and specific.
3. Greater awareness of own bodily responses and feelings.
4. An ability to sense other's feelings, moods, and needs. (Hammond *et al*, 1977, pp. 97–136)

If the nurse possesses empathy, she shows awareness of the uniqueness and individuality of the client. She is involved with sharing in the feelings of the client. She cares about the client as a sentient being like herself. If the client is perceived as an object, he is immediately put on the defensive. However, if the client perceives that the nurse cares about him and how he feels, the relationship will bring forth trust and open communication. Hammond *et al* declare that to really be empathic, the helper has to listen so well that she can act as intended, perceive and accept the inner feelings and experiences of the client as the client experiences them, and can paraphrase feelings, ideas, and intentions to the client's satisfaction.

Two essential actions are necessary for a nurse to develop empathy: (1) awareness and acceptance of self as a feeling person open to own experiences, and (2) the ability to listen to each message of the client, identify the feelings associated with it, and respond to the feelings of the client. Thus, what empathy involves is far more than the cognitive or thinking part of the self. It involves the acceptance that we are feeling beings, with emotions frequently of more than one kind at a time. In effective communication, the feelings of the client perceived and accepted by the nurse are known to self and the client.

Respect

The principle of respect in the nurse-client relationship is that in order for the client to experience his right to exist as an other, the nurse must demonstrate a receptive attitude that values the client's feelings, opinion, individuality and uniqueness (Hammond *et al*, 1977, pp. 170–203). Respect is the act of giving particular attention, consideration, or an act of giving high or special regard or esteem (Webster, 1949, p. 722). Hammond and colleagues accept the definition that respect is the nonpossessive caring for and affirmation of another's personhood as a separate individual. Respect builds self-esteem and self-image. In the nurse-client relationship, respect is demonstrated when there are equality, mutuality, and shared thinking about strengths and problems.

Hammond and associates (1977, pp. 170–207) offer the following guidelines for the nurse to follow in responding with respect to clients:

1. The nurse needs to show a high level of commitment to understand by her willingness to fully explore subjects of importance to the client. This requires a great deal of skill in verbal communications.
2. The nurse needs to convey acceptance and warmth by being nonjudgemental. Nurses must develop a high level of immunity to being embarrassed, shocked, dismayed, or overwhelmed by the client's behavior (however offensive it might be). This requires a great deal of skill in nonverbal communications.
3. The nurse needs to welcome the opportunity to relate to different individuals and feel enriched by the relationships. This requires freedom from prejudice.
4. The nurse must believe in the capacity of others to change.

Respect by the nurse affirms the strengths and problem-solving capabilities of the client.

Genuineness

Genuineness, used synonymously with authenticity, is supported in the nursing principle: Positive therapeutic outcomes for the client are enhanced when the nurse in the helping relationship acts with genuineness. In defining authenticity, phrases such as "being actually and precisely what is claimed," "genuine," "good faith," and "sincere" are used. Genuineness is "sharing of self by behaving in a natural, sincere, spontaneous, and real, open, non-defensive manner" (Hammond *et al,* 1977, p. 204). The genuine nurse would act unrehearsed and noncontrived. It has been argued that neutrality is the essence of the nurse's behavior in a helping relationship (Rogers, 1951). Others argue that neutral behavior often has the appearance of being depersonalized, thus is ambiguous and leads to anxiety on the part of the client, who may not get a clear message of how he stands with the nurse.

Guidelines for the effective use of genuineness that are applicable to the nurse in the nurse-client relationship are:

1. Avoid early self-disclosure until the client demonstrates a readiness to respond positively to your disclosure.
2. As trust is established, the nurse can become more open and spontaneous while adhering to the principles of empathy and respect.
3. Avoid using self-disclosure in order to manipulate, give advice, or influence for your own goals. If empathy and respect accompany authenticity, such personal motivations are not likely. (Hammond, *et al,* 1977, pp. 204–227)

To summarize, effective changes in clients occur when the nurse uses a high degree of positive regard, demonstrates congruence between who she is and what she is, demonstrates congruence between verbal and nonverbal communication, and infers accurately the inner world of the client by listening well and understanding the subjective and objective world of the relationship as it changes over time. Internalizing the principles of empathy, respect, and genuineness make it possible for the nurse to demonstrate these behaviors and experience satisfaction in the nursing process.

HELPING RELATIONSHIPS—THE NURSE AS HELPER

The "nurse-client relationship is a helpful, purposeful interaction between an authority in health care, the nurse, and a person or group with health care needs" (Murray and Zentner, 1979, p. 129). The nurse as an authority in health care recognizes her expertise in the promotion, maintenance, and restoration of health and the prevention of illness. The nurse also accepts her obligation to society to share her abilities with clients in need of nursing services. Although the nurse in the United States today usually is not directly employed by the client, she nevertheless is professionally accountable first to the client who is the recipient of her services and then to herself and her employer and other health team workers. It is the nurse's responsibility to fulfill a helper role regardless of the specific parameters and purposes of each relationship. The nurse must validate that the client knows the areas of concern for which he is ready to seek help, and assume that they will mutually share the responsibility for the outcomes of the nursing process. The nurse further assumes that the client can achieve an improved state of health. The helping role is viewed as a facilitative one in which the professional nurse uses herself and her expertise as a therapeutic tool to assist clients to more successfully develop responses to resist or overcome threats to their health.

Rogers (1958) set the following essential conditions of a helping relationship that are applicable to the nursing process:

1. The individual is able and expected to be responsible for himself.
2. Each individual (nurse and client) have a strong drive to become mature and to be socially responsible.
3. The climate of the helping relationship is warm and permits the expression of both positive and negative feeling.
4. Limits, mutually agreed on, are set on behavior only, not on attitudes.
5. The helper communicates understanding and acceptance.

The characteristics of helping as developed by Rogers have positively influenced many health professionals and have continued to be refined and reformulated in improving their practice.

The Client as the Petitioner

Discussing the foundation, purposes, responsibilities and rights in the nurse-patient relationship, Curtin (Curtin and Flaherty, 1982) examines the situation of the patient (synonymous with client in this text) who is a petitioner, a seeker of help. She describes how infringement on human autonomy is the first outcome for the person/family who experiences illness or threats to health. The person who perceives such a threat is forced to change from an independent role to a petitioner role if the person is to get help. Curtin declares that the more personal or the more threatening the disclosure, the harder it is for one to petition. She maintains that both the loss of independence and the obstacle of vulnerability cited above need to be overcome by the professional serving as an advocate for the client. Curtin believes that nurses are particularly sensitive to the need for advocacy for clients and can indeed accept the value system of the client and "act in behalf of" the petitioning client. Professional nurses who serve as advocates accept the premise that disease, illness, or perceived threats to health interfere with a person's ability, but not the person's right to make choices.

Curtin (Curtin and Flaherty, 1982) further analyzes how the petitioner role of the client creates an imbalance of power between the professional and the client unless the professional structures a collaborative relationship. The professional who needs to exercise power and receives satisfaction from others' dependency will demonstrate more unjustifiable patronizing behavior to the client than the professional who is committed to an advocacy role with the client. Curtin states, ". . . tragic errors may occur unless patients are permitted–indeed, assisted–to become full partners in the development, design and implementation of their own care" (Curtin and Flaherty, 1982, p. 93). To negate the dangers inherent in the client's need to assume the petitioner role, the professional nurse must act as an advocate and a change agent in the helping relationship. This means the nurse must readily provide information, share power equitably, encourage the client to assume responsibility for his own health, and diligently work to preserve the integrity of the client and self.

The Nature of Helping in Progressive Stages of the Nurse-Client Relationship

The purposes and functions of the nurse-client relationship vary as interaction proceeds through predictable sequential stages. Although the nurse in a helping relationship always enacts the roles of facilitator, advocate, and coordinator in the relationship, functions and purposes evolve throughout the relationship. The facilitator helps clients move toward greater health. The advocate protects the client from stress inherent in the petitioner role and acts on behalf of the client in promoting the client's access to and use of health care delivery services. The coordinator attempts to organize and articulate all the services related to the client's health care needs being met.

The knowledge base needed to act as a helper in the nursing process was largely developed and shared by Dr. Hildegard Peplau over 30 years ago. Her book, *Interpersonal Relations in Nursing,* represented a thorough analysis of Harry Stack Sullivan's interpersonal theory in psychiatry and gave nursing a sound conceptual model for practice. Although nurse scholars have developed other models or evolved changed forms of the interpersonal model, Peplau's contribution about the phases of the nurse-patient relationship remains applicable. Following is a brief summary of the phases and their purposes with associated functions of the nurse in each phase (Peplau, 1952).

> *Phase of Orientation*: The purposes of the phase of orientation include the introduction of nurse and client, the elaboration of the client's need to recognize and understand his difficulty and the extent of need for help, the acceptance of the client's need for assistance in recognizing and planning to use services that professional personnel can offer, the agreement for client to direct energies toward the mutual responsibility for defining, understanding, and meeting productively the problem at hand, and the clarification of

limitations and responsibilities in the delivery system environment. When the nurse and the client validate understanding of the client's need for help and the acceptance of resources to meet those needs with feelings of shared responsibility and a sense of trust, they move into a new phase of the relationship.

Phase of Identification: The purposes of the phase of identification include the provision of the opportunity for the client to respond to the helper's offer to assist, the encouragement of the client to express what is felt in order to reorient feelings and strengthen positive forces in the client, and to provide opportunity for the nurse and the client to clearly understand each other's preconceptions and expectations.

Phase of Exploitation: The purposes of the phase of exploitation include the full use of the nurse-client relationship to mutually work on the solution to problems and the changes needed to improve health and the provision of opportunities for the client to explore earlier experiences and behaviors and to have emerging needs met.

Phase of Resolution: The purposes of the phase of resolution include the provision of opportunity for the formulation of new goals, the encouragement of gradual freeing of the client from identification with the nurse, and to promote the client's ability to act more independently.

Overlapping in various stages, the following roles of the professional nurse tend to emerge as the nurse promotes growth (change) in the client:

1. Phase of Orientation:	Stranger
2. Phase of Identification:	Unconditional mother surrogate
	Resource person
	Counselor
	Teacher
	Leadership
	Surrogate
3. Phase of Exploitation:	The adult support person in new enactment of above roles
4. Phase of Resolution:	Same adult roles

It should be noted that the nurse moves back and forth in some of these roles in the various phases. Essentially, however, as client's needs are met, more mature needs arise, thus the need for more "mature" roles.

In the stranger role, the nurse is an individual unknown to the client. Peplau points out how essential it is for the nurse in this role to accord the client respect and positive interest to promote open communications. A surrogate is a substitute figure who, in the client's mind, reactivates the feeling generated in earlier relationships. The nurse's responsibility in that role is to help the client to become aware of likenesses and differences and to differentiate the nurse as a person. Permitting clients to reexperience old feelings, the nurse acting as surrogate sets up the opportunity for growth experiences. The resource person role involves the nurse in providing specific information, usually formulated in relation to larger problems. The teaching role in the nursing process involves the nurse in sharing information and promoting the client's learning through experience and requires the development of novel alternatives with open-ended outcomes in the nurse-client relationship. The leadership role involves the nurse facilitating the client's work on the solution of problems. The counselor role incorporates all of the activities associated with the promotion of experiences leading to health. The counselor helps a client become aware of his health behaviors, evaluate them, and plan how to improve them. Counseling focuses primarily on how the client feels about himself and what is happening to him (Peplau, 1952).

Mutuality in Responsibility and Decision-Making

All of the specified roles above represent elements of empathy, respect, and genuineness. Communication in these role relationships will evolve from diagnostic interactions to therapeutic interactions and eventually to educative and supportive interactions as the client moves from illness to a higher level of health. The absolute element of all of these roles is mutuality in responsibility and decision-making if both the nurse and the client are expected to experience growth and satisfaction in the nursing process.

Communication and the Phenomenon of Anxiety

Social systems are characterized by continual interaction between its components. This means that every person involved in the communication process *affects and is affected by* every other person in the communication field. Rogers calls this phenomenon reciprocy (Rogers, 1970, p. 97). Reciprocal relationships are the basis of the nursing process. The fact that the nurse has the potential to affect the client, as well as to be affected by the client, offers the nurse the potential to assist the client to change behaviors in the direction of improved health. Such nurse-client exchanges can be very powerful in problem-solving and decision-making situations that determine the nature and direction of change. The nature of change includes alternatives of cognitive repatterning (using new information to increase understanding), affective adjustment (using the relationship to become aware of, accept, and express feelings), and the synthesis of cognitions and feelings in interpersonal repatterning (using the relationship to learn to interact with others in the social system). The direction of change can be toward greater or lesser health. Obviously, the professional nurse wants to affect the direction of change toward greater health.

Every social system has expected role behavior on the part of its constituents. The way one communicates is greatly affected by one's perceived role in the system. "Roles are structures that are imposed on behavior" (Berlo, 1960, p. 153). There are three aspects of role one needs to understand in trying to positively affect "the other" in a relationship: role prescription, role description, and role expectations. Berlo (1960, p. 153) defines these aspects:

1. Role prescription: the formal, explicit statement of what behaviors should be performed by persons in a given role.
2. Role descriptions: a report of the behaviors that actually are performed by persons in a given role.
3. Role expectations: the images that people have about the behaviors that are performed by persons in a given role.

In the ideal relationship between the nurse and the client, there is congruence between the role prescriptions, descriptions, and expectations. Together the nurse and the client have agreed on the structure and dynamics of their purposeful communication. When there are differences between the prescriptions, descriptions, and expectations of role behavior between the nurse and the client, communication breakdowns occur. As noted in an earlier part of this chapter, the helping role of the nurse takes different forms in the various stages of the relationship. In the continually evolving relationship, it is necessary for the nurse to assume responsibility for keeping role-behavior prescriptions, descriptions, and expectations closely related. According to Berlo (1960, p. 156), this is done by the persons in the social system periodically validating what it is that each is to do in the relationship, agreeing on accurate prescriptions of behavior of each, and being able to expect what will happen before it happens. Congruence in role relationships in the social system reduces uncertainty. Uncertainty and ambiguity lead to increased tension and discomfort in the system. Such tension in human systems leads to dissipation of energy and less ability to use the energy exchanged for purposes of improving health. In interpersonal systems, such tension is often called anxiety.

Anxiety is the tension state of the human resulting from the actual or anticipated negative appraisal of the significant other human in the communication process. Prolonged or intensive anxiety ties up available energy. Thus, energy is less available to the system for decision-making or problem-solving that are necessary for purposeful change to healthier role behaviors.

A principle commonly accepted today is that the tension state of anxiety in one person is readily communicated, thus, engenders anxiety in the other person(s). Sullivan (1953) attributes great power to the tension of anxiety in the interpersonal growth, development, and ability of the individual in all stages of life. The actual or anticipated negative appraisals by others that lead to anxiety are perceived as threats to one's self-image. If the anxiety is limited in amount and duration, it simply leads to an increased state of alertness, mediation through physiologic reactions, and behavior to reduce the tension. However, if the state of anxiety is not limited in amount or duration, the level of alertness and successful tension-reducing behaviors are decreased. In fact, Sullivan (1953, pp. 151–154) postulates that learning occurs through an anxiety gradient. That anxiety gradient is from mild to severe degrees. With a mild degree of anxiety, the client is able to focus energies on most of what is really occurring. If anxiety is moderate, the client has limited ability to focus on what is really occurring and tends to distort reality. When anxiety is severe, the client cannot focus energies on what is really happening, thus cannot react effectively in problem-solving or decision-making. Since the effective nursing process requires both the nurse and the client to be able to focus on what is really happening, it is essential to control anxiety in the communication process.

The professional nurse has two primary responsibilities in controlling anxiety: to be aware of one's own feelings of anxiety in order to structure interactions in such a way that limited anxiety is empathized to the client and to use effective strategies for intervening in client's anxiety. Such strategies are usually called "therapeutic." Intervention in client's anxiety is based on the nurse recognizing the presence of anxiety in the client. Once the tension state is recognized in the client, the nurse intervenes according to the following procedure: (1) Help the patient to recognize his anxiety; (2) help the patient to gain insight into his anxiety; and (3) help the patient to cope with the threat behind his anxiety (American Journal of Nursing Company, 1965, p. 146). The techniques to help clients recognize, gain insight into, and cope with threats of anxiety are discussed in the following section.

Communication Strategies for Helping Clients

Listening is the most important therapeutic technique in the process of effective communication. Sundeen (1976, p. 89) states that it is devastating to the formation of a helpful relationship if the nurse fails to listen. Listening transmits the message that "you are of value to me" and "I am interested in you." Long and Prophit (1981, p. 6) suggest that one cannot encourage self-disclosure, increase feelings of self-worth, promote increased understanding, increase satisfaction with interaction, or encourage problem-solving and appropriate decision-making without listening. Therapeutic communications are characterized by these very behaviors, thus, the nurse must "listen effectively" in order to pursue the goal of helping the client. How does one know the nurse is listening? Long and Prophit (1981, p. 6) evaluate communication through the criteria of the following nurse behaviors that all reflect effective listening. The nurse:

1. Stops talking or at least talks one at a time and does not interrupt.
2. Gets rid of distractions.
3. Looks at the person who is speaking.
4. Searches for the main point (both thoughts and feelings).
5. Evaluates how the message was given.
6. Assesses what is avoided.
7. Evaluates the intensity of emotions being expressed.

In order for the nurse to listen effectively, the nurse must use verbal communication techniques that facilitate verbal and nonverbal expressiveness of the client. Such techniques are generally referred to as "therapeutic communication techniques" (Table 13–1).

The nurse must respond empathically, attempt to extend the client's meaning, and respond with respect and authenticity in order to be helpful to clients. What does the nurse do to show empathy? The empathic nurse attends carefully, listens intensely, responds reciprocally to verbal and nonverbal messages, uses appropriate language, times responses appropriately, clarifies and confirms ideas, explores the world from the client's point of view, and paces verbal and nonverbal behavior to the abilities of the client. What does the nurse do to help the client understand and/or problem-solve? The nurse identifies relationships and makes connections based on knowledge, states implicit assumptions, conceptualizes trends and patterns, verbalizes implied feelings, thoughts, goals, and attitudes, summarizes appropriately, explains purposes of activities, identifies nonverbal meanings, and assumes responsibility for her role in the nursing process. What does the nurse do to show respect? The nurse verbalizes a clear commitment to understand, conveys acceptance, clearly affirms the worth in the client as a unique person, and affirms the strengths of the client and the client's ability to assume responsibility for self. Such a nurse will help the client to strengthen self-identity. Strengthening self-identity is heard in phrases like "You have . . ." and You do . . ." How does the nurse respond with authenticity? The nurse is consistent in responding with real thoughts and feelings and resists all urges to "play-act," is clear on owning ideas and feelings emanating from the self, and permits self to share emotions with clients. The nurse who is authentic will say, "I feel," "I think," or "I believe" (Sundeen, 1976; Long and Prophit, 1981; Hammond *et al,* 1977; Pasquali *et al,* 1981; Berlo, 1960; and Hein, 1980).

All of the above therapeutic activities on the part of the professional nurse re-

TABLE 13-1. Techniques of Therapeutic Communication

Technique	Definition	Example
Using broad opening statement	Initiating the discussion by allowing the client to determine what will be discussed	"Is there something you would like to tell me?"
Using general leads	Indicating that nurse is listening and is interested in what client is saying	"Yes," "Oh?" "And then . . .," "Go on."
Reflecting	Repeating all or part of the client's words	Client: "I am terribly worried." Nurse: "Terribly worried?"
Sharing observations or perceptions	Stating to the client your perceptions or observations	"You're grimacing when you turn." "You seem to be in pain."
Acknowledging the client's feelings	Verbalizing acceptance and understanding of client's feelings or thoughts	"It must be extremely upsetting to you to be confined."
Selective reflecting	Directing back to the client what the nurse believes to be main idea client has stated.	Client: "It's too much! I will never be able to go home!" Nurse: "Too much?"
Using silence	Maintaining an attentive, expectant silence to promote reflection.	Silence conveys sadness, distress, anger, contemplation.
Giving information	Providing client with information to answer questions or dispel misinformation.	"When you wake up, you will be in the recovery room, where the nurse will . . ."
Clarifying	Requesting that client make his meaning clear	"I'm not sure that I understand . . ."
Verbalizing implied thoughts and feelings	Verbalizing implied thoughts and feelings to verify nurse's impression of the client.	Client: "I think this is going to do the trick." Nurse: "You are eager to get discharged, aren't you?"
Validating	Requesting the client to validate that need has been met.	"Are you feeling better now?"

(Modified from Nurse-Patient Interaction, Instructor's Manual, pp 87–91. Cosa Mesta, Calif, 1970)

quire the ability to listen. Listening shows the ability of the professional nurse to place the needs of the self secondary to the needs of the client (Sundeen, 1976, pp. 89–90). The use of therapeutic techniques is based on the belief by the nurse that the client has the ability to be responsible for self and to solve problems. The nurse facilitates the client's efforts to solve problems, express self, and improve health status. The client shares equally in both the responsibility and accountability for the nursing process.

Communication Strategies That Are Hurtful to Clients

The failure to listen is the most hurtful communication behavior the nurse can exhibit. When the nurse fails to listen, the message communicated to the client is: "You are not of value to me," or "I am not interested—actually, I'm bored" (Sundeen, 1976, pp. 89–90). Other nurse behaviors that are not helpful to clients are being judgemental (*i.e.,* putting nurse's values, beliefs, and perceptions above the client's); making stereotyped responses (*i.e.,* negating the uniqueness of the client by stating platitudes and cliches); and changing the subject (*i.e.,* stating nonverbally to the client that the topic will be chosen by the nurse and that what the nurse thinks is more important than what the client thinks) (Sundeen, 1976, pp. 89–90).

Blocks to therapeutic communication have been summarized in Table 13–2.

Why do nurses use hurtful communication techniques with clients? Generally, one can assume that the nurse who communicates nontherapeutically has some need to behave regressively. This need, accompanied by increasing anxiety, sometimes leads to one seeing self as superior and is expressed in negative actions such as moralizing, rejecting, or reacting with hostility. Defensive behavior is common in regressive states. For example, one might demonstrate denial, unconsciously evading or negating the real factors in a situation. In regressive states, one might also see distortions, rote habitual actions, dogmatic responses, loss of control, the act of making unvalidated assumptions (jumping to conclusions), parroting, inappropriate timing, and the act of making poor judgements. These behaviors are significant components of nontherapeutic strategies or hurtful communication behaviors of the nurse. Since therapeutic communication is essential for effective professional nursing practice, it is imperative that professional nurses evaluate their communication techniques and seek help if a pattern of nontherapeutic behaviors is demonstrated. In actual nurse-client situations, it is suggested that the nurse let her own feelings be the guide to evaluation. The feeling of persistent anxiety or tension is perhaps the best cue of unwitting communication in a nonhelpful way.

Outcomes of Helping Relationships

Two major client outcomes are desirable goals for the nurse-client relationship: increased understanding by the client of how better personal responsibility and accountability for health can be achieved (learning) and perceived satisfaction in the relationship. In terms of nurse outcomes, knowing that the client is adequately prepared to solve problems is the desired outcome. If the client is adequately prepared, he is free to choose, to put forth energy, and to assume greater responsibility for his own health.

In the nurse-client relationship, change occurs in two ways: as an outcome of learning in terms of the information gained and understood and as an outcome of

TABLE 13–2.   Techniques of Nontherapeutic Communication

Technique	Definition	Example
Using reassuring cliches	Reassuring the client to reduce own anxiety rather than to base reassurance on facts	"Don't worry. Everything is going to be all right."
Giving advice	Telling the client what to do —imposing own opinions and solutions	"I think you should do . . ."
Giving approval	Verbalizing the nurse's and concepts of right and wrong	"I think that is the right thing to do. You have a good attitude."
Requesting an explanation	Asking the client to immediately explain feelings or actions.	"Why are you doing this?"
Agreeing with the client	Introducing nurse's opinion of what is correct or incorrect.	"That's the correct solution. I agree with your view."
Expressing disapproval	Indicating disapproval of the client's feelings or acts.	"That's bad. You should not feel that way."
Belittling the client's feelings	Equating client's feelings with those felt by nurse and other people.	"I know how that is. Lots of us have had that . . ."
Disagreeing with the client	Contradicting the client—sharing a negative judgement.	"No, that's not the way it is. You are wrong."
Defending	Responding defensively to a client's criticism.	"I don't understand. Ms. Jones is a top-notch nurse."
Making stereotyped comments	Using social cliches or trite phrases.	"It's a nice day, isn't it?"
Changing the subject	Directing the focus of the conversation away from the client.	"I almost forgot. I meant to tell you . . ."

(Modified from Nurse-Patient Interaction, Instructor's Manual, pp. 91–96. Cosa Mesta, Calif, 1970)

learning in terms of the interpersonal experience in the nursing process. Both expressions of growth are facilitated by the nurse-client relationship characterized by open and helpful communication. Change, according to Munn and Metzger (1981, p. 3), means moving from old ways that have been tested and have become comfortable to new ways that are unknown and somewhat threatening. The quality of communication plays the paramount role in change. When change and its effects are not communicated clearly, the change cannot be understood. Lack of understanding leads to resistance. For change to be effective, communication content and process must consider the following factors:

1. One must receive communication of full information.
2. One must be forewarned or prepared for change.
3. One should be consulted in advance to discuss the necessity for change and the several alternatives possible.
4. Change activities should not ignore established norms or customs of those affected.
5. In communicating with the client, the nurse must consider, in detail, exactly how the change will occur, every step that will be taken to promote change, and every change strategy to be used.
6. In communicating with the client, the nurse must give sufficient consideration to the problems that are likely to arise and cite alternative ways to deal with the problems.
7. Communicating about change should not reflect, in any way, criticism of the past. Criticizing the past is a remarkable stimulant for resistance to change.
8. Promote nursing process in which the interaction is directed toward getting clearly verbalized and validated how one feels about the change.
9. Therapeutic communications always need to be characterized by a theme of both the nurse and the client understanding what can be done about their feelings. (Munn and Metzger, 1981)

Hunsaker and Alessandra (1980, pp. 140–141) have proposed a schema for self-evaluation of communication patterns of people in management positions. They raise a number of questions that are clearly applicable to the evaluation of communication in the nursing process:

1. Did I comprehend each point made?
2. Did I make judgements of the word before the speaker was through speaking?
3. Did I make decisions in my own mind while he/she was still speaking?
4. Did I hunt for evidence that would prove the speaker right? wrong?
5. Did I hunt for evidence that would prove myself right? wrong?
6. Did I become upset while listening?
7. Did I generally jump to conclusions while listening?
8. Did I let the client speak at least 50% of the time?
9. Did I understand the words in terms of their intended meanings?
10. Did I restate ideas and feelings accurately?
11. Did I study voice, posture, actions, and facial expressions as the client talked?
12. Did I listen between the lines for unspoken meanings behind the words?
13. Did I really try to listen to the client?
14. Did I really want to listen to the client?
15. Did I really show the client I was, in fact, motivated and interested in listening to him?

The nurse should continually evaluate her own communication behaviors. In addition to self-evaluations by such schema as that described above, the nurse should consistently evaluate the effectiveness of the communication with the client. Feedback should be sought from the client about what has been said and about how the client feels the relationship is going. The value of the nurse-client interactions should be explored at intervals in order to promote mutual benefits to nurse and client. A focus on "how are we doing" states to the client that the nurse values the client and cares how the communication affects him.

Communication is such an important medium for the nursing process that most professional programs of study include intensive special study of the communication process as well as the continual development of communication strategies in every course in professional nursing. This chapter serves as a beginning reference, describing the content aspects of communication as well as the factors associated with the process of communication.

REFERENCES

American Journal of Nursing: Anxiety: Recognition and intervention. Programmed instruction. Am J Nurs 65:129–152, 1965

Berlo DK: The Process of Communication. New York, Holt, Rinehart & Winston, 1960

Carkhoff R: Helping and Human Relations, vol I. New York, Holt, Rinehart & Winston, 1969

Carkhoff R: Helping and Human Relations, vol II. New York, Holt, Rinehart & Winston, 1969

Ceccio JF, Ceccio CM: Effective Communication in Nursing Theory and Practice. New York, John Wiley & Sons, 1982

Curtin L, Flaherty MJ: Nursing Ethics: Theories and Pragmatics, pp 87–90. Bowie, Md, Robert J Brady, 1982

Hall ET: Proxemics in a cross cultural context. *In* Bennis WG et al (ed): Interpersonal Dynamics: Essays and Readings on Human Interaction, ed 3, pp 78–90. Homewood, Dorsey Press, 1973

Hammond DC, Hepworth DH, Smith VG: Improving Therapeutic Communication. San Francisco, Jossey-Bass, 1977

Hein EC: Communication in Nursing Practice, ed 2. Boston, Little, Brown, 1980

Hunsaker PL, Alessandra AJ: Art of Managing People. Englewood Cliffs, NJ, Prentice Hall, 1980

Long L, Prophit P: Understanding/Responding—A Communication Manual for Nurses. Monterey, Calif, Wadsworth Health Science Division, 1981

Munn HE Jr: Metzger N: Effective Communication in Health Care. Rockville, Md, Aspen Systems, 1981

Murray RB, Zentner JP: Nursing Concepts for Health Promotion, ed 2. Englewood Cliffs, NJ, Prentice-Hall, 1979

Nurse-Patient Interaction, Instructor's Manual. Cosa Mesta, Calif, Concept Media, 1970

Pasquali EA, Alesi EG, Arnold HM et al: Mental Health Nursing: A Bio-Psycho-Cultural Approach. St Louis, CV Mosby, 1981

Peplau H: Interpersonal Relations in Nursing. New York, GP Putnam's, 1952

Pluckham ML: Human Communication: The Matrix of Nursing. New York, McGraw Hill, 1978

Rogers CR: Client-Centered Therapy: Its Current Practice, Implications and Theory. Boston, Houghton Mifflin, 1951

Rogers CR: Characteristics of a helping relationship. Personnel and Guidance J 37:6–16, 1958

Rogers ME: An Introduction to the Theoretical Basis of Nursing. Philadelphia, FA Davis, 1970

Smith VM, Bass TA: Communication for Health Professionals. Philadelphia, JB Lippincott, 1979

Sullivan HS: The Interpersonal Theory of Psychiatry. New York, WW Norton, 1953

Sundeen SJ, Stuart GW, Rankin ED et al: Nurse-Client Interaction. St Louis, CV Mosby, 1976

Sutterly DC, Donnelly GF: Perspectives in Human Development. Philadelphia, JB Lippincott, 1973

Taylor A, et al: Communicating. Englewood Cliffs, Prentice-Hall, 1977

Travelbee J: Interpersonal Aspects of Nursing ed 2. Philadelphia, FA Davis, 1971

Twaddle AW: Sickness Behavior and the Sick Role. Boston, GK Hall, 1979

Webster N: Webster's New Collegiate Dictionary, ed 2. Springfield, G & C Merriam, 1949

Chapter 14

Leadership

THOUGHT QUESTIONS

1. How does leadership differ from management?
2. What inputs might affect the outcomes of leadership?
3. How can the nurse deal with the conflicting demands of relationships and task accomplishment?
4. What is the relationship between leadership and professional nursing roles of change agent and contributor to the profession?

"Leadership has been seen as the focus of group processes, as a personality attribute, as the art of inducing compliance, as an exercise of influence, as a particular kind of act, as a form of persuasion, as a power relation, as an instrument in goal attainment, as an effect of interaction, as a differentiated role, and as initiation of structure" (Bass, 1981, p. 584). For example, leadership has been defined as:

"Interaction between members of a group that initiates and maintains improved expectations and competence of the group to solve problems or attain goals" (Bass, 1981, p. 584).
"Influencing individuals or groups to take an active part in the process of achieving agreed-upon goals" (Epstein, 1982, p. 2).
The translation of innovative ideas into action (Moloney, 1979, p. 12).

In this chapter nursing leadership is defined as a process of interpersonal influence through which a client is assisted in the establishment and achievement of goals toward improved well-being.

Leadership can be applied at many different levels of systems complexity: individual, family, groups of clients or professional colleagues, or the larger society. The purposes of leadership may also vary from improved health status and potential with individual or family clients; or increased effectiveness and satisfaction in providing care of professional colleagues; to changed attitudes and expectations related to the nursing profession of citizens and legislators. This chapter focuses on leadership with the individual client rather than on "team leading" or organizational change. Leadership in promoting the nursing profession is discussed in Chapter 17, "Contributor to the Profession Role."

In much of the literature, leadership is associated with group interaction within an organizational setting. Thus there is confusion between leadership and management. Management has been defined as "the use of delegated authority within the formal organization to organize, direct, or control responsible subordinates . . . so that all service contributions are coordinated to attain a goal" (Yura *et al,* 1981, p. 75). Management is an assigned, legitimately designated responsibility associated with a position or role. "Managers are appointed, have a legitimate power base, and utilize power to either reward or punish. Their influential capacity derives from the authority inherent in their formal position" (Moloney, 1979, p. 11). Managers are primarily interested in organizational goals. However, since their authority comes from their subordinates as well as their superiors, managers must validate their power base and ensure that their goals are congruent with those of the people whom they manage.

Moloney (1979, p. 12) has suggested that "leadership is often referred to as a function of management." For example, "leading . . . has to do with managerial and coordination activities and is but one vital aspect of the management process. Controlling, organizing, planning, and budgeting comprise other areas of the manager's responsibility." Douglass and Bevis (1983, p. 3) state that "good managers are better if they are also good leaders; however, good leaders may or may not have the knowledge and skills to be managers."

In contrast we consider leadership and management to be two *different,* although often complementary, roles. Both roles are important for the nurse functioning within an institutional setting; however, only leadership will be discussed in this chapter. The next section considers a variety of theories about leadership, followed by a discussion of behaviors that comprise effective nursing leadership.

LEADERSHIP THEORIES

Leadership Traits

The earliest theories about leadership were based on the belief that a person was born with leadership characteristics. The belief that leadership qualities were passed on in the genes became the basis for royal succession. With time, however, it was recognized that leaders, or "great men," existed outside of the ruling classes. Efforts were made to define leadership through identification of the qualities possessed by these "great men." This approach evolved into an attempt to identify the qualities, or traits, that characterize leadership so that they could be taught to others.

A number of qualifications have been suggested as desirable traits for a leader to possess. These include more intelligence than the group being led, initiative, creativity, emotional maturity, energy, drive, good health, self-confidence, strong communication skills, persuasion, perception, helpfulness, tolerance for ambiguity, ability to motivate morale, trustworthiness, persistence, above average height, loyalty, tactfulness, being entrepreneurial, introspective, and courageous (Claus and Bailey, 1977; Bernhard and Walsh, 1981; Yura *et al,* 1981; Marriner, 1978). However, since no traits or qualifications have been identified that are universal for all leaders, the emphasis has shifted from the identification of what a leader is to clarification of what a leader does. This has led to a focus on styles of leadership.

Leadership Styles

Early work by Lewin, Lippitt and White (1946), indicated that leadership behavior could substantially influence group climate and outcomes. The patterns or styles they used were labeled authoritarian, democratic, and laissez-faire. These styles were conceptualized on a continuum from a highly controlling and directive type of leadership to a very passive, inactive style. Discrimination between authoritarian and democratic leadership was based on four factors: (1) sharing of decision-making (2) concern for followers, (3) maintenance of social distance, and (4) use of punishment and coercion.

Later research has focused on two major, and bipolar, factors that affect leadership style. These factors were originally given the labels, initiating structure (task related) and consideration (relationship related). *Consideration* is "the degree to which the supervisor shows concern, understanding, warmth, and sympathy for the feelings and opinions of his subordinates, and the degree to which he is considerate of their needs and welfare and willing to explain his actions. *Initiation of structure* subsumes behaviors that are related to the assignment of roles and tasks within the group, scheduling work assignments, defining goals, setting work procedures and standards, and evaluating the work of subordinates" (Fiedler, 1974, p. 48).

Leaders who function within a bureaucratic setting must balance their needs with the expectations of the institution. The need for accomplishment of tasks and the development of relationships varies in different people and is influenced by the setting. Each of the three theories described below projects a different view of the relationship between style (as determined by task and relationship orientation) and leader effectiveness.

Blake and Mouton's Managerial Grid

Blake and Mouton took two leadership factors, concern for production and concern for other persons, and developed a grid of possible combinations. The possible interactions were considered possible leadership styles.

The grid adapted for nursing is shown in Figure 14-1. The horizontal axis indicates concern for production of hospital services. The vertical axis indicates concern for staff members as people. Each is a 9-point scale, with 1 representing a minimum concern, 5 symbolizing an intermediate degree of concern, and 9 representing maximum concern. There are 81 possible combinations represented on the grid, each of which "is a theory about how the leader thinks about the relationship between the care given patients and the staff responsible for giving the care" (Blake *et al*, 1981, p. 3).

The theories in the corners are the most distinctive theories and the ones seen most often in practice. In the lower right corner is the style of a 9,1 oriented nurse with high concern for delivering hospital services (9) coupled with little or no concern for staff as individual persons with thoughts or feelings (1). In the upper left corner is the 1,9 oriented theory, where a minimum concern for administering hospital services is joined with a maximum concern for staff nurses and other hospital personnel. In the lower left corner is the 1,1 oriented strategy where concern for both services and staff are at a low ebb. In the upper right corner is the 9,9 oriented position. This couples high concern for delivery of services with high concern for staff as individuals.

Blake and Mouton believe that it is possible for a person to change leadership style. However, they believe that regardless of the situation, the 9,9 style of leader-

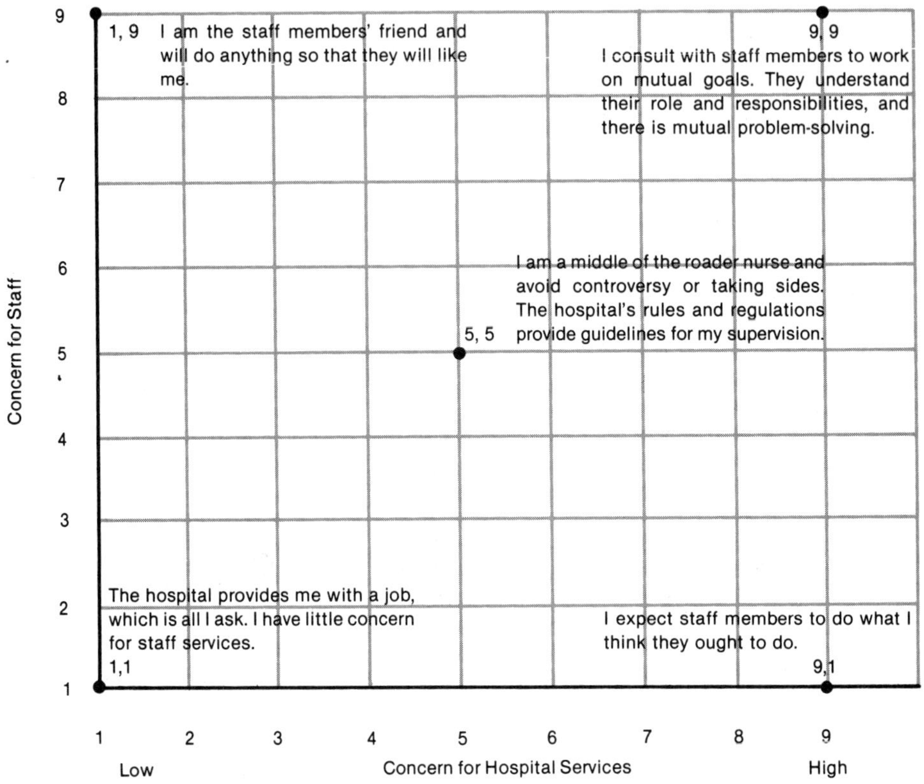
1, 9 I am the staff members' friend and will do anything so that they will like me.
9, 9 I consult with staff members to work on mutual goals. They understand their role and responsibilities, and there is mutual problem-solving.
I am a middle of the roader nurse and avoid controversy or taking sides. The hospital's rules and regulations provide guidelines for my supervision.
5, 5
The hospital provides me with a job, which is all I ask. I have little concern for staff services.
1,1
I expect staff members to do what I think they ought to do.
9,1
Concern for Staff
1
2
3
4
5
6
7
8
9
Low
Concern for Hospital Services
High

Figure 14–1. The nurse administrator grid (Blake R, Mouton J, Tapper M: Grid Approaches for Managerial Leadership in Nursing, p 2. St Louis, CV Mosby, 1981. Used with permission)

ship is the best, and the one for which everyone should strive. The high valuing of hospital goals as well as staff needs is certainly desirable. However, this theory does not provide guidance for the situation when one or the other concern must take precedence.

Hersey and Blanchard's Life Cycle Theory

Hersey and Blanchard also believe that "no one leadership behavior or style is effective in every situation. The forces within the leader, the group members, and the situation determine which leadership style a leader uses" (Bernhard and Walsh, 1981, p. 58).

Two factors of leader behavior are described. *Task behavior* is "the extent to which a leader organizes and defines the roles of individuals and members of her group by explaining what activities each is to do as well as when, where, and how tasks are to be accomplished. It is further characterized by the extent to which a leader defines patterns of organization, formalizes channels of communication, and specifies ways of getting jobs accomplished" (Hersey et al, 1976, p. 18). *Relationship behavior* is "the extent to which a leader engages in personal relationships with individuals or members of her group; the amount of socioemotional support and psychologic strokes provided by the leader as well as the extent to which the leader engages in interpersonal communications and facilitating behaviors" (Hersey et al, 1976, p. 18).

Task and relationship behavior can be plotted on two separate axes similiar to the Blake grid, as shown in Figure 14-2. The figure demonstrates relationships among:

1. The amount of direction (task behavior) a leader gives.
2. The amount of socioemotional support (relationship behavior) a leader provides.
3. The maturity of her followers or group. Maturity, which is determined in terms of a specific task, is related to the capacity of the group to set attainable goals, their achievement motivation, willingness and ability to take responsibility, and their education and experience (Hersey et al, 1976, p. 19).

The life cycle theory implies that "the difference between the effective and the ineffective (leadership) styles is often not the actual behavior of the leader, but the appropriateness of this behavior to the situation in which it is used" (Hersey et al, 1976, p. 18). Hersey et al believe that "when working with people who are low in maturity in terms of accomplishing a specific task, a high task style (quadrant 1) has the highest probability of success; whereas in dealing with people who are of average maturity on a task, moderate structure and moderate-to-high socioemotional style (quadrants 2 and 3) appear to be the most appropriate; and a low task and

Quadrant 3 High relationship and low task	Quadrant 2 High task and high relationship
Quadrant 4 Low task and low relationship	Quadrant 1 High task and low relationship

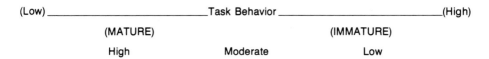

(Low) _____Task Behavior_____(High)

    (MATURE)   (IMMATURE)

    High   Moderate   Low

Figure 14-2. Life cycle theory: effective styles. (Hersey P, Blanchard KH, LaMonica EL: A situational approach to supervision. Superv Nurs 5:20, May 1976. Used with permission)

low relationship style (quadrant 4) has the highest probability of success working with people of high task maturity" (Hersey, et al, 1976, p. 19).

The concept of task maturity is unique to Hersey and Blanchard, and offers a rationale for alteration of leadership style in relationship to the capacities of the client. They suggest that successful leaders are those who can adapt their behavior so that it is appropriate to the unique demands of each situation.

The Reddin 3D Theory of Leader Effectiveness

Reddin believes that there are four basic styles of leader behavior, again based on the degree of emphasis on orientation to tasks (TO) or orientation to relationships (RO). Since any of these styles could be effective in certain situations and ineffective in others, he divided each basic style into a more effective equivalent and a less effective equivalent, resulting in eight managerial styles (Fig. 14-3). The eight leadership styles are defined in Table 14–1 (Reddin, 1970, pp.41–43).

The *executive* is a leader who uses a high-task orientation and a high relationships orientation in a situation where such behavior is appropriate. This leader is more effective, perceived as a good motivating force who sets high standards, treats everyone somewhat differently, and prefers team management.

The *compromiser* is a leader who uses a high-task orientation and a high relationships orientation in a situation that requires a high orientation to only one or neither. This leader is less effective, is perceived as a poor decision-maker, as one who allows various pressures in the situation to influence him too much, and as avoiding or minimizing immediate pressures and problems rather than maximizing long-term production.

The *benevolent autocrat* is a leader who uses a high-task orientation and a low relationships orientation in a situation where such behavior is appropriate. This leader is more effective, and is perceived as knowing what he wants and how to get it without causing resentment.

The *autocrat* is a leader who uses high-task orientation and a low relationship orientation in a situation where such behavior is inappropriate. This leader is less effective, perceived as having no confidence in others, as unpleasant, and as interested only in the immediate task.

The *developer* is a leader who uses high relationships orientation and a low-task orientation in a situation where such behavior is appropriate. This leader is more effective, perceived as having implicit trust in people and as being primarily concerned with developing them as individuals.

The *missionary* is a leader who uses high relationships orientation and a low-task

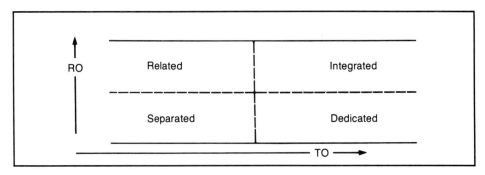

Figure 14–3. Four basic styles of leader behavior. (Reddin WJ: Managerial Effectiveness, p 12. McGraw-Hill, 1970. Reproduced with permission of the publisher)

TABLE 14–1.   Eight Leadership Styles Derived From the Four Basic Styles Used
Effectively and Ineffectively

When Used Inappropriately and Therefore Less Effectively	Basic style	When Used Appropriately and Therefore More Effectively
Compromiser	Integrated	Executive
Deserter	Separated	Bureaucat
Autocrat	Dedicated	Benevolent Autocrat
Missionary	Related	Developer

Reddin WJ: Managerial Effectiveness, New York, p 40. McGraw-Hill, 1970. Reproduced
with permission of the publisher)

orientation in a situation where such behavior is inappropriate. This leader is less
effective and is perceived as being primarily interested in harmony.

The *bureaucrat* is a leader who uses low-task orientation and a low relationships
orientation in a situation where such behavior is appropriate. This leader is effective, perceived as being primarily interested in rules and procedures for their own
sake, as wanting to control the situation by their use, and as conscientious.

The *deserter* is a leader who uses low-task orientation and a low relationships orientation in a situation where such behavior is inappropriate. This leader is less effective and is perceived as uninvolved and passive or negative.

"Managerial style, with its connotations of effectiveness, simply cannot be defined solely with reference to behavior. It always must be defined with reference to
the demands of the situation" (Reddin, 1970, p. 44). Reddin, like Hersey and
Blanchard, believes that an individual must be flexible and match the appropriate
behavior to the situation.

In summary, more leader activity, regardless of style, is usually associated with
more satisfaction and effectiveness. Participative leadership enhances decision quality and is more satisfying, but it may be less conductive to productivity than directive leadership (Bass, 1981, p. 324). It has been shown that the "best" leadership
style "tends to depend on the leader's personal characteristics as well as situational
contingencies such as characteristics of the followers and the organization and task
goals and constraints within which the leadership occurs" (Bass, 1981, p. 332).
Thus, from a consideration primarily of the leader's style of behavior, the emphasis
has shifted to theories that consider the interaction between the leader and the environment within which the leader functions. Three examples of these so-called situational theories are described below.

Situational Theories

Fiedler's Contingency Theory

"The performance of a group is contingent upon both the motivational system
of the leader and the degree to which the leader has control and influence in a particular situation, the 'situational favorableness' " (Fiedler, 1974, p. 73). Fiedler
identifies three major variables that contribute to a leader's influence and control:
(1) interpersonal relations between the leader and followers (follower's acceptance

of leader), (2) structure of the task and the degree to which tasks are clear cut, and have unambiguous goals and procedures, and (3) formal authority of position (ability to punish or reward members). "The interpersonal relationship between the leader and his group members is likely to be the most important single variable which determines his power and influence. . . . The degree to which the task requirements are spelled out determines in large part the leader's authority to give instructions and to evaluate performance" (Fiedler, 1974, pp. 64, 66). These variables contribute to the situational favorableness. Fiedler believes that a leader's effectiveness varies, depending on "situational favorableness." He believes that it is very difficult for an individual to change leadership style, since it is so strongly influenced by the leader's personality. Therefore, he stresses changing elements of the situation such as leader–member relationships or the structure of tasks in order to increase the effectiveness of the leader in a particular situation.

Fiedler has developed an instrument to assess the motivational system of the leader, an index of the leader's reactions to her least preferred co-worker (LPC). "LPC is an index of a motivational hierarchy, or of behavioral preferences, implying that some goals are more important to the individual than others" (Fiedler, 1974, p. 74). According to Fiedler a leader with a high LPC perceives her least preferred co-worker in a more favorable, more differentiated manner, has as a basic goal to be engaged in relationships, and has secondary goals of status and esteem. In contrast the leader with a low LPC rating has a basic goal to accomplish the task. Her self-esteem is derived from achievement.

Fiedler uses the LPC rating of the leader to predict leadership effectiveness in a particular type of situation. "Leadership effectiveness depends upon the leader's style of interacting with his group members and the favorableness of the group-task situation. Specifically, low LPC (least preferred co-worker) leaders who are primarily task-motivated perform best under conditions that are very favorable or very unfavorable for them. Relationship-motivated leaders perform best under conditions that are of moderate favorableness" (Fiedler, 1974, p. 81).

This theory has received a great deal of criticism because of questions about what the LPC is really measuring. In general, however, Fiedler's theory is helpful in emphasizing the importance of the interaction between the leader and the situation in determining leader effectiveness.

Path-Goal Theory

Path-goal theory is an interpretation of motivation theory as applied to leadership. The theory is based on the belief that "the force on an individual to engage in a specific behavior is a function of his expectations that the behavior will result in a specific outcome, and . . . personal satisfaction or utility that he derives from the outcome" (House, 1971, p. 322). In other words, this theory is concerned with how the nature of the task affects whether initiation of structure, consideration, or both affects satisfaction and effectiveness.

It is assumed that individuals are basically goal-directed and that they will attempt to behave in a way that they perceive will lead to their goals. The leader acts to identify the best "path" to the desired goal, and helps to facilitate that path. Actions of the leader might include providing support, removing obstacles in the way of completing the task, and increasing personal payoffs for goal achievement. The focus is on the leader to modify her behavior and accomodate to the scope of the goal desired and the follower's expectations and perceptions. This theory has implications for leadership behavior, especially when actions are combined with approaches suggested by other situational theories.

One limitation of path–goal theory, however, is that it tends to consider interactions between the leader and the situation as if "the situation" were composed of only one variable, client motivation. In most situations a variety of variable interactions may affect the leadership process.

At the present time there is no one theory that is predictive for leadership effectiveness in a variety of situations. Effective nursing leadership requires an eclectic choice of principles from a number of different theories. Client motivation and experience are two inputs that can affect the system. In addition the organization may have expectations for task achievement (organizational input). The leader who can modify her style in relation to the other system inputs, has the greatest potential for achieving effectiveness and client satisfaction. The development of a systems approach that considers the multiple inputs and influences that may affect the nurse-client interaction, offers the best hope for predictive theory for nursing leadership.

THE NURSE AS A LEADER

"Effective leadership is a learned process" (Douglass and Bevis, 1983, p. 340). It requires an understanding of the needs and goals that motivate people, the cognitive ability to use the leadership process, and the interpersonal ability to influence others.

Components of Leadership

Motivation

A number of factors may motivate an individual at any point in time. Past experiences and behavior, current psychologic and physiologic needs, and goals for the future may all have an influence. In addition, the family and the work place hold certain expectations of the individual that affect his motivation and behavior. Too often the health professional attempts to impose goals and behavior on the client without assessing or appreciating the client's motivation. Effective leadership, on the other hand, is based on intervention to meet the *the client's* goals and uses strategies based on *the client's* motivation. This philosophy requires thorough assessment and planning with the client before intervention strategies are applied.

This philosophy can also be applied when working with groups of colleagues within an institutional setting. In this case, the assessment process must include identification of organizational goals in addition to those of the individual members of the group. This is a more complex situation than the one that focuses on individual client change. However, the process remains the same. The likelihood of success in leadership is enhanced when the needs of followers are met at the same time that incentives are provided to motivate them to work toward goals of the leader or the organization.

Authority

Authority has been defined as "the right to take actions" (Claus and Bailey, 1977, p. 11), or, "the right to give commands, enforce laws, or exact obedience" (Douglass and Bevis, 1983, p. 340). However, authority is based on an interactional relationship, and can only be exercised effectively if it is accepted by subordinates or followers. The follower is expected to indicate acceptance of the leader's authority by complying with her wishes or instructions.

Formal authority is a constant right that is vested in a position. This type of authority is associated with status and is conferred by the organization within which the individual is functioning. For example, a supervisor (or in some cases a head nurse) has the authority to assign work times for the staff working on "her" units. This is a legitimate use of authority, and subordinates are expected to conform. *Functional* authority on the other hand, is based on personal qualities. It is "comprised of elements related to job responsibilities and areas of competence" (Yura *et al*, 1981, p. 41). For example, a primary nurse has the authority to design plans of care with certain assigned patients. Other nurses will accept that authority if they believe that she is competent. Some of the qualities that might comprise functional authority include effective problem-solving and decision-making, actions based on knowledge and relevant information, effective channels of communication, a high degree of creativity, effective use of managerial and human relations processes, and recognition of the need for personal and professional growth (Claus and Bailey, 1977, pp. 11–12).

Communication

The nurse–leader is also the coordinator of communication. Leadership takes place through a relationship between the nurse and the client. "The interaction between the nurse–leader and an individual client is a specific type of relationship, often called a therapeutic relationship. . . . The interaction between the nurse–leader and another member of the health care organization is also a specific type of relationship, ideally a collaborative relationship" (Bernhard and Walsh, 1981, p. 65). Essential in both types of relationships is the ability to establish open communication based on mutual trust. (See Chapter 13, "Communication and Helping Relationships").

Influence

"Authority implies the right to make decisions affecting the behavior of others. . . . Influence indicates a mutual and reciprocal relationship affecting the behavior of those to be influenced. . . . The individual using influence may advise, suggest, discuss, persuade, or propagandize, but he does not exercise authority. He affects the behavior of another indirectly" (Yura *et al*, 1981, pp. 66–67).

Nursing leadership was defined earlier in this chapter as a process of interpersonal influence through which a client is assisted in the establishment and achievement of goals toward improved well-being. Through a relationship between the nurse and the individual or group client, goals toward improved health and a process for their achievement are negotiated. The nurse assumes leadership by initiating, facilitating, and successfully terminating her influence in the process. A number of behaviors that are needed for effective leadership are discussed in the next section.

Nursing Leadership Behaviors

Demonstrating Expertise in the Nursing Process

Yura *et al* (1981, p. 96) identify four behaviors that are related to demonstrating expertise in the nursing process: deciding, relating, influencing, and facilitating, as diagrammed in Figure 14–4.

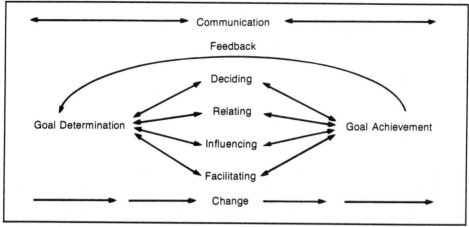

Figure 14–4. Nursing leadership process. (Yura H, Ozimek D, Walsh MB: Nursing Leadership: Theory and Process, p 97. New York, Appleton-Century-Crofts, 1981. Used with permission of the publisher)

Decision-making requires a sound basis of knowledge and skills for making judgements; relating is based on trust and respect; influencing aims to establish and implement plans; and facilitating is based on intellectual and interpersonal skills rather than personality alone. These behaviors are appropriate during all phases of the nursing process.

Assessing. The variables that should be assessed are related to the client, the nurse–client relationship, and the environmental situation. Some of the factors that must be considered include:

1. The status and potential for health of the client
2. The client's health goals
3. Strengths and weaknesses of the client in achieving his health goals
4. Client needs
5. Available resources (including significant others)
6. Goals of the nurse and their congruence with the client's goals
7. Knowledge and skill of the nurse relative to the client's goals
8. Openness and adequacy of communication between the client, nurse, and significant others
9. Environmental influences that impact on the situation.

A therapeutic relationship based on trust and respect between the client and the nurse will provide the vehicle for influencing and facilitating desired client behaviors. Relating, a critical element in communication, is used to initiate and maintain an appropriate flow of information. Deciding, an application of knowledge and judgement, is used to analyze and organize data as they are collected, which moves the process into the planning phase.

Planning. The essence of the planning phase is to negotiate jointly agreed-upon goals with the client and appropriate strategies to accomplish the goals. These purposes require judgement and decision-making ability (deciding), ability to influence the client toward goals that promote well-being, ability to facilitate the planning process through the therapeutic relationship, and communication with professional colleagues and client support systems (relating). Once a plan is agreed upon, elements of the intervention phase begin.

Intervening. Leadership during the intervention phase of the nursing process is based on all four of the interpersonal and cognitive skills. The nurse must be able to maintain a helping relationship with the client, have the knowledge and skills needed to implement the planned strategies, and adapt her behavior on the basis of responses from the client or unexpected influences from the environment. The use of legitimate authority may be appropriate, but the nurse's "will" should not be imposed. Rather, the judicious use of rewards (and limited use of punishments) should be an incentive to help the client continue toward the agreed-upon goal(s).

Evaluating. Yura *et al* (1981, pp. 188–198) suggest a number of criteria for evaluation of nursing leadership. A few pertinent questions are indicated below:

1. Does the leader demonstrate a mastery of the nursing process?
2. Does the leader demonstrate sensitivity to the impact of self on others, leading to effective use of self?
3. Does the leader demonstrate mastery in the use and determination of verbal and nonverbal communication?
4. Can the leader initiate, continue, and terminate effective relationships?
5. Can the leader effectively modify her own behavior and that of others?
6. Can the leader delegate action to be accomplished by selected knowledgeable persons?
7. Is the leader able to develop resources as needed to facilitate action?
8. Does the leader demonstrate accountability and morality in application of the leadership process?

Leadership behaviors of relating, deciding, influencing, and facilitating are used to demonstrate expertise in the application of the nursing process. These behaviors assist the nurse to obtain and share knowledge, set priorities among goals mutually with the client, and determine, implement, and evaluate strategies for accomplishing the mutually agreed-upon goals including providing teaching-learning experiences that are appropriate to the client's capacity and level of well-being.

Collaborating with Other Health Professionals

Professionals may base their expectations of patients and of health team members on stereotypes reflecting lack of knowledge and openness to experience. For example, the physician may expect a compliant nurse who is respectful of his authority, and consequently become angry if the nurse demonstrates independent judgement. The nurse may expect the physician to be aloof and demeaning, and be threatened if he seeks collaborative decision-making. The patient is often treated as the passive object of care rather than as a participant in decision-making. Stereotypic expectations of health professionals are also held by the patient, who may expect a task orientation (tempered by kindness) from the nurse, and a relationship orientation (while others carry out his orders) from the physician.

Professionals may also have a great deal of difficulty dealing with the conflicting demands of accomplishing tasks while maintaining rewarding and effective relationships. Some professionals may opt to accomplish the demands of the job, and assume a distant manner to avoid time-consuming relationships.

True collaboration can only be accomplished when there is a willingness to risk open communication and avoid sterotypic actions. Self-confidence provides a basis for respect for the abilities of others. Only when no one is threatened can people learn and grown through dialogue and debate. Mutuality, applied to relationships between health team members as well as between the client and individual members of the team, provides the foundation for the blending of unique contributions from all participants toward improvement of client well-being.

Coordinating and Managing Conflict

Most nurses work in bureaucratic settings. Conflict is intrinsic in the various expectations inherent in the work situation. The organization holds expectations that are related to efficient and cost-effective task accomplishment. The nurse holds expectations that are related to personal characteristics, role socialization, and reflected appraisals from co-workers and supervisors. These reflected appraisals may be supportive of the desires and strengths of the individual nurse or they may provoke additional pressure on areas of weakness or lack of confidence. Many nurses are dedicated to trying to help others, and face guilt if the ideal is not reached. The nurse may react by working harder and harder, perhaps even substituting work for a satisfying social life. Many of these factors can lead to burnout.

"Factors contributing to burnout include conflict between needs and accomplishment, unrealistic dedication, use of work as a substitute for a satisfying personal life, an authoritarian management style, and inability to delegate authority and responsibility and to say no to unreasonable demands" (Clark, 1982, p. 91). Some desirable approaches to the prevention or alleviation of burnout include

1. Opening up communication with oneself and others
2. Ensuring adequate nutritional intake
3. Relaxing
4. Finding physical outlets for stress
5. Establishing peer and mentor support systems
6. Clearly defining responsibilities in relationship to peers and subordinates
7. Decreasing workload through negotiation and redistribution
8. Learning how to say no when necessary or desirable
9. Cutting down on nonproductive activities
10. Developing contingency plans
11. Setting realistic goals that are likely to result in success (Clark, 1982)

Using and Delegating Authority

Nurses have traditionally been more comfortable with formal authority than with authority derived from personal qualities. This dependance on the trappings of position (*e.g.,* starched uniform, cap with stripes) and hierarchy (*e.g.,* "orders" and lines of command) are a legacy from the earliest days of organized nursing. Undue reliance on chain of command encourages lack of independent responsibility and risk taking and perpetuates the image of the nurse as dependent on the orders of others (even other nurses). The nurse may then, in turn, treat the client as a subject of formal authority, by demanding compliance with her "orders." The inappropriate use of authority is an attempted use of power to control the behavior of others.

Functional authority, on the other hand, is based on competence that is recognized and respected by clients, peers, and colleagues. Functional authority provides expert and legitimate power. It leads to creative and highly professional practice and personal growth by the individual, and contributes to the evolving professionalism of nursing.

Using Power

We have taken the position that leadership in promoting change in client behavior is best accomplished by appropriate use of authority and influence, rather than through application of power. The use of power to affect change in variables affecting the profession is discussed in Chapter 17, "Contributor to the Profession Role."

Acknowledging Accountability and Responsibility

Burns insists that the leader must be accountable not only for her own actions and those of her followers, but also for maintaining a morally based value system. "The ultimate test of moral leadership is its capacity to transcend the claims of the multiplicity of everyday wants and needs and expectations, to respond to the higher levels of moral development, and to relate leadership behavior—its roles, choices, style, commitments—to a set of reasoned, relatively explicit, conscious values" (Burns, 1978, p. 46).

This charge obligates the nurse to a moral as well as a cognitive evaluation of desired goals and appropriate strategies for their accomplishment. It requires that the nurse–leader maintain full disclosure and open communication with clients and co-workers. It also implies that there may be situations where the nurse may have to refuse involvement because of her moral convictions.

SUMMARY

Effective nursing leadership is critically needed at all system levels. Through expert and ethical use of leadership behaviors in conjunction with nursing and change processes, clients can be assisted toward the achievement of their goals for improved health.

REFERENCES

Bass BM: Stogdill's Handbook of Leadership. New York, The Free Press, 1981

Blake R, Mouton J, Tapper M: Grid Approaches for Managerial Leadership in Nursing. St Louis, CV Mosby, 1981

Bernhard LA, Walsh M: Leadership: The Key to the Professionalization of Nursing. New York, McGraw-Hill Book, 1981

Burns JM: Leadership. New York, Harper Colophon Books, 1978

Clark CC: Burnout: Assessment and intervention. In McConnell EA (ed): Burnout in the Nursing Profession. St Louis. CV Mosby, 1982

Claus KE, Bailey JT: Power and Influence in Health Care. St Louis, CV Mosby, 1977

Douglass LM, Bevis EO: Nursing Management and Leadership in Action. St Louis, CV Mosby, 1983

Epstein C: The Nurse Leader: Philosophy and Practice. Reston, Reston Publishing, 1982

Fiedler FE: Leadership and Effective Mangement. Glenview, Scott, Foresman, 1974

Hersey P, Blanchard KH, LaMonica EL: A situational approach to supervision. Superv Nurs 7:17–20, May 1976

House RJ: A path-goal theory or leader effectiveness. Adm Sc Quar 16:321–338, September 1971

Lewin K, Lippit R, White RK: Patterns of Aggressive Behavior in Experimentally Created "Social Climates." In Harriman PL (ed): Twentieth Century Psychology. New York, The Philosophical Library, 1946

Marriner A: Theories of leadership. Nurs Leader 1:13–17, December 1978

Moloney MM: Leadership in Nursing: Theories, Strategies, Action. St Louis, CV Mosby, 1979

Reddin WJ: Managerial Effectiveness. New York, McGraw-Hill, 1970

Yura H, Ozimek D, Walsh MB: Nursing Leadership: Theory and Process. New York, Appleton-Century-Crofts, 1981

Chapter 15

The Professional Nurse
as Change Agent

THOUGHT QUESTIONS

1. How do Lippitt's phases of change relate to the nursing process?
2. How does the classical design theory as applied to hospitals affect professional nursing practice?
3. What is meant by the change agent role?
4. What factors affect the choice of strategies for change?

Change is all around us. Some changes, like the seasons of the year, or the cycle of light and dark, are completely predictable. Other changes, like the phenomena of the weather, or unexpected events, appear to be more random and unpredictable. People respond to change in different ways. Some people seem to seek frequent changes and thrive on the unexpected, while others are most comfortable when daily activities are consistent and controllable. Readiness for change can vary from day to day, and in response to how fast it seems that change is occurring. For example, a person may feel bored or restless when daily events seem predictable. However, when changes occur very rapidly the person may show signs of stress and resistance.

As a change agent the professional nurse works with the client to identify when and what change is needed, and helps to facilitate desired change to promote better health. This chapter examines types of change and theories that attempt to explain how change occurs. The content describes ways that people respond to change, factors that affect resistance to change, and strategies that can facilitate desired change in the health of clients.

TYPES OF CHANGE

Haphazard

There are a number of different kinds of change. Haphazard change is generally random and completely unpredictable. An example of this kind of change is the movement of a tornado. It is impossible at this time to anticipate where, when, or even whether it will touch down on land.

Spontaneous

Spontaneous change occurs in response to natural, uncontrollable events. For example, a body cell may change spontaneously in what is called a mutation. Although the elements leading to spontaneous change are understood and predictable, some degree of the timing of the change is unpredictable, as is the way that the altered cell will function. Nursing intervention may not be possible for haphazard or spontaneous change because of their unpredictability.

Developmental

In developmental change one stage or phase leads into another in a more or less orderly fashion. The stages are sequential and have various identifiable characteristics. Many theorists believe that people grow through developmental change. The process of maturing is viewed as a succession of sequential stages that are predictable and characteristic. Since developmental stages occur naturally, the role of the nurse is to help the client to modify his response to the change, and to assume control over the direction of developmental changes. (For more information about stages of development, see Chapter 7, "Theories as a Basis for Practice.")

Planned

The last type of change is planned change. Planned change "results from deliberate and conscious actions taken to adjust the operations of a given system to meet the demands of the situation" (Lancaster and Lancaster, 1982, p. 6). Thus, planned change is deliberate and is entered into with conscious intent. The nurse and the client mutually identify areas where change is desired and/or needed and then proceed to implement and evaluate the change.

DEFINITIONS

Change

Change has been defined as "the relearning on the part of an individual or group (1) in response to newly perceived requirements of a given situation requiring action, and (2) which results in a change in the structure and/or functioning of social systems" (Zaltman and Duncan, 1977, p. 10). The emphasis on modification of a system is reflected in the definition of *planned change* as an "intended, designed or purposive attempt by an individual, group, organization, or larger social system to influence directly the status quo of itself, another organism, or a situation" (Lippitt, 1973, p. 37).

Planned change involves a deliberate process that has direction. The purpose is the improved functioning of the system. Any change causes a lack of equilibrium that affects the entire system. In the process of establishing a new equilibrium, the system may have to establish new behaviors, attitudes, and/or relationships. Thus, any planned change is a complex intervention that requires knowledge, anticipation of consequences, and skillful action on the part of the nurse acting as an agent of change.

THEORETICAL FRAMEWORKS _____

Individual and Group Change

Developmental Model

There are two basic models of change. The developmental model assumes that goal-directed growth and change is natural. The model is concerned with the identification of successive phases or stages and with the turning points or critical events that characterize change. In this model the agent of change operates from outside the system to diagnose any existing blockages to change, and to help shape the client's response. The agent then "gets out of the way" of the change forces, and allows change to occur (Chin, 1976, p. 101).

Systems Model

The systems model emphasizes stability of the system, which is derived from integration or equilibrium of the components of the system. Tensions and conflict create structural stress that must be resolved. Emphasis is placed on the organization, interaction, interdependency, and integration of the parts and elements. In this model the agent of change begins as an outsider to the system, but then moves into the system through a relationship with the client. Interventions either reduce tension in order to facilitate restoration of equilibrium, or increase tensions and conflict in order to facilitate creativity, innovation, and social change. Particular emphasis is placed on interdependent interaction between the change agent and the client (Chin, 1976, pp. 100–101).

Lewin's Theory. Lewin's theory of planned change fits within a systems model. He described a process consisting of three aspects: "unfreezing, (if necessary), the present level L1, moving to the new level L2, and freezing group life on the new level. Since any level is determined by a force field, permanency implies that the new force field is made relatively secure against change" (Lewin, 1951, pp. 228–229).

Schein's Theory. Schein (1969) later described Lewin's three steps as unfreezing, changing, and refreezing.

Unfreezing refers to the processes involved in overcoming resistance to change. In most people there are a number of personal and social factors that help to stabilize existing behaviors and beliefs. Thus, when change is needed often the person must be motivated to change. The client must recognize and accept the need or benefit of a change. Changing refers to the processes that lead to new behaviors and a cognitive redefinition. This is the stage that focuses on the actual change. Refreezing refers to the ways in which the new patterns become stabilized and integrated into the person's cognitive and social structures. In this stage, reinforcement, through positive feedback, encouragement, and constructive criticism can be a driving force to facilitate the change. However, attention must also be paid to restraining forces that might impede the change cycle. The change is more likely to persist if driving forces can be added or opposing ones diminished (Zaltman, 1973; Lancaster and Lancaster, 1982).

Lippitt's Theory. While Lewin described three stages of planned change, Lippitt's theory (1973, p. 52) of planned change includes seven phases (Table 15-1).

TABLE 15–1.   Comparison Between Lewin and Lippitt's Change Phases and the Nursing Process

Lewin	Lippitt	Nursing Process
Unfreezing	1. Diagnosis of the problem	Assessing
	2. Assessment of motivation and capacity for change	
	3. Assessment of change agent's motivation and resources	
	4. Selecting progressive change objectives	
Moving to a new level	5. Choosing the appropriate role of the change agent	Planning
	6. Maintenance of the change once it has been started	Intervening
Refreezing	7. Termination of a helping relationship	Evaluating

Phase I—Diagnosis of the Problem.   In phase I the change agent has the task of identifying and diagnosing any existing or potential problems. Through assessment of the client, the client's significant others, and the environment, data are collected. These data are then shared for validation with the client and key people in the situation. The client must share the nurses' perception that a problem exists and that change is desirable, or the change process will not be successful.

If a client does not recognize the existence of a need, the nurse should identify the perceived problem and needed change. The client will be influenced by his perception about his ability to use a particular change, about the degree of commitment that will be required, and by the degree of control he will have over the change process. These factors may all selectively influence a client's perception and retention of the information shared with him. The nurse is unlikely to be successful if she tries to impose her opinion on the client. Rather, the major goals in this phase should be to create or stimulate perception of a problem and solution, and to shape the client's perceptions in a way that the change agent believes to be desirable.

Phase II—Assessment of the Motivation and Capacity for Change.   People usually have some resistance to change. Habits are behaviors that have become comfortable, and thus the anticipation of change creates discomfort. A person is more likely to seek or be open to change if he feels deprived by a felt unmet need and if he perceives control over the change process. Thus, the nurse should try to actively encourage the client to be concerned about solving his problem.

Six categories of people have been identified based on their readiness to accept change. The first group, the innovators, are venturesome and curious. They are usually the "pacesetters," eager and enthusiastic about new experiences. The second group are the early adopters of change. They are respectable, well-established members of their social group, and often sought for guidance. They may demonstrate moderate enthusiasm for the change, according to the readiness of the group. The third group are the early-majority adopters. These people are deliberate in their actions, and accept change before most people. They are often willing and dedicated to the change, but are rarely leaders. Late-majority adopters, the fourth group, are skeptical and need pressure from their peers to accept change. They cannot be counted on for support although they are not active dissidents. Laggards, however, in group five, are suspicious of change and discourage others from participating. They are often traditionalists, negative, and socially isolated from the social group. Rejectors, in group six, openly reject the change and encourage others to do so also (Rogers and Shoemaker, 1971, pp. 183–185). "Change can be advanced and resistance minimized by identifying and soliciting the support of the active acceptors, locating and neutralizing the active rejectors, and persuading the uncommitted to accept the change" (Lancaster and Lancaster, 1982, p. 14).

Social support can be very helpful in increasing motivation for change. The person is much more likely to act in a way that is consistent if there is congruence between the person's attitudes and social support. A client may seek legitimation, or reinforcement for an action that is being considered. The nurse can demonstrate the social acceptability (legitimacy) of a proposed change by bringing the client into contact with others who have successfully adopted the change.

Phase III—Assessment of Change Agent's Motivation and Resources. The change process is often time consuming and difficult, and requires commitment on the part of the nurse and client. Personal resources are an important aspect for consideration. The nurse must have the appropriate knowledges and skills to follow through until the change is successfully implemented. She also must have a relationship with the client that is based on trust and respect. She must be aware also of her personal motivation for wanting to promote a particular change. Is her motivation genuine concern for the well-being of the client, or is she influenced by desire for recognition, power, or possibly change simply for the sake of change?

Resources are also crucial elements for assessment. A particular modification may be needed and highly desirable, but it may not be feasible because of the lack of adequate supplies, personnel, money, or time. For example, a desired modification in the scheduling of hospital staff may not be feasible because of inadequate staffing on one or more shifts. A change in a client's job in order to reduce stress may not be possible if the client's family is dependent on the income from the present position.

Phase IV—Selecting Progressive Change Objectives. The phases of the change process to this point have been concerned with decision-making about whether or not a particular change is needed, desired, and feasible. At this point the decision-making shifts to consideration of how to implement the specific change.

A strategy composed of steps to be taken, by whom, and according to what timetable must be established. This plan should set specific goals, with deadlines that establish the time by which the objectives should be achieved. It also may be desirable to design a trial period to test the proposed plans. At the end of the trial period, the goals, methods, and timetable can be reassessed and modified if necessary.

Phase V—Choosing an Appropriate Change Agent Role. Change strategies are actually implemented during this phase. The change agent may function in a variety of different ways, depending on the particular situation. In some cases she may function as an expert role model by demonstrating how a particular skill should be performed, or she may function as a teacher, group leader, caretaker, or catalyst. Frequently, the nurse change agent acts as a facilitator of change by promoting effective communications and helping to maintain the process toward the preset goals.

It is important that the nurse, the client, and others involved in the change process have the same expectations of each other's roles. If, for example, the client expects the nurse to do a procedure for him, and if the nurse perceives her role as that of a teacher and facilitator, it is obvious that there will be conflict and misunderstandings that could jeopardize the success of the project. The nurse needs to validate her perceptions frequently with the client in order to ensure that communications remain open.

Phase VI—Maintenance of the Change. Once the change has been implemented, it must be maintained. This is an especially delicate phase in the process. It takes time before the new procedure or process feels comfortable, and some people may wish to return to the "old ways." Expectations may be unrealistic, and it may appear that the desired outcomes are not being realized, when, in fact, they have not had sufficient time to be demonstrated. The change agent may act to support the change and to reenergize the client's commitment to continue the change.

It is helpful to guard against the desire to implement too much change too quickly. Each aspect of change must be assimilated and accepted before the new equilibrium allows the system to consider additional changes. If a large change appears to be needed, it may be desirable to break the change into smaller pieces for implementation.

Phase VII—Termination of the Helping Relationship. The client must be the one who actually maintains the change. The change agent must slowly withdraw from the situation, allowing the client to take over all aspects of the change.

At this point it will become clear if the client and key others have been involved fully in the process, and if they have the power and authority to maintain the change. Unless they are committed to the change, it will not succeed.

The change agent should keep the client informed about when the relationship will be terminated, and whether there will be any future relationship between the nurse and the client. Joint evaluation of the process and its outcomes is desirable before the relationship is terminated. Through joint assessment of the significance of the relationship, both the nurse and the client can focus on the strengths gained, rather than on a sense of loss at its termination. It may also be helpful to develop a written summary of the change project to help ensure its survival, and as a source of information for future reference.

Organizational Change

While Lewin and Lippitt's theories are applicable to both individual and group clients, there are additional theories that are particularly applicable to organizational change.

There are a number of conceptual models of organizations. One is that an organization is an autocracy. In this view, one person has primary knowledge and power, with others in a subordinate relationship. Another view is that of the organization as a bureaucracy. Here, control is through policy, which governs the behavior of hired assistants. Jobs are structured and efforts are compartmentalized.

Organizations may also be viewed as federations, which are voluntary associations of completely autonomous organizations. The recently revised structure of the American Nurses Association (ANA) is based on this view of federated state associations. There is also the egalitarian view, which emphasizes professional interdependency based on common ethics and free communications. This type of organization is often decentralized, with emphasis on the self-direction and self-discipline of the member. A final view is that of the organization as an interaction of component systems, adapting dynamically to change (Lippitt, 1973, pp. 276–284).

Classical Design Theory

The classical design theory is based on a view of the organization as a bureaucracy and on the assumption that there is one absolutely best way to organize to accomplish the goals of the organization. Basic concepts of this theory include:

1. Division of work—The primary goal, efficiency, can be increased by keeping limits on the amount of specialization allowed. Instead of concern with the functions best performed by individuals, this approach focuses on full use of categories of employees. The nurse, for example, would be expected to do clerical work and transport patients rather than employing other workers especially to do these tasks.
2. Hierarchy—Management is organized into levels. This creates a vertical pyramid of authority with a relatively small number of people responsible to the top administrator.
3. Unity of command—This concept is related to hierarchical organization. It means that no one individual should have more than one supervisor at any one time.
4. Span of control—This concept limits the number of people who report to any one administrator to the number that can effectively be managed.
5. Departmentalization—In order to facilitate an appropriate span of control within the hierarchy, people are organized into units based on function. For example, there might be a nursing service, a dietary service, and so forth. Within each department, the organization is hierarchical.
6. Comprehensive system of rules, procedures, and policies—This approach requires that all expectations are clearly understood and followed. As many eventualities as possible are covered by the rules and regulations that are usually written and available to each unit.

The classical design theory, which has been applied widely to hospitals, aims for efficiency of effort in order to reduce costs. However, several problems are created. Incentives for individual creativity and innovation are lost, and individuals may well be subordinated to the welfare of the organization. In addition, there is an inherent tendency toward order and the status quo, which reduces the flexibility to respond with needed change (Lippitt, 1973).

Systems Theory

As an alternative view, the systems theory focuses on the interdependency of the parts that make up the organization. The major types of input to the system of organizational behavior are the (1) environment, which presents constraints, demands and opportunities; (2) resources available to the organization; (3) history that explains key events and decisions that have an effect on current functioning; and (4) strategy, which is "the set of key decisions about the match of the organization's resources to the opportunities, constraints, and demands in the environment within the context of history" (Nadler, 1981, pp. 192–193).

The output of the system includes the performance of individuals and groups who contribute to the performance of the organization. All the parts of the system are interrelated, and change in any one component will affect all other components. The system aims for a state of balance, but it is capable of adjusting to change.

Nadler describes a process for organizational change based on the systems theory. His model involves assessment of the current state of the organization, design of the desired future state of the organization, and implementation of the plan in a transition state.

The first step for the change agent is to identify and surface dissatisfaction with the current state. If people are satisfied with the way things are, they will not be motivated to change. On the other hand, the greater the pain and dissatisfaction with the current state, the greater the motivation to change and the less the resistance to change. Thus, as action steps to motivate change, the agent may need to "unfreeze" the organization by making people receptive to change. Strategies may include creation of dissatisfaction with the status quo, building in participation in the change, giving participants time and the opportunity to disengage from the present state, and building in rewards for the desired behavior.

Success in the transition stage depends on a clearly developed and communicated image of the future. The change agent needs to make use of multiple and consistent leverage points to promote movement toward the desired outcomes. Consistency of sequence of structural changes is also important so that everyone involved in the process understands what is happening. It may be helpful to have a "transition manager," who takes care of the organizational arrangements. It is critical that key power groups are involved in the process and assure their support.

All of the preceding theories are concerned with processes to promote change despite resistance. The next area of content will examine the concept of resistance.

RESISTANCE

Resistance may be defined as "any conduct that serves to maintain the status quo in the face of pressure to alter the status quo" (Zaltman and Duncan, 1977, p. 63). It is not simply the lack of acceptance or the reverse of acceptance. It is active behavior whose goal is to prevent the proposed change from occurring.

A cycle of resistance in a situation of successful change has been proposed. This cycle has five stages. In the first (early) stage resistance may appear massive and undifferentiated. By the second stage the forces for and against the change can be identified. In the third stage resistance is mobilized to crush the proposal. The resistance is either overcome or the strength of the opposers is substantially reduced. By the fourth stage the supporters are in power with the others considered a nuisance. The fifth stage finds few adversaries, with these individuals isolated from the group. (Watson, 1973, pp. 118–119).

Cultural Factors

In order to deal more effectively with resistance, nurses need to understand factors from a number of areas. One such area is that of cultural barriers. The change agent may demonstrate cultural ethnocentrism. Without being consciously aware of it, the nurse may believe that her own cultural patterns are the best. Unless she is aware of this prejudice, she may try to change a client's behavior to conform to her own cultural beliefs regardless of how appropriate the new behavior may be in the client's culture. The particular change may be incompatible with a trait that is deeply imbedded in the client's culture. In addition, the relative values held by the change agent are not necessarily shared by the client. For example, the nurse might not understand the resistance of an Oriental family to the institutionalization of an aged member unless she were aware of the veneration of age in that culture.

Social Factors

Social barriers may also assume great importance. Many social groups maintain complex interdependencies, and reject outsiders. Many groups maintain customary and expected ways of behaving, called norms. Changes, especially those believed to be contradictory to norms, are best introduced by group decision so that change can occur throughout the entire system. The change agent also needs to be aware of the hierarchy of the group. If the group is stratified, change can be introduced with the assistance of those in power, but "grassroots" change is very difficult in such a system. Essential to any change is free communication, with mutual trust and supportive interpersonal relationships between the change agent and the group.

Organizational Factors

Organizational factors may also be powerful barriers. The proposed change may be perceived as a threat to power or influence. Change should be initiated with the support of the top power structure. Openness and potential for change are related to the perceived need for change. The resistance will be greater when both the need for change and the perception of openness to and potential for change are low. High need for change may create anxiety and lead to a perception that change is not possible. A supportive climate can reduce anxiety and increase the openness to change.

Psychologic Factors

Psychologic factors are major barriers to change. Most people need a certain degree of stability and security, and change presents unknowns that cause anxiety. People seek a comfortable level of stimulation, and then try to maintain it. Thus, conformity and commitment can be powerful forces working against change.

Change that is imposed (*e.g.,* illness) reduces the individual's sense of autonomy and self-control. There may also be lack of a common perception of the cause of a mutually perceived problem, leading to different ideas of how to remedy the situation. Lack of clarity about behaviors that are needed may also cause resistance.

People typically develop patterns for coping that may include "1) efforts to manipulate aspects of the external environment to facilitate goal achievement; 2) efforts to come to grips with inner conflicts that cannot be resolved in direct or conscious ways; 3) efforts to find meaning and order in the environment; 4) efforts to enhance one's self esteem and to actualize one's self concept; 5) efforts to relate one's self to important others in the environment" (Kelman and Warwick, 1973, p. 25).

Because of selective perception and retention people do not hear or remember things with which they disagree. In addition, familiar habits become comfortable and are preferred. Many people lean toward complacency, especially when a change is perceived as threatening.

Zaltman and Duncan have proposed a framework for the identification of forms of rejection of ideas for change (Table 15–2). An awareness of the reasons for particular responses can help the nurse plan specific activities to modify rejection of change by the client.

Avoiding Resistance

In view of these various sources of resistance, a critical step in facilitating change involves unfreezing, in Lewin's terms, or overcoming resistance, so that the client can be open to new patterns. Two broad categories of strategies might be feasible. One involves challenging or undermining the supports for existing patterns of behavior and attitudes. This can be done through confrontation with information that raises questions about previously held truths. In an extreme example, in "brainwashing," social support for the individual's self-concept, beliefs, attitudes, and values is withheld while divergent information is promoted. The other category of approach is to minimize anxiety. Reassurance and diversion are two strategies that might reduce the client's perception of threat from the proposed change. In the examples given in Table 15–2 the nurse might combine these strategies by presenting information in a nonthreatening way.

Table 15–3 summarizes various factors that are involved in setting a climate in which change can occur.

The previous discussion about change theories and principles have frequently referred to the role of the nurse as a change agent. This role is addressed in the following section.

TABLE 15–2.   Framework for the Identification of Forms of Rejection

Form of Rejection	Cause of Rejection	State of Subject	Anticipated Responses
Ignorance	Lack of dissemination	Uninformed	"The information is not easily available"
Suspended judgement	Data not logically compelling	Doubtful	"I want to wait before I try it"
Situational	Data not materially compelling	Comparing	"Other things are just as good"
		Defensive	"Regulations will not allow it"
		Deprived	"It costs too much"
Personal	Data not psychologically compelling	Anxious	"I don't know if I can"
		Guilty	"I know I should do it"
		Alienated	"It will never work"
Experimental	Present or past trials	Unconvinced	"I tried this once and it didn't work"

(From Zaltman G, Duncan R: Strategies for Planned Change, p 87. New York, John Wiley & Sons, 1977. Used with permission of the publisher)

TABLE 15–3.   Factors Involved in the Climate for
                           Change

Perceived need for change	Extent to which client experiences a problem
Openness to change	Readiness to accept change
Potential for change	Capacity to accept and implement change
Perceived control over the change process	Extent of influence client feels he has on selection and implementation of the change
Commitment to change	Recognition of the importance of taking action in response to a problem

(From Zaltman G, Duncan T: Strategies for Planned Change, p. 243. New York, John Wiley & Sons, 1977. Used with permission of the publisher)

THE CHANGE AGENT ROLE

A change agent is "any individual or group operating to change the status quo in a system such that the individual or individuals involved must relearn how to peform their role(s)" (Zaltman and Duncan, 1977, p. 17). More specifically, "the change agent generates ideas, introduces the innovation, develops a climate for planned change by overcoming resistance, and marshalling forces for acceptance, and implements and evaluates the change" (Lancaster and Lancaster, 1982, p. 20).

The Change Agent's Cognitive Style

An individual's mode of problem-solving and decision-making develops through formal education and experience, and tends to be relatively consistent. Evaluation of information refers to processes commonly used in reaching a decision about a problem. It has been hypothesized (Jung, 1953) that there are two basic ways of reaching a decision—thinking and feeling. Thinking persons tend to approach a problem by structuring it in terms of the scientific method, which leads to a rational solution. Feeling types, on the other hand, make decisions based on personal considerations. Feeling types tend to personalize a situation by stressing its individual uniqueness (Slocum, 1978).

Information gathering essentially relates to the process by which the mind organizes many bits of stimuli into a coherent whole. Again, according to Jung (1953), individuals can take in data from the environment by either sensation or intuition. Sensing types typically take in information through their senses and are most comfortable when attending to details and specifics. In contrast, intuitive types typically take in information by looking at the whole situation. These types tend to concentrate on hypothetical possibilities of the situation rather than on hard facts and details.

The Change Agent's Communication Style

Communication style refers to the way in which a person conveys a message to others. The concept of style differentiates the way in which a message is presented from the apparent content or substance of the communication. There is evidence that an individual's communication style can affect the effectiveness and social success of interpersonal communication (Miller, 1975).

This "method" of communication tends to remain fairly consistent for each individual. "Some people appear to have a narrow or rigid orientation to all or nearly all other people. They tend to respond to nearly all others in about the same way. On the other hand, many persons have a wider repertoire of responses, and can appropriately react in different ways to differing interpersonal behaviors of others" (Giffin and Patton, 1974, pp. 66–67).

Miller (1975) indicates a number of personal characteristics and attributes that may contribute to a person's communication style. These include self-esteem, self-acceptance, confidence, facial and vocal qualities (tone, vocal inflection, rate, momentum, and duration of speech), ability to stimulate emotions, friendliness, and amount of dominance (talkativeness, aggressiveness, and outgoingness). It has been found that there is an optimal level of talkativeness at which a person who contributes somewhat more than his share is perceived by others in the most favorable light (Miller, 1975, p. 8), and that style is more important than content in affecting judgements of interpersonal distance (Leginski and Izzett, 1973, p. 301).

Bradley and Edinberg (1982, pp. 54–64) describe a number of dimensions that they believe contribute to communication style. These include:

1. Congruence, or how well the words, body language, tone of voice, and so forth, fit together with each other. The message sent should be congruent with the internal feelings and beliefs of the message sender or the recipient will sense the discrepancy.

2. Defensiveness, or the use of defense mechanisms by the message sender to defend against anxiety. Defense mechanisms may include denial (negation of an uncomfortable impulse or truth), projection (placing inner conflicts on others), rationalization (making up excuses to explain behavior), reaction formation (acting the opposite of how one feels), or repression (putting uncomfortable thoughts out of awareness). Defense mechanisms may be used when the recipient unconsciously perceives a message as an attack on his self-worth. The defense mechanism protects his ego, but can then distort the interpersonal communication.

3. Openness, or the ability to listen, understand, and accept criticism or differences between people.

4. Self-disclosure, or the ability to talk about one's own feelings and perceptions directly and honestly. The timing and content of the communication must be appropriate however.

5. Acceptance, or the ability to allow others the freedom of their feelings and beliefs even if they are different from one's own. This includes responding to others without judging them, and avoiding blaming others for what they do even if the behavior is "wrong."

It appears that one's reaction to another person may be substantially influenced by the style of communication apart from the content of the communication *per se*. Therefore, in order to facilitate effective communication, it is important for the change agent to be aware of the way in which she is perceived and to be open to the possible need for attention to her style of communication.

Categories of Change Strategies

Change strategies can be categorized by their theoretical rationale.

Empirical–Rational

The empirical–rational category assumes that people will act in a way that is rational and in their own self-interest. These strategies are therefore aimed at educating people to their available options, assuming that the person will change behavior because he knows the new behavior will be desirable. For example, inservice education may include a demonstration of the latest techniques available for a particular task, with the expectation that nurses will then apply that knowledge to improve their care.

Normative–Reeducative

The normative–reeducative category assumes that sociocultural norms are fundamental to a person's behavior. Thus, in addition to rationality and intelligence, change must involve modifications of attitudes, values, skills, and significant relationships. This is the basis for the belief that the change process must be based on mutuality and collaboration between the client and the change agent. This allows for the problem-solving and personal growth that is believed to be needed to promote effective change.

Power–Coercive

The third category is that of the use of power-coercive strategies. These are based on the use of power. It is believed that despite the need for knowledge, and for modification of attitudes and values, change will only occur when it is supported by power. This rationale is the basis for much political action, and may imply the use of legitimate channels of authority or violent, nonsanctioned methods (Chin, 1976).

Zaltman and Duncan discuss four types of change strategies: facilitative, reeducative, persuasive, and power.

Facilitative

Facilitative strategies are used to make the client aware of the availability of help in sufficient detail and clarity that he knows exactly what is available and where and how assistance may be obtained. Facilitative strategies are appropriate when there is openness to change, but are relatively ineffective when resistance is expected. Examples of this type of strategy are simplifying data, providing feedback, and providing the necessary tools to help the client to recognize a problem; providing multiple potential solutions; and involving the client and others in the decision-making process. This produces a greater commitment to change, but the agent must be sure that there are sufficient resources, commitment, and capability to maintain the change after the agent has withdrawn from the process.

Reeducative

Reeducative strategies are based on empirical–rational theory. Relatively unbiased presentation of fact is assumed to provide a rational justification for action. This type of strategy is necessary when effective use of an advocated change requires skills and knowledge that the client does not possess. It is also desirable when resistance is prevalent and based on inaccurate information, and when the change involved is a radical departure from past practices and there is a great deal of uncertainty about the ability to successfully perform the new practices. However, in themselves, reeducative strategies are inadequate to bring about change unless there is a strong felt need and a strong motivation to satisfy that need.

Reeducative strategies work slowly, and thus are feasible only when time is not a pressing factor. Examples of reeducative strategies are creating awareness that a problem exists by indicating how much better off the client could be, connecting symptoms with causes to aid in problem identification, and demonstrating alternative possible solutions to an identified problem. Reeducative strategies heighten awareness of a problem and a possible solution, but do not heighten the need or motivation to change. This requires persuasive strategies.

Persuasive

Persuasive strategies attempt to bring about change partly through bias in the manner in which a message is structured and presented. Reasoning, urging, and inducement through incentives are examples of this type of strategy.

Persuasive strategies are more effective for those who are less open to change, and can be used to increase both attitudinal and behavioral commitment. Knowledge about the client can help the agent to be more persuasive, especially in combating resistance to change. A persuasive strategy is indicated when the proposed change is risky, not amenable to limited or small scale trial, is technically complex, has no clear relative advantage, and must be implemented in a short time. In a situation where the change agent has limited resources with which to initiate and sustain a change, these strategies are especially useful.

Power

Power strategies imply the use of coercion. They typically result in compliance, which indicates a low level of commitment to the change, but leads to adoption of the induced behavior because the target expects to gain specific rewards and avoid punishment by conforming.

Power strategies may be necessary if the client or target group has limited resources and is generally unwilling to allocate available resources to the continued implementation of a change. However, forced compliance requires surveillance to maintain the change. This is not an appropriate approach if the goal is to produce a self-sustaining change.

In most situations a variety of strategies may be appropriate. In the awareness stage of promoting change, reeducative strategies may be desirable. At the adoption stage facilitative strategies increase in importance. Persuasive strategies are most useful at the evaluative stage (Zaltman and Duncan, 1977 pp. 90–165).

Implementing Change Within the Nursing Process

The promotion of change is an important component of providing nursing care. The nurse does not "put on a different hat," when acting in the change agent role. Rather, principles and strategies to promote change must be integrated into all phases of the nursing process.

Assessment Phase

The assessment phase of the nursing process involves the identification of characteristics about the client, including his openness and motivation for change. The client's culture and social group are important sources of data about possible biases. Influences of the client's family, significant others, and the environment should also be considered.

The relationship between the nurse and the client is critical to the success of the process. Trust must be established. The nurse should assess the degree of congruence between her values and those of the client. If there are basic differences, it may not be possible for the nurse to be an effective agent for change with that particular client.

The principle of mutuality must be an integral part of the relationship. As data are collected, the nurse should validate the accuracy of her perceptions with the client. The client must have the same perception of a problem as does the nurse, and must understand that it is his responsibility to decide whether or not to implement possible solutions. The client should know what the nurse expects of him, and he should be able to share his expectations of the nurse. The client must be an informed and equal participant from the beginning of the change process.

Planning Phase

One of the greatest potential problems in the planning phase is the lack of clearly defined goals. This can lead to ambiguity, uncertainty, and anxiety. The nurse and the client must be clear about the objectives for change that she has identified, and be sure that the client and other key people are informed, understand, and accept the goals. This involvement will facilitate commitment to support the change process.

An important component of the planning phase is the identification of potential support systems for the client to facilitate the proposed change. Time is an important resource that is often overlooked. The amount of time that is available to implement and support the change has a major influence on strategies that should be used. Setting a trial period for the change can be an effective technique to reduce resistance. Key influential people are a resource that should be cultivated to develop allies although the informal structure can be very effective as well.

Personal characteristics of the change agent are essential to the development of relationships that inspire confidence, avoid defensiveness, and create support for the change process. Such qualities include respect for others, the ability to empathize, and genuineness in interactions. The specific roles assumed by the change agent are influenced by her special abilities and personality.

It is critical that the plan be developed in detail, and include goals, intervention and communication strategies, time-table, and evaluation methods.

Implementation Phase

The implementation phase includes the process of instituting the change strategies, and then maintaining the change once it has begun. The change agent has to maintain a balance between leading and developing the capabilities of the client and significant others to promote continuation of the process. At this time nurturance, constructive criticism, positive feedback, and rewards for progress may be helpful strategies.

Recall of strategies to avoid or reduce resistance is important at this phase. Communication is critical so that everyone knows his role. Self-esteem, autonomy, and sense of security must be promoted. Conflict should be avoided, while an open atmosphere is maintained. It is probably realistic to assume that optimal rather than minimal time will be needed to promote change in a manner that does not increase resistance.

A major potential error that can be made is to attempt too sweeping a change too quickly. If major change is needed, it is desirable to break the process into several stages. The simplest solutions should be used whenever possible. The agent should always have contingency plans ready if the original plan hits unanticipated snags.

Evaluation Phase

The evaluation phase involves a judgement about whether or not the change process has been successful. This decision requires assessment of the effectiveness of the change process in relation to the objectives for change. Effectiveness is a subjective dimension that concerns attitudes toward the process of change. Degree of adoption of the change is more objective, and relates to whether the change has made a measurable impact and been continued.

There should be a process of evaluation during all the phases of the nursing process. The possibility of the plan not working must be anticipated, and there should be a way to reverse the process or implement alternative plans if needed. The plan must be open to revision during all phases, and the change agent should be aware in advance of what modifications she is willing and able to make.

If the change has been adopted and internalized, the change agent is ready to terminate the relationship and withdraw from the scene. She should ensure that the client and key others have the ability to maintain the change. She should also determine, in collaboration with the client, if she will have any future contact with the client.

The nursing process, as discussed in this section, has focused on the role of the nurse in promoting change in the health of an individual client. The nursing process is just as applicable when the change involves groups or larger systems. There are more variables to assess, and a larger number of interrelationships for which to plan, but the principles and process remain the same.

SUMMARY

This chapter has set the conceptual framework for and explored the role of the nurse as a change agent. Change principles, as part of the nursing process, permit the nurse to work in collaboration with the client to propose, implement, and maintain changes that will promote his health.

REFERENCES

Bradley JC, Edinberg MA: Communication in the Nursing Context. New York, Appleton-Century-Crofts, 1982

Chin R: The utility of systems models and developmental models for practitioners. *In* Bennis WG, Benne KD, Chin R (eds): The Planning of Change, ed 3, pp 90–102. New York, Holt, Rinehart & Winston, 1976

Giffin K, Patton B: Personal Communication in Human Relations. Columbus, Merrill, 1974

Jung C: Collected works (Vols 7,8,9, Part 1). Read H, Fordham M, Adler C (eds): Princeton, Princeton University Press, 1953

Kelman HC, Warwick DP: Bridging micro and macro approaches to social change: A social-psychological perspective. *In* Zaltman G (ed): Processes and Phenomena of Social Change, pp 13–59. New York, John Wiley & Sons, 1973

Lancaster J, Lancaster W: Concepts for Advanced Nursing Practice: The Nurse as a Change Agent. St Louis, CV Mosby, 1982

Leginski W, Izzett R: Linguistic styles as indices for interpersonal distance. J Soc Psych 91:291–304, 1973

Lewin K: Field Theory in Social Science. Connecticut, Greenwood Press, 1951

Lippitt GL: Visualizing Change: Model Building and the Change Process. La Jolla, University Associates, 1973

Miller LD: Perceptual accuracy as a function of communicator style in dyads. Unpublished Dissertation. University of Michigan, 1975

Nadler DA: Managing organizational change: An integrative perspective. J Appl Behav Sc 17:191–211, 1981

Rogers EM, Shoemaker FF: Communication of Innovations: A Cross-Cultural Approach. New York, Free Press, 1971

Schein EH: The mechanisms of change. *In* Bennis WG, Benne KD, Chin R (eds): The Planning of Change, ed 2. New York, Holt, Rinehart & Winston, 1969

Slocum JW Jr: Does cognitive style affect diagnosis and intervention strategies of change agents? Group Organ Stud 3:199–210, June 1978

Watson G: Resistance to change. *In* Zaltman G (ed): Processes and Phenomena of Social Change, pp 117–131. New York, John Wiley & Sons, 1973

Zaltman G, Duncan R: Strategies for Planned Change. New York, John Wiley & Sons, 1977

Chapter 16

The Role of Client Advocate

THOUGHT QUESTIONS

1. What are the beliefs a nurse must hold in order to be an effective client advocate?
2. What are the responsibilities of the nurse in the role of client advocate?
3. What is the reason for assuring mutuality between nurse and client in the conduct of advocacy?
4. What are the essential human rights the nurse must respect in the conduct of the advocate role?
5. What are the changes in society today that support the need for the nurse to be a client advocate?
6. Why are reimbursement and employment considered to be problematic for the nurse's assumption of the client advocate role?

If the professional nurse believes that the client has a right to a nurse-client relationship based on mutuality, shared respect, consideration of information and feelings, and full participation in the problem-solving related to his health and health-care needs, the nurse believes in advocacy. If the professional nurse believes that it is the professional's responsibility to ensure that the client has access to the health care delivery systems appropriate to his needs, the nurse believes in advocacy. If the professional nurse believes that the client is responsible for his health and that the nurse is responsible for mobilizing and facilitating the strengths of the client in achieving the highest level of health possible, the nurse believes in advocacy.

One role of the professional nurse that has evolved along with the development of practice based on nursing theory is the client advocate role. Nurses have always acted as advocates for clients to some extent. Advocacy for the client was given highest priority unless it conflicted with advocacy for the physician or advocacy for the employing institution. As nursing has perceived itself as an autonomous profession rather than a dependent subsystem of medicine, the nature of advocacy has changed. Today the nurse attempting to act in the role of client advocate accepts the obligation to keep the client first in priority at all times. The ability to be an advocate for the client without being an adversary of others in the health care delivery system is the challenge for the nurse who is a client advocate today.

The purpose of this chapter is to explore the meanings of advocacy, its ethical bases, clients' needs for advocacy, and the challenges and rewards of the nurse serving as a client advocate.

THE MEANINGS OF ADVOCACY

The selection of the client advocate as a professional role for nursing is made within the context of the purpose of nursing, beliefs about humans, and the needs of the public for health care. Because the role of client advocate involves a process of influencing others, it may be considered a leadership role. Through leadership behaviors the nurse attempts to influence the client. According to Tappen (1983, p. 67), "... every attempt to influence others has some kind of purpose. ..." The process of influencing others and its purpose is directly related to the way the leadership role is defined. The dictionary definition of advocacy is "the action of pleading for, or supporting" (Webster, 1976, p. 32). The advocate is defined as "one that pleads the cause of another ... one that argues for, defends, maintains, or recommends a cause or proposal" (Webster, 1976, p. 32). These definitions, without further operationalization, would lead one to believe that nurses acting as advocates assume an active position and the client assumes a passive position. Based on the assumption of nursing science that man is always capable of growing and developing, nurses have operationalized the advocate role to focus on the "supporting" aspect of advocacy and the advocate behavior of "maintaining or recommending a cause," that cause being health and every person's right to have adequate health care.

The theoretical basis for advocacy in the nurse-client relationship is that man is viewed in an organismic way rather than a mechanistic way. Fawcett (1984, pp. 10–11) describes the characteristics of organicism:

1. The person is holistic—is an integrated organized entity who is not reducible to discrete parts.
2. Parts have meaning only within the context of the whole.
3. The person is an active organism rather than a reactive one.
4. The person is capable of qualitative and quantitative change.

With this view of the person and the view that life is characterized by change, through which growth and realization of potential is possible, the advocate has a strong rationale for assisting the client to take action on his own behalf, to actively assume responsibility for his health and decisions about it, and that the nurse both mobilizes and supports the client's potential (Fawcett, 1984, p. 12).

Simms and Lindberg (1978, p. 5) state: "Advocacy is a special kind of responsibility. It means to be accountable for one's care. It means to be the patient's spokesperson, if needed. It means to deliver excellent care." Kohnke (1982, p. 145) specifies advocacy in nursing as "the act of informing and supporting a person so that he can make the best decisions possible for himself." Curtin asserts that nurses must act as human advocates, thus the client advocate is really a human advocate. "We must—as human advocates—assist patients to find meaning or purpose in their living or in their dying. . . . Whatever patients define as their goal, it is their meaning and not ours, their values and not ours, and their living or dying and not ours" (Curtin, 1979, p. 7). It is clear in at least the latter two descriptions of advocacy that the nurse in the client advocate role serves the client in supportive ways, acts on behalf of the client, and gives full or at least mutual responsibility in decision-making for the client. Our view is that through the advocacy role the nurse participates with the client and professional peers in the advancement of processes that ultimately promote health. Essential to all these processes are collaborative relationships. Collaboration means shared responsibility for planning, problem-solving, and evaluating with clients and others in the health care delivery system. Following is a brief discussion of the leadership behaviors that constitute the role of client advocate.

Emphasis on Mutuality

Evidence is abundant that decisions made for people by other people without participation of those affected or those who have the expertise to make the most informed judgements are less likely to be understood or workable. Nurses have the expertise in health and nursing's ability to help people achieve health. Clients have the expertise in understanding and evaluating their situation. They have control of their lives and their health. Thus, it is entirely appropriate that decisions affecting health be made by the client with full informational support, empathy, and respect from the nurse. Mutuality means that the nurse and the client together describe fully the health situation of the client, agree on the direction and nature of change that the client would like to make, explore alternative ways to achieve the mutually agreed on goals, and then work together as the client implements the changes. The advocate at this stage makes sure that technical and informational supports are provided for the client and assists the client in gaining access to the health care services that are needed. In almost every nurse-client situation one can identify, it is possible to focus on the strength of the client and to reasonably expect that the client can be responsible. For example, in work with bereaved parents following the death of a child, nurses found the potential for positive growth in significant numbers (Miles and Crandall, 1983). The researchers pointed out that focusing on the growth potential in bereaved parents was in no way meant to minimize the pain of grief, rather to help them find meaning in their lives at the time. How does emphasis on mutuality enter into this nursing situation? It is important because two essential elements of mutuality are respect and sharing. Respecting the client's right to make the decisions about working on finding meaning while at the same time emphasizing their ability to be responsible for themselves, the nurse sets up a relationship that is based on mutuality. The nurse empathizes with the parents, showing understanding of the pain from loss, respects the strengths of the parents, and gives choices to the family as they mutually establish a goal of reducing the pain of grief and searching for meaning in their lives.

The most important factor in mutuality is that the nurse and the client are seen as equally able and responsible for the outcomes of the nursing process. Their areas of expertise vary, but their authority and significance in the relationship are equal. One's potential can be more fully realized in a relationship characterized by mutuality.

Emphasis on Facilitation

The advocate assumes that every client has strengths and that the job of the nurse is to help the client to use those strengths to achieve the highest level of health possible. Moccia and Pfordresher (1983, p. 146) quoted a nurse, Janice Veliko, who clearly reflects advocacy by raising the following question: "Given a medical diagnosis of cancer, how can I help this patient to choose between different treatments, to be pain free, to continue family responsibilities, to continue to enjoy living?" Kohnke (1982, pp. 145–146) and Clark (1977, p. 8) suggest that such emphasis on facilitation in the advocacy process requires that the advocate take responsibility to "make sure they (client) have all the necessary information to make informed decisions" and to "support clients in the decisions they make." King (1984, p. 17) suggests that an effective way of facilitating growth in self and others is through values clarification, that is, the nurse would help the client think through issues and develop a personal value system that would aid with decision-making. Hames and Joseph (1980) suggest that facilitation is effected through helping the client understand the tasks before him, ensuring that the client experience some success when he is trying to accomplish something, providing an environment that is conducive to learning (one of trust and respect), and offering informational and emotional supports.

Emphasis on Protection

Client advocates are increasingly becoming aware of their responsibility to protect clients. Commonly, nurses are called on to examine their roles in protecting the patient's right to live or die. The Bandmans report that nurses are commonly caught in an ethical dilemma between physicians and incurably ill or hopelessly disabled persons. The advocate must determine what actions to take in terms of protecting the patient from either forced treatments or withholding treatment. The Bandmans conclude that morality tends to support a person's right to live over letting others decide that the person's life is not worth living, that the welfare of others is not necessarily in conflict with a person's right to die, and that there are cases in which the nurse can legitimately decide to protect a patient's wish to end life (Bandman and Bandman, 1979, pp. 30–33).

Perhaps the greatest need for the nurse to act as protector is the need to change a condition or situation in the health care delivery system in which the client is either given inadequate care or the environment poses some hazard. Quite simply, this protective role means that the nurse is obliged to monitor the quality of care and to be responsible for intervening when harmful behaviors are observed in any health care worker. This does not mean that one acts as an adversary to a colleague, rather that the client is protected and efforts are made to resolve the conflict resulting from the protection need of the client (Mauksch and Miller, 1981, p. 41).

Emphasis on Coordination

The most widely accepted role of the client advocate is the coordinator. It is usually acceptable for the nurse to articulate the relationships between the various health care workers caring for the client. Since the nurse is the one professional who is focusing on the client's whole response to his health situation, the nurse can use the coordination responsibilities to ensure that the client has access to all parts of the delivery system that are needed and that the various services are offered at a time, place, and costs that are reasonable for the client.

ETHICS OF ADVOCACY

Ethics, the science of moral values, guides the practice of nurses. According to Mooney (1980, pp. 7–8), six ethical issues, personhood, rights of the person, consent, rights of society, distributive justice, and personal integrity are considered in all the conceptual models for nursing. As a profession that offers services to people, nurses must be concerned about adherence to a code of conduct. That code reflects the professional's sense of right and wrong and the profession's acceptance of the responsibilities vested in it by society. The code for nurses is included in Chapter 3, "Socialization for Professional Practice." Personhood, rights of the person, consent, and distributive justice and personal integrity all address ethical behaviors in the nurse–client relationship. The rights of society address the ethical relationships between the nurse and the client and society at large.

Autonomy—Personal Liberty

Davis defines autonomy as a form of personal liberty. As such, autonomy is the basis for the rights of individuals. It is accepted in our culture that autonomy represents the right of the individual to make his own decisions, to be independent, and to be self-reliant. In health care institutions, these personal rights of individuals may frequently be violated. In illness the person is often forced into a position of dependence and that, erroneously, is sometimes equated with lack of ability to make decisions (Davis, 1982, pp. 218–221).

By law, patients are to be advised of their rights whenever they are admitted to any health care institution. The most important feature of the rights established for all patients is the respect for autonomy. The patient is personally free to make choices and decisions. Because illness sometimes interferes with the ability to actively take control of decision-making, the nurse advocate can play a vital rôle by guarding the patient's rights for choices and decisions when he is in less control of self and environment.

Human Rights and Needs

Curtin, noted authority on ethics in nursing, has challenged nurses to look at the daily disrespect to which patients are subjected. Examples of that disrespect are falsely reassuring a child that something is not going to hurt when it is bound to be painful, carrying out procedures without explanation, and distributing unequal treatment to different persons, among many others. Curtin defines human rights as "a person's just due" (Curtin, 1982, p. 4), and states that, "If human beings have any natural rights at all, they have the right to be recognized and respected as human beings" (Curtin, 1982, p. 7). Humans have needs that must be met in order to continue to exist. What is our obligation to meet those needs? Most would agree that it is the individual's right to have basic or fundamental needs met. It is also the individual's right to make choices not to have needs met. Curtin indicates that the limits of the individual's freedom to choose are that the individual may choose not to exercise a given right, but nurses, like everyone else, are not free to make that decision for other humans (Curtin, 1982, p. 10).

Responsibilities

If one believes in the autonomy of the individual and respects the rights of that individual to make choices and decisions, one assumes certain obligations. Those obligations are part of professional responsibility. Nurses are morally obligated to carry out professional duties in relation to the rights of clients (Curtin, 1982, pp. 17–18). According to Aroskar (1984, p. 5), nurses are becoming more ethically responsible, taking an interest in resource allocation that is equitable to all (distributive justice). Chenevert asserts that we need a bill of responsibilities as well as a bill of rights. Examples of rights tempered with responsibility are:

1. Where there is the right to speak, there is the responsibility to listen.
2. Where there is the right to have problems, there is the responsibility to find solutions.
3. Where there is a right to cry, there is a responsibility to dry tears. (Chenevert, 1983, p. 53)

Further responsibilities for the professional nurse are cited at the end of this chapter.

NEEDS FOR ADVOCACY

"Current nursing practice mandates a morally responsible professional who is an advocate for the client and a guardian of client rights," says Omery (1983, p. 2). It is clear that nurses have many experiences with clients in which they must make moral judgements. These judgements must be made from moral values about things like justice or utility rather than the rules of those in authority. Integrating the advocate role helps the nurse keep the rights of the client in the foreground in decision-making.

Changes in Population

Several changes in the population point out the need for nurses to be advocates. Demographic changes in the population alone support the need for the role. The proportion of people who are over 65 is increasing every year. One thing that happens to older people is that they do not appear to be respected for their abilities, rather they are commonly treated as disabled. The nurse advocate would guard against that and would assist them to get the health care they need and to be able to make choices and decisions about their goals and how to achieve them.

Another factor calling for the advocate role of the nurse is that the public nursing serves has become increasingly sophisticated and active. Knowledge is rapidly diffused to the public. This knowledge and the sense of outrage at the rapidly and ever-increasing costs of health care have led to the consumers taking charge of the decisions about health care. There is an emphasis on self-care and a challenge to the past elitism of the health care professional. The consumer expects to participate in the decisions rather than be issued directives about what he must do to achieve health. Advocacy is needed to help clients participate in health care decisions (Curtin, 1982, pp. 80–82).

Changes in Technology

Perhaps the greatest need for client advocacy arises out of the rapidly expanding technology. Great strides have been made in the development of health care technology. Diagnostic and therapeutic equipment have assisted greatly in the prevention and treatment of health care problems. The moral issue that has arisen is related to the high costs of that technology. Costs lead to an ethical dilemma: who shall get the benefits of this expensive technology? Nurses have great opportunities to assist clients to have the advantages of the improved technical supports and to ensure that care is distributed in a just and equal manner. Needs for access for all to the best care possible supports the need for the client advocate.

Changes in the Profession

With the growth and development of moral responsibility as a legitimate responsibility of nursing has come nurses' interest in public policy, particularly health policy. Aiken says that nurses are interested in influencing policy because they see in their day-to-day activities how significantly nursing and the public are influenced by policies and programs related to health. She says that nursing has recognized the need to participate in shaping policies aimed at removing financial barriers to health care, improving the quality of nursing care available, ending the shortage of nurses, improving nurses' economic rewards, expanding nurses' independent roles within the delivery system, and developing new roles outside the hospital (Aiken, 1982, pp. 5–7). Clearly these concerns demonstrate that advocacy is needed for the profession as well as for the public. Professional gains made in all the concerns cited above will serve to fulfill the public's need for an advocate to assist them to achieve better health care.

The three changes noted that support the need for advocacy, change in the population, change in technology, and change in the health professions, have a common denominator, which is escalating costs. Walker (1982, p. 131) says that there is widespread concern about costs, resulting in a movement to reduce unnecessary hospitalizations and diagnostic and therapeutic procedures. Nurses acting as advocates could play a significant role in protecting clients from such unnecessary costs by providing them with the informational support necessary to make wise decisions and helping them to understand their rights.

THE CHALLENGES AND REWARDS OF THE NURSE SERVING AS A CLIENT ADVOCATE

Noting the need for role restructuring in the health care system, Jacox (1982, pp. 88–97) advises that reconstruction must be considered in three areas: (1) the work itself—acknowledging and emphasizing the knowledge and judgements required for professional practice; (2) working conditions—including when and how the nurse works; and (3) where the role of the nurse is placed in the total organization—considering where the nurse is placed in the decision-making structure.

Assuming the client advocate role challenges the present structure of the health care delivery system, all three areas noted by Jacox require restructuring in order to successfully meet that challenge. The accepted view of the work of nursing needs to be adjusted to give credence to the facilitative, protective, and coordinating functions as well as the present restorative functions of the nurse. Emphasis needs to be placed on the knowledge and skills necessary to assist clients to increase competency in assuming responsibility for their own health. In such a restructured system, the nursing staff would be supported in:

1. The development of understanding of the *responses* of clients to various threats to health and development of strategies to respond effectively to clients' responses.
2. The refinement and further development of health promotion and illness prevention abilities as well as restorative abilities.
3. The re-evaluation of belief systems about the independent versus dependent role of clients and self.
4. The assumption of collaborative responsibility for monitoring the effectiveness of the delivery system as well as the independent responsibility for evaluating the effectiveness of the nursing interventions in responding to the client's health needs.
5. The implementation of interdisciplinary dialogue with all professional workers sharing equal responsibility and authority for meeting the health needs of clients.
6. The provision of opportunity for all members of the team to evaluate effectiveness in collaboration in order to avoid the establishment of adversary relationships.

Work would be viewed in terms of professional responsibilities implicit in the categories cited above. The challenge to professional nursing to restructure the work of the nurse as an advocate includes gaining acceptance and emphasis of the following role behaviors for professional nurses. The professional nurse would be expected to:

1. Interact with the client in a manner and quantity that permits exploration of his personal responses to his health or threats to health, evaluation of the environmental circumstances in which he exists, identification of strengths and limitations, identification of resources perceived to be needed, and clear allocation of responsibilities of client and nurse that ensures the client's assumption of responsibility for his health and the nurse's assumption of responsibility for the informational and interactional supports needed.
2. Prepare for and implement teaching programs needed by clients.
3. Update techical skills as new therapeutic techniques and equipment are made available for health care.
4. Discuss beliefs about abilities of clients with professional peers in an effort to evaluate own values about independence and dependence in various states of health.
5. Update nursing care plans in an effort to evaluate outcomes of nursing care.
6. Participate in nursing research as a consumer and assist in nursing studies conducted in the setting.

7. Identify all units of the delivery system needed to be involved in the client's care.
8. Coordinate efforts of the multiple health care workers involved in the care of the client.
9. Assess the adequacy of efforts of all workers involved in care according to the stated needs of the client.
10. Resolve conflicts that might occur in relation to advocacy efforts for the client by respecting the position of all involved, gathering data that describes the whole system of client/environment, promoting expression of conflicts, participating in the problem-solving process, and allowing the client to make decisions based on data rather than advice from others.
11. Recognize and show appreciation for the contributions of team members to the health care of clients.
12. Periodically discuss and evaluate the quality of the interactions of members of the health care team and evaluate own interpersonal effectiveness with clients and team members.

Fulfillment of these work role behaviors reflect the professional nurse's commitment to client advocacy as a legitimate role.

For restructuring the working conditions for themselves, nurses must be advocates for professional colleagues and selves. It has been suggested in the chapter on research that an effective method for gaining control over practice is to develop and use data as a basis for recommending changes. Data, rather than opinion, gives a group strength. Advocacy for anyone is more effective if the advocate is working from a position of strength, armed with data and the belief that what one is trying to accomplish is not only worthwhile for self, but vital to the quality of care that one is able to deliver.

For nursing to be able to effectively carry out the role of client advocate, restructuring the health care delivery system in terms of where the nurse is placed in the total organization is necessary. In most delivery systems, advocacy efforts are challenged by the nurse's lack of equality in authority. Equality in responsibility is more likely to be evident between health care disciplines. There is agreement that each discipline is fully responsible and accountable for its own practice. However, as noted throughout the book, authority is more commonly dispersed in a hierarchical manner in which nursing may occupy a position of disadvantage. Therefore, nurses attempting to operate as client advocates in an hierarchical system will be more effective if they both learn to negotiate the hierarchy and to develop image building strategies that promote the significance of their advocacy work. If the need for equal authority to fulfill the advocate's role is perceived as important, the nurse must demonstrate the effectiveness of the advocate's work (such as improved client outcomes and the accomplishment of serving more people at costs that are affordable) and the improvement in satisfaction and retention of nurses. The public's support cannot be underestimated. A public image of the nurse as competent and appreciated for advocacy efforts will result in public support. Public support is one of the most powerful forces for change in society. Thus, nursing can use the public to help restructure the health care delivery system. As nurses gain the respect of the public it serves, the more likely they are to gain the respect of interdisciplinary peers. Such respect is necessary to change the position of nursing in the delivery system to ensure full participation in decision-making. To fulfill the responsibilities of a client advocate, the nurse must participate in decision-making.

Problems Associated with the Advocate Role: Reimbursement, Employment, and Differences in Values

"The excellent nurse, without always realizing it, lets you know that she's constantly protecting her right to nurse her patients" (Hodgman, 1979, p. 24). Such advocacy efforts are not without problems and constraints. The fact that most of the nursing care that is done today occurs within the boundaries of hospitals and extended care facilities creates some problems for the client advocate. The nurse is an employee of an institution, not the client. Most advocate relationships are characterized by the advocate being in the direct employ of the client. This employee status presents conflicts for nurses when there appears to be a question of priority or a choice between what is perceived to be best for the client and what is institutional policy and expectation. A process for dealing with this challenge is suggested at the end of this chapter. The professional person is obligated to assign priority to the client. Assuming that obligation may put the employee, the nurse, at risk.

Kohnke suggests that there are ways to reduce the risks as an employee when conflict occurs between the nurse in a client advocate role and the institution. She suggests that the nurse must be very knowledgeable about the law, the system, and how to handle interactions with clients (Kohnke, 1982, pp. 147–148). Most important is that the client is the decision-maker.

Zusman, a physician and head of an advocacy program, suggests that the advocate sometimes encounters values conflicts. To deal with these values conflicts, he believes the advocate acts responsibly if she adheres to the following guidelines:

1. Demonstrate concern for the patient's total situation.
2. Recognize the difference between needs and wants in a person under stress.
3. Recognize the widespread effect a change in the patient's situation may have on others.
4. Balance the patient's needs against others.
5. Negotiate to resolve conflicts in order to avoid adversary relationships. (Zusman, 1982, p. 49)

Zusman presents the idea that perhaps nurses should not always be advocates in his admonition, "Think twice about being a patient advocate" (Zusman, 1982, p. 46). We agree with the suggestion that the nurse should seriously consider the risks of being an advocate, however, we suggest that the choice is not really between being or not being an advocate. It is between assuming the advocate role by collaborative processes or operating as an adversary to those with whom conflict occurs. Clearly, collaboration is the preferred choice.

Effectiveness of the Role in Changing the Public Image of the Nurse

Whenever the client perceives that the nurse has not only truly acted on his behalf to ensure adequate health care but has also respected his ability to assume responsibility for his own health and make his own decisions, the client grows in feelings of personal worth and competence and the nurse gains respect and appreciation for professional services. The fact that the advocate offers informational support is an indication to the client that nursing is a scholarly activity. The fulfillment of the advocacy role with clients, therefore, gives the nurse excellent opportunities to influence the image of nursing that society holds. It offers the nurse the opportunity to portray an image of a professional person who brings "about a good result . . . and as giving selfless attention to a client's affairs" (Camilleri, 1981, p. 407). That image is desirable and highly acceptable to the public. Camilleri adds that such acceptance by society leads to legitimation of the professional role. That legitimacy allows the nurse to practice in a way that is specific to nursing and gives decision-making power. If nurses do not use this legitimate power to "control" clients, but rather use it to share power and responsibility with clients, they will grow in autonomy and gain better control of their practice (Camilleri, 1981, pp. 407–408).

As nurses gain control of their practice and integrate more autonomous perceptions of self, they present to the public an image of competent professional workers. That positive appraisal sets the stage for significant opportunities for nursing. As the image of competence and collaboration grows, nurses will be accorded respect for their abilities. Hopefully, that respect will facilitate nurses' participation in planning and policy-making bodies that afford the opportunity to positively influence the health of society.

When nursing services are perceived to make a positive difference, which they should if nurses *act* as advocates, the demand for nursing services should increase. That increased demand for services should reaffirm the worth of the practitioner and support nursing in its goal of excellence in health care.

REFERENCES

Aiken LH: The impact of federal health policy on nurses. *In* Aiken L (ed): Nursing in the 1980s—Crisis–Opportunities–Challenges. Philadelphia, JB Lippincott, 1982

American Academy of Nursing Task Force on Nursing Practice in Hospitals: Magnet Hospitals—Attraction and Retention of Professional Nurses. Kansas City, American Nurses' Association, 1983

Aroskar M: Ethics are important in allocating health resources. Am Nurse 16:5, 1984

Bandman EL, Bandman B: The nurse's role in protecting the patient's right to live or die. Adv Nurs Sci 3:21–36, 1979

Camilleri DD: Governance and the health care system. *In* McCloskey JM, Grace HK (eds): Current Issues in Nursing. Boston, Blackwell Scientific, 1981

Chenevert M: STAT—Special Techniques in Assertiveness Training, ed 2. St Louis, CV Mosby, 1983

Clark CC: Nursing Concepts and Processes. New York, Delmar, 1977

Curtin L: What are human rights. *In* Curtin L, Flaherty J (eds): Nursing Ethics: Theories and Pragmatics. Bowie, Md, Robert J Brady, 1982

Curtin L: The commitment of rights: Responsibility. *In* Curtin L, Flaherty J (eds): Nursing Ethics: Theories and Pragmatics. Bowie, Md, Robert J Brady, 1982

Curtin LL: The nurse as advocate: A philosophical foundation for nursing. Adv Nurs Sci 3:1–10, 1979

Davis AJ: Ethical issues in nursing. *In* Lancaster J, Lancaster W (eds): Concepts for Advanced Nursing Practice—The Nurse as a Change Agent. St Louis, CV Mosby, 1982

Elliott JE, Osgood GA: Federal nursing priorities for the 1980s. *In* Aiken L (ed): Nursing in the 1980s—Crisis–Opportunities–Challenges. Philadelphia, JB Lippincott, 1982

Evans D, Fitzpatrick T, Howard-Ruben J: A district takes action. Am J Nurs 83:52–54, 1983

Fawcett J: Analysis and Evaluation of Conceptual Models of Nursing. Philadelphia, FA Davis, 1984

Fleming JW: Consumerism and the Nursing Profession. *In* Chaska NL (ed): A Time To Speak. New York, McGraw-Hill, 1983

Flaherty MJ: The nurse—institution relationship. *In* Curtin L, Flaherty MJ (eds): Nursing Ethics: Theories and Pragmatics. Bowie, Md, Robert J Brady, 1982

Hames CC, Joseph DH: Basic Concepts of Helping—A Wholistic Approach. New York, Appleton-Century-Crofts, 1980

Hamilton MS: Mentorhood: A key to nursing leadership. *In* Hein EC, Nicholson MJ (eds): Contemporary Leadership Behavior: Selected Readings. Boston, Little, Brown, 1982

Hodgman EC: Excellence in nursing. Image 11:22–27, 1979

Jacox A: Role restructuring in hospital nursing. *In* Aiken L (ed): Nursing in the 1980s—Crisis–Opportunities–Challenges. Philadelphia, JB Lippincott, 1982

King EC: Affective Education in Nursing. Rockville, Aspen Systems, 1984

Kohnke MF: The nurse as advocate. *In* Hein EC, Nicholson MJ (eds): Contemporary Leadership Behavior: Selected Readings. Boston, Little, Brown, 1982

Mauksch IG, Miller MH: Implementing Change in Nursing. St. Louis, CV Mosby, 1981

Miles MS, Crandall EK: The search for meaning and its potential for affecting growth in bereaved parents. Health Values: Achieving High Level Wellness 7:19–23, 1983

Moccia P, Pfordresher K: If nurses had their way. Ms 11: 104–106, 146, May 1983

Mooney MM: The ethical component of nursing theory. Image 12:7–9, 1980

Omery A: Moral development: A differential evaluation of dominant models. Adv Nurs Sci 6:1–17, 1983

Pilette PC: Mentoring: An encounter of the leadership kind. *In* Hein EC, Nicholson MJ (eds): Contemporary Leadership Behavior: Selected Readings. Boston, Little, Brown, 1982

Simms LM, Lindberg JB: The Nurse Person. New York, Harper & Row, 1978

Smitherman C: Nursing Actions for Health Promotion. Philadelphia, FA Davis, 1981

Styles MM: On Nursing—Toward a New Endowment. St Louis, CV Mosby, 1982

Tappen RM: Nursing Leadership: Concepts and Practice. Philadelphia, FA Davis, 1983

Walker DD: The cost of nursing care in hospitals. *In* Aiken L (ed): Nursing in the 1980s—Crisis–Opportunities–Challenges. Philadelphia, JB Lippincott, 1982

Webster: Websters Third New International Dictionary. Springfield, G&C Merriam, 1976

Zusman J: Think twice about being a patient advocate. Nurs Life 2:46–50, 1982

Chapter 17

The Contributor to the Profession Role

THOUGHT QUESTIONS

1. What factors have affected the current image of nursing? How can nurses help to further improve the image of the profession?
2. What is the difference between use of influence to change client health patterns and the use of power to change the health care delivery system?
3. What are the pros and cons of educational mobility? What should be done to clarify the numerous current levels of educational preparation for registered nurse practice?
4. Is third-party reimbursement for nurses desirable? What strategies should be used to accomplish legislative approval?
5. What are the positive factors affecting nursing research and the development of nursing science? What are the implications for further efforts by the profession?

The health care delivery system is in a period of transition from a disease-oriented to a health-oriented system of care. Because of the developing consensus within nursing that it is unique in its purpose of maximizing health potential, the nursing profession should appropriately assume responsibility for significant contributions within the evolving delivery system.

However, at the present time, the power of the nursing profession to influence external events is limited by lack of unity and preoccupation with internal conflicts. This chapter examines three major areas: the influence of nursing on the practice arena, nursing manpower, and the development of nursing science. The concepts of power, autonomy, collaboration, and accountability are viewed as critical to the development of unified professional influence.

PROFESSIONAL NURSING INFLUENCE ON THE PRACTICE ARENA

The Image of Nursing

There is much evidence that nurses lack a professional self-image that contributes to a lack of a collective image for the profession. "Traditional, prescribed role behaviors have been internalized by nurses, with consistent performance and reinforcement of these behaviors preventing any real formation of more progressive attitudes" (Weiss and Remen, 1983, p. 86).

Nursing and Sex Stereotypes

The development of nursing as a profession, dating from the mid-19th century, is intimately connected with the Victorian concept of the role of women. In fact, in her definition of the nursing role, Florence Nightingale emphasized the dependence and subordination of nurses (female) to physicians (male).

Nurses, primarily women, are strongly influenced by social definitions of what a woman is and what she ought to be. In our society, girls have been socialized into preparation for the roles of wife and mother, while boys were prepared for the role of active participant in the world of work and public activity. "Females are to be nurturing, empathizing, noncompetitive responders who meet others' needs, while males are aggressive, competitive, analytic decision makers who initiate ideas, take risks, and lead others" (Yeaworth, 1978, p. 72). Women have tended to accept these values as if they were inborn, rather than imposed.

"The skill of successful nurturing, however, is not coextensive with dependence" (Eisenstein, 1982, p. 101). This packaging of the qualities of femininity — nurturance, dependence, passivity, and subordination — is particularly damaging to the self-concept of women. The competent nurse needs the ability to nurture and care for patients to be sure, but she also needs the ability to make decisions, administer, organize, and lead others.

The result of this gender stereotyping has been the internalization by many women of the concept that a woman must choose between her natural tendency toward nurturing a family, or to compete like men in the world of work. As a result many female nurses have viewed the work of nursing as a "preparation for marriage," rather than a career, and demonstrate little identification with the profession. In a study of nurse career patterns, the National League for Nursing (NLN) found that 16% of respondents were involved in nonnursing work 15 years after graduation, and 43% were not working. (On the positive side, 67% indicated that if they were starting their education again they would again choose nursing) [Knopf, 1983, pp. 75–76].

Many nurses "drop out" to raise a family, or work primarily to supplement family income. Johnson and Vaughn (1982, p. 499) found that the proportion of nurses not actively employed in nursing remained relatively constant at about an annual average of 30% between 1972 and 1977, and decreased to about 25% in the 3-year period 1977 to 1980. When nurses move in and out of the job market the emphasis is placed on job security and subservience to avoid "rocking the boat." The lack of professional identification seems to prevent nurses from forming a "cohesive supportive nursing alliance with one another" (Weiss and Remen, 1983, p. 83). This lack of cohesion is easily exploited by the employing institution.

Despite a high patient to nurse ratio, rotating shifts, reassignment to "cover" other units, and constant change in patient assignments, some nurses, isolated from collective power to change the situation, will make do and maintain the status quo.

Willingness to accept second class status, to be less powerful than and placed under the authority of men has been a major obstacle to the development of a professional image and autonomy. The assumption that nursing, because it is women's work, is therefore second class in status is a powerful barrier to recruitment, retention, and improvement of the image of the profession.

Lack of Professional Identity

Many nurses have a great deal of difficulty articulating the professional domain of nursing. This uncertainty about what nursing contributes as a profession reinforces the image of the nurse as a "helper" or physician adjunct. In a study by Weiss and Remen (1983, p. 84) it was found that there is a "general tendency among nurses to reduce their professional expertise to personal bias." Nurses "behaved as if it was not acceptable for them to have professional opinion, and although "they verbally expressed a desire for greater recognition, greater power, and expanded professional rights, (they) visibly displayed their discomfort with responsibility" (Weiss and Remen, 1983, p. 85). "Through both word and gesture, nurses communicated subservience to the ideas and wishes of physicians" (Weiss and Remen, 1983, p. 85).

Roberts (1983) has analyzed nursing from the perspective of oppressed group behavior. Within this perspective, the values and norms of the dominant group (in this case medicine) lead to power and control. Inability to revolt against the powerful group leads to a "submissive aggression syndrome" among those with less power. This leads to "horizontal violence" manifested by internal conflict and fear of change. Leadership in the powerless group is characterized by "hatred of its own kind," desire to be like the oppressor, and rigid, controlling, and coercive behavior. Roberts suggests that nurses need to discover and value the "lost culture of nursing," and communicate its attributes through grass roots leadership.

Nursing has shown a "collective failure to adequately differentiate from medicine and firmly establish a separate professional identity" (Rogers, 1981, p. 479). Nurses tend to "identify the most responsible actions as the realm of the physician, and tend to devalue their own profession's abilities" (Weiss and Remen, 1983, p. 86). Nurses frequently are unable to identify the unique contribution of nursing to client health, "the diagnosis and treatment of human responses to actual or potential health problems" (American Nurses' Association Social Policy Statement, 1980, p. 9).

One of the most distinguishing characteristics of nursing is that it involves practices that are nurtrative, generative, or protective in nature. They are developed to meet the health needs of individuals as integrated persons rather than as biological systems. The nurtrative or nurturing behaviors provide comfort and therapy in the presence of illness or disease and foster personal development. The generative behaviors are oriented to development of new behaviors and modification of environments or systems to promote health-conducive adaptive responses of the individuals to health care crises or problems. The protective behaviors involve surveillance, assessment, and intervention in support of adaptive capabilities and developmental functions of persons. These nurse behaviors are responsive to people with conditions diagnosed and treated by nurses as they apply theory in order to explain and to guide nurse action in practice." (American Nurses' Association Social Policy Statement, 1980, p. 18)

"To be for nursing does not mean we need be against physicians or administrators" (Rogers, 1981, p. 481). Nurses need to come to terms with themselves as professionals with a body of knowledge and skills that are different from and complimentary to those of the medical profession. Until nursing appreciates and promotes the value of its practice, the profession will continue to be dominated and manipulated by others. For example, the current emphasis on cost containment in the health care delivery system could have major deleterious effects on nursing practice, especially in institutional settings.

Financial Issues

The United States spent $321 billion on health care in 1982. Medicare, the single largest payer of personal health services, spent $51 billion in 1982, and has been experiencing a 19% average annual increase in its expenditures (Davis, 1983, p. 67). Health care costs have been doubling every 5 years, based largely on increases in hospital costs. "The percent of the gross national product spent on health has grown from 6.2% in 1975 to 9.5% in 1980 and is expected to jump to 11.5% by 1990" (Kalisch and Kalisch, 1982, p. 94).

Variables that have influenced the continuing increase in health care expenditures are:

1. Higher health expectations among larger numbers of consumers.
2. Greater demand for a growing number of medical techniques and procedures.
3. A greater willingness on the part of a growing number of health care providers to give each patient the most and the best.
4. Increased expansion of beds, facilities, and services by hospitals seeking organizational prestige.
5. A tendency for third-party payers to reimburse uncritically for health care services." (Kalisch and Kalisch, 1982, p. 95).

A large part of health care cost escalation has been caused by the current structure of health care financing. Physicians and hospitals have a monopoly on health care costs, supported by third-party reimbursement schedules through Medicare, Medicaid, and private insurance payments. As medical specialization and technologic discoveries have increased the costs of diagnosis and treatment of disease, the costs have been passed on to the consumer. Since the salary costs for nursing personnel are hidden in the total hospital bill, the consumer is unaware that they have declined as a percentage of hospital expenses since 1968 (Fagin, 1982, p. 60). Registered nurses' salaries constituted only 11% of hospital costs in 1983 (Am Nurse, 1983). "The way in which nursing services are delivered prevents clients and colleagues from identifying a constant, accountable, and knowledgeable nurse provider" (Fagin, 1982, p. 57).

A number of studies have demonstrated that nurse practitioners can provide care as well and sometimes better than physicians, tend to elicit a positive response from their clients, and are generally cost-effective. For example, studies have shown that "nurse-midwifery achieved major reductions in prematurity and neonatal mortality, decreases in percentage of low birth-weight babies born, and increases in the number of babies born symptom free" (Fagin, 1982, p. 57). In another example, the frequency and length of stay of hospitalization of chronically ill elderly patients were markedly reduced when nurse practitioners provided their care (Fagin, 1982, p. 57). These data support the need to open the system and increase professional competition in the provision of health care. "Not only are their direct costs lower than those of physician providers, but the cost of ancillary services is greatly reduced when nurses are the primary carers" (Fagin, 1982, p. 59). In addition, nursing can have a major impact on the design of programs of health promotion and disease prevention that can ultimately reduce reliance on high-cost technologic interventions.

Current societal factors that reduce the likelihood of major changes in reimbursement systems include the rapid increase in the supply of physicians (Tailor, 1982), and a concurrent slowdown in the growth of total new dollars entering the health care system in the 1980s. These factors predict a growing pressure on the average earnings of physicians. Under the circumstances, they are likely to strenuously resist any efforts by nursing to provide competitive care, especially to "paying customers." At the same time the federal government, already struggling to bring the current system of reimbursement under some control, is unlikely to increase public liability by providing for fee-for-service reimbursement for nurse practitioners.

In fact, efforts toward cost containment in existing reimbursement systems have a real potential to threaten current support for quality nursing care. The change in medicare hospital and medical reimbursement from a per diem to a cost per discharge fee is known as diagnostic related groups (DRG). In this system, which began in October 1983, the patient population is divided into major diagnostic categories (MDC) and then subdivided into diagnostic related subgroups (DRG). Formulas permit adjustments for age of patients and presence or absence of complications. The hospital and medical income are based on prospectively established rates determined by the average cost per DRG, which are then multiplied by the number of patients discharged.

Significantly, nursing services are not directly reimbursed. Thus, the mix of nursing personnel needed to provide patient services is likely to be determined in large measure by criteria of cost-effectiveness rather than by standards of "quality nursing care." Directors of nursing services are required to provide a data base to justify the costs of nursing services, including the time required to achieve specified patient outcomes. In this climate it will be difficult to support the use of more highly educated (and hopefully, better paid) nurses in hospital patient care unless it can be documented that their care results in shorter hospitalizations, less complications, or less cost for auxillary personnel. There is no advantage to the hospital for reduced admissions or increased patient satisfaction with care!

On the other hand, third-party reimbursement has already been mandated in at least one state (Maryland) for nurse midwives and nurse practitioners without direct physician supervision (Griffith, 1982). One strategy that may help to encourage movement of other states toward direct third-party reimbursement of services provided by nurses is to stress the cost savings for the consumer that nurses can provide. As Maraldo (1982) says, "would not consumers and nurses alike be better served if nurses could deliver quality care *at a reasonable price?*" A percentage of the rate received by the physician would provide a dramatic demonstration of lower health delivery costs, based on the rationale that physician's fees are inflated and not that nurses provide less valuable service than do physicians. Nurses have also been encouraged to seek reimbursement for services already covered by insurers rather than attempting to obtain reimbursement for unique services (Griffith, 1982). This strategy increases the direct competition with physicians, but has the advantage of precedence, since "nurses have succeeded in receiving third-party payments for their services in cases where they have offered the same service for less in the "'substitution of other providers'" (Maraldo, 1982, p. 3). Direct third-party reimbursement for nursing services, a necessary component of autonomous nursing practice, is going to be difficult to attain. However, there is evidence of real progress on other fronts in the movement to foster truly professional, collaborative, and autonomous nursing practice within various care environments.

Developing Professional Influence

A person's feeling of being able to influence events through personal effort has been called political efficacy (Larsen, 1982). This approach has shown that if individuals believe that they can make a difference and can influence events in their lives they are likely to participate actively in trying to get what they want. Thus political efficacy is related to the perception of power.

Power

Power "represents the actual ability to control the behavior of other persons" (Moloney, 1979, p. 69). Power is defined as "the potential a person has to guide, direct, control or alter the behavior of others" (Yura *et al*, 1981, p. 48). It can be thought of as "potency or mastery, and the hallmark of power is effectiveness" (Kalisch and Kalisch, 1982, p. 2).

The two essentials of power are motive and resource (Burns, 1978, p. 12). It is assumed that the individual with power possesses something that is valued and can be manipulated by being increased or decreased by one person with respect to another. Power can be measured by the degree of production of the desired effects. For example, the threat of disapproval is often an effective source of power. If a child behaves because he fears his parent's withdrawal of affection, the parent has power.

There are a number of theories for determining who has power in a given context:

1. *Resource* theory indicates that the balance of power is on the side of the person who has the greatest resources. For example, if the nurse has the expertise to resolve a client's problem, the nurse has power.
2. *Exchange* theory views power in relation to an exchange of rewards and costs. For example, a nurse can have power in relation to a physician, by assisting him with procedures, following his medical orders, and so forth. In response, the physician can have power in relation to the nurse by rewarding her with praise in front of colleagues, the patient, or the administration.
3. *Decision-making* theory explains power in terms of who makes the final decision. Many students attribute power to their faculty because of their grade-granting authority.
4. *Systems* theory assumes that all system components are interdependent, and that power relationships involve more than simple cause and effect. For ex-

ample, a nurse may cause pain while giving an injection. When she tries to give the same patient another injection, her potential power based on possession of resources may be decreased by the patient's ability to say no. According to this theory it is not possible to look at one single exchange and determine who is exercising power (Kalisch and Kalisch, 1982, pp. 16–18).

It has been suggested that there are four sources of power: legitimate authority, control of rewards and punishment, identification, and persuasive communication (Yura *et al,* 1981, p. 59). French and Raven (1959, pp. 155–156), on the other hand, described five bases of power:

1. *Reward* power is based on the person's perception that the social agent has the ability to mediate rewards for him. The reward, which may be praise, recognition, status, or money, is a positive sanction. The director of nursing who can offer a raise in pay based on merit performance is using reward power as an incentive.

2. *Coercive* power is based on the person's perception that the social agent has the ability to mediate punishments for him. The punishment, which may be a threat or the withholding of a reward, is a negative sanction. It is usually used to punish noncompliance. The physician who threatens to report a nurse for "insubordination" is attempting to use coercive power. It may be effective if the nurse perceives that the complaint will have negative consequences. A high degree of threat is less productive than moderate or mild threats (Bass, 1981, p. 186).

3. *Legitimate* power is based on the person's perception that the social agent has a legitimate right to prescribe behavior for him. This is the same as authority that is vested in a role, position, or office, and is based on norms and expectations that are accepted and recognized by members of the organization. The supervisor who asks a nurse to work a double shift in an emergency is using legitimate power.

4. *Referent* power is based on the person's identification with the social agent. Often this kind of power is based on personal characteristics that the individual wants to emulate. Staff nurses may assume referent power in relation to student nurses who want to be "just like them."

5. *Expert* power is based on the person's perception that the social agent has some special knowledge or expertness. Groups tend to defer to the perceived and the actual expert. The patient usually perceives the nurse as an expert and, therefore, complies with her instructions.

Several other sources of power have been added to the above list. *Informational* power involves the ability of the agent to give good reasons for the recipient to behave as prescribed. "If the recipient sees these as valid, and if the information is consistent with the recipient's value system, then he or she complies" (Stevens, 1983, p. 11). This type of power is very similiar to expert power. *Associative* power is derived from a close alliance with a powerful individual or group. For example, membership in the American Nurses Association (ANA) provides power for the individual nurse because of the collective power of the organization. *Hierarchical* power is based on a boss-subordinate relationship within an organization. This type of power often is based on legitimate power with associated reward or coercive power.

The French and Raven classification has been criticized because the various bases of power were not defined in a conceptually parallel way. "Thus reward power and coercive power are defined in terms of resources available to the influencer. Referent and legitimate power are described in terms of the characteristics and motives of the target person. Finally, expert power depends on characteristics of the influencer and resources he or she possesses" (Bass, 1981, p. 191).

Another type of classification of sources of power is the differentiation between personal, interpersonal, and organizational power. Power can be derived in the form of affection, sympathy, recognition, consideration, or secure relationships. In personal power strength is a key element. Claus and Bailey (1977, pp. 43–47) describe it as a kind of dominance through strength and resiliency, energy, self-confidence, and action. Interpersonal power is derived from the moral support, joint problem-solving and team spirit, and feeling of pride often associated with a group. Organizational power is related to controls and authority in a formal structure, where individual needs are matched to needs of the organization.

"Coercive, reward, and legitimate power bases are organizationally controlled, whereas the referent power (attractiveness) and expert power bases are controlled by the individual leader" (Moloney, 1979, p. 71). It has been found that "subordinates are more satisfied when their superiors exercise expert and referent power (due to their person) than when they exercise reward, coercive or legitimate power (usually due to their position)" (Bass, 1981, p. 178). In addition, "groups are better satisfied and more productive when high-power positions are occupied by individuals scoring high in personal dominance" (Bass, 1981, p. 178).

Nurses need to assume power in order to exert professional leadership. Expert power should be used to affect the organizational climate within which nurses work, using nursing knowledge to promote desirable change. For example, knowledge of rhythm theory and research on the effects of shift changes present a strong rationale for changes in staffing patterns to avoid shift rotation. Associative power could be used to affect salaries and benefits, develop influence in the determination of policies, and assume authority for participation in the management of client care. Legitimate power should be used to affect the quality of the support systems available to the nurse in client care. For example, the head nurse has a legitimate right to expect the availability of sufficient administrative and technical assistance so that staff nurses' energies and time are not dissipated in nonnursing activities. Nurses can apply referent power to mobilize community resources in support of desired change.

As individuals, nurses must maintain their competence by continuing professional growth. Continuing education, whether or not for a credential, is necessary to keep up with rapid change in knowledge and its application to care. The professional must also be an activist in the work setting and the nurses' own community, setting an example as a change agent and advocate for client health.

However, nurses have the most potential power when they unite, using the power of numbers and associative power with the consumer to generate support for desired policies. As the largest group of health care providers, nursing has the power to modify the health care delivery system, promote funding for health promotion and illness prevention, and enhance the prestige of the profession. "Unity of purpose and conguence of motivation foster causal influence far down the line" (Burns, 1978, p. 439). The collective power of nurses exercising expert power with clients and interpersonal power with unified purposes on the system could be a major force toward change in the delivery of health care. It is unfortunate that until now nursing has chosen not to use that power.

Collaboration

Health care is a "composite of planned care provided by interdependent professions whose members collaborate with individuals and groups being served" (ANA Social Policy Statement, 1980, p. 13). "Collaboration means true partnership, in which the power on both sides is valued by both, with recognition and acceptance of separate and combined spheres of activity and responsibility, mutual safeguarding of the legitimate interests of each party, and a commonality of goals that is recognized by both parties" (American Nurses' Association Social Policy Statement, 1980, p. 7).

Nurses have had difficulty collaborating even with colleagues within the nursing profession. For years nursing educators and nursing service administrators have not been able to resolve differences of opinion about how students should best be educated in order to provide effective care. Kramer says, "nurse educators have lost both their perception of realistic professional nursing practice and their power to influence nursing practice in the work setting . . . " Nursing service has an "unrealistic vision of what is possible and lack of differentiation between ideal and deliverable" (Kramer, 1981, pp. 646, 651). Should new graduates be able to "hit the ground running," or is an orientation period of 3 to 12 months an appropriate expectation? Do new graduates "make up" for lack of confidence and limited technical skills on graduation with depth in analytical and leadership skills after the orientation period? Answers to these questions vary since little research data are available.

Collaborative nursing practice with other health care professionals requires that nurses develop confidence in their clinical competence and assume responsibility for decisions. Nurses must be assertive in their interpretation of appropriate nursing roles. This involves knowledge of facts, confidence, and the ability to keep one's ego out of the discussion. Ideally, interdependent collaborative relationships between nurses and other professionals would be characterized by "more equitable distribution of data collection about the client, joint decision making, a mutually agreed upon division of labor, and unified goal achievement" (Mauksch, 1981, p. 35). However, collaborative practice also assumes that the members of the partnership have autonomy in their practice.

Autonomy

Autonomy is a concept that is related to the independence, identity, and authority possessed by members of the occupation. Mundinger (1980, p. 7) has identified four reasons why nursing has been slow to identify and practice autonomous therapies: (1) "Nursing's close alliance with medicine, (2) nurse's employee status and secondary access to clients, (3) apprenticeship education, and (4) lack of definitive and permanent health outcomes." Critical to all of these is the need to articulate and demonstrate the unique and valuable contributions that nurses can make to health. Unfortunately, it is the technical components of care that are the most visible and predictable in outcome. It is important that nursing identify outcome measures based on comprehensive assessments and interventions that promote optimum health of clients, and demonstrate the effectiveness of nursing care.

Autonomy means to be "self-directed and accountable directly to clients" (Mundinger, 1980, p. 152). In the present health care delivery system, most nurses work for hospitals rather than for clients. Most people value what they choose and contract for. Thus, nurses must help clients to identify and value nursing services as specific, valuable contributions to their health. It is hoped that clients will then demand the services that only autonomous nursing practitioners can provide.

The profession needs to develop consensus about the areas in which only nursing can provide the expertise that people need. Nursing can work to establish a monopoly over the areas that have been claimed. DeSantis (1982), suggests that care of clients with chronic disease, in treatment programs for drug abuse and alcoholism, and those in need of preventive care are possible areas to begin to carve out exclusive control. She suggests that nursing should offer to develop less expensive forms of health care services than currently exist, and develop outcome measures to demonstrate cost-effectiveness. Another population in great need of health promotion to decrease illness and its effect on life-style are the aged. If such areas of influence are to be maintained however, nurses must be assertive, willing to assume risks, and accept accountability for their own autonomous actions.

Accountability

Accountability means to be answerable for one's own actions. This is the ultimate risk-taking. "Instead of being reaction oriented, assertive techniques are action-oriented and can help one achieve a sense of personal power, independent decision-making ability, and autonomy" (Henderson, 1981, p. 596). Nurses must be willing to influence others through the assertion of competence as an expression of professional self-worth. If nurses are to assume professional status, the greatest risk is to take no risks at all (Henderson, 1981, p. 597).

However, if nurses are to be able to exert expert power and be accountable for their actions, nursing practice must be based on valid and reliable knowledge derived from research. Too many practitioners continue to base their actions on intuitive or rote rationales, rather than on protocols verified by research data. In addition, there are some who resist changing practice, even when data are available. The anti-intellectualism that has affected nursing in the past must be replaced by increased emphasis on the conduct, dissemination, and use of sound research. Practice-based research is especially critically needed.

Professional nursing has been discussed from the perspective of autonomous, accountable, collaborative practice. Yet, the profession remains engrossed with internal struggles mainly related to manpower considerations. These concerns are discussed in the following section.

NURSING MANPOWER INFLUENCES

Before World War II nursing education was primarily financed by the private sector. However, since the war, as the number of diploma schools (financed by hospitals) has decreased, and the number of associate degree programs (financed mainly by state and local tax dollars) has increased, nursing education has increasingly been supported by public monies. Since 1970 baccalaureate degree programs in nursing have been almost evenly divided between private and public institutions.

The first comprehensive federal legislation to provide funding for nurse education was the Nurse Training Act of 1964, which aimed to prevent future shortages of nurses. Nurse training acts have been renewed in successive years, with almost $1.6 billion appropriated between 1962 and 1982. The primary impetus for continued funding was the perpetual "need" for more nurses than were available in the labor force. However, in the late 1970s, Congress mandated the Institute of Medicine to study need, supply and demand for nurses to determine whether the federal government should continue "its specific support of generalist nursing education in order to assure the adequacy of their supply?" (Institute of Medicine Study, 1983, p. 1). A full study committee was constituted in 1981, and the recommendations were published in 1983. Some of the data from the Institute of Medicine study are discussed below.

Changes in Health Care Delivery

During the 1970s there were widespread reports of a shortage of registered nurses to staff hospitals and nursing homes. Although large numbers of registered nurses joined the work force, there was a dramatic growth in the demand for nursing services. Increasingly, complex technology led to a growth from 3,200 intensive care unit beds in 1971 to 68,000 beds in 1980 (IOM Study, 1983, p. 56). The average length of stay in acute care hospitals decreased, resulting in an increased amount and intensity of nursing care needed by acutely ill patients. At the same time there was a tremendous growth in ambulatory care, and per capita community hospital admissions rose by 10%. The effect of these changes in health care delivery was an increased demand for numbers of experienced nurses to provide care for seriously ill patients.

Changes in Educational Preparation

During the decade between 1970 and 1980 there was a dramatic shift from diploma graduates (who comprised half of the total in 1970) to associate degree graduates (who made up almost half of the 1980 graduates). During that same period, the proportion of baccalaureate degree graduates grew steadily, from one fifth of the annual total in 1970 to one third in 1981 (IOM Study, 1983, p. 55).

In 1980 20% of practicing registered nurses held an associate degree as the highest level of educational attainment, 51% held a diploma, and 29% held a baccalaureate degree or higher. The projection for 1990 is that 36% of practicing registered nurses will hold a baccalaureate degree or higher, 28% will have an associate degree, and 36% will have diploma preparation as their highest level of educational attainment (IOM Study, 1983, p. 77).

The Western Interstate Commission on Higher Education (WICHE) developed criteria to assess the need for nurses with various types of educational preparation that has been used by a number of states to review their manpower needs. Based on these criteria, the IOM Study concluded that "there will be a much higher proportion of diploma and associate degree graduates than the WICHE judgement of need projection anticipates." Also, by 1990, "the educational system will have produced a much lower supply of registered nurses with baccalaureate and advanced degrees than the WICHE process projected" (IOM Study, 1983, p. 79) [Table 17–1].

There are a wide range of opinions among professional experts about what are appropriate and necessary nurse staffing goals in different parts of the country. Table 17–1 indicates the judgements of professional experts in nine states about required staff for inpatient hospital services, compared with the criteria for staffing developed by the WICHE National Panel of Expert Consultants.

The manpower data from the IOM Study raise a number of issues:

TABLE 17-1. Expert Panels' Judgement of Required Nursing Staff for Hospital Inpatient Services, US and Nine States, Using WICHE Methodology

	FTE Staff per 100 Patients				Ratio			Hours per Patient per Day			Educational Preparation					
	RN	LPN	Aide	Total	RN	LPN	Aide	RN	Total	%RN	Doctorate	Master's	Baccalaureate	Associate Degree/ Diploma	Associate Degree	Diploma
National panel	49.0	12.0	12.0	73.0	10.0	2.4	2.4	2.4	3.6	67.0	—	—	50.0	50.0	—	—
Alabama	73.9	39.9	0.0	113.8	10.0	5.4	0.0	4.2	6.5	65.0	—	7.5	60.0	—	20.0	12.5
Colorado	81.0	20.0	0.0	101.0	10.0	2.5	0.0	4.0	5.0	80.0	—	—	50.0	50.0	—	—
Mississippi	40.0	20.0	30.0	90.0	10.0	5.0	7.5	2.0	5.0	40.0	—	5.0	20.0	75.0	—	—
New Hampshire																
General units	32.3	22.6	0.0	54.9	10.0	7.0	0.0	1.6	2.7	59.0	—	3.0	55.0	42.0	—	—
Primary care	48.5	29.1	0.0	77.6	10.0	6.0	0.0	2.4	3.8	83.0	—	3.0	55.0	42.0	—	—
Ohio																
General units	79.0	37.0	6.0	122.0	10.0	4.7	0.8	3.9	6.0	65.0	—	—	60.0	—	15.0	25.0
Pediatrics	92.0	43.0	7.0	142.0	10.0	4.7	1.0	4.5	7.0	65.0	—	—	60.0	—	15.0	25.0
Rhode Island	48.0	15.0	—	63.0	10.0	3.1	—	2.4	3.1	77.0	—	6.0	35.0	59.0	—	—
West Virginia	47.5	15.7	6.0	69.2	10.0	3.3	1.3	2.3	3.4	68.0	—	—	20.0	—	30.0	50.0
Wisconsin	80.0	0.0	20.0	100.0	10.0	0.0	2.5	3.9	4.9	80.0	—	5.0	20.0	—	75.0	—
Wyoming	78.0	15.0	15.0	108.0	10.0	1.9	1.9	4.0	5.5	73.0	—	—	50.0	50.0	—	—

(Modified from data in Kearns JM, Cooper MA, Uris PF: Comparison of the rationale and criteria for staffing developed by the National Panel of Expert Consultants with those developed by panels of eight states [revised February 1981]. Boulder, Colorado, Western Interstate Commission for Higher Education, 1980, and Institute of Medicine Study, p 82, and Wyoming Nursing Manpower Plan 1982–1986, Wyoming Department of Health and Social Services, 1982, p. 17).

Levels of Education

Are all present forms of nursing education needed or desired? Documented changes in the health care delivery system toward increasingly acutely ill patients in hospitals supports the need for a sound theory data base for nursing care judgements. At the same time, increasing costs of hospitalization mandate changes in the delivery system to provide ambulatory care to maintain health and prevent disease. Both of these emphases can best be provided within baccalaureate nursing education. Yet, the perpetuation of the "a nurse is a nurse" mentality creates the impression of a sufficient supply of nurses at a time when the number of nurses being prepared at the baccalaureate level is woefully inadquate. The profession must develop acceptable criteria for differentiating between types of nursing preparation as a rationale for the need for support to the baccalaureate level of generalist education. In addition, help should be given to diploma schools to phase out in favor of programs organized within institutions of higher education. All of nursing should support the immediate establishment of only two *kinds* of education within registered nursing, with movement toward clarification of educational patterns for two *levels* within nursing.

How should the products of AD and BS levels of nursing education be differentiated? There are at least two significantly different philosophies underlying the "leveling controversy. One position is based on a belief that baccalaureate education is an additive process. Proponents of this position believe that the critical components of professional practice can be taught at the AD level, and that other knowledge and skills (*e.g.*, leadership, research and health maintenance roles) can be added later. This position is related to a view of the BS graduate having skills that are somehow "more than" rather than "different from" the AD graduate. Another position is based on a belief that baccalaureate education is a synthesis of liberal and professional content that prepares a practitioner with a different critical thinking process and a different conceptualization of roles than the AD graduate.

Belief in the "additive" philosophy has led to an increase from 29 to 84 "RN only" programs between 1971 and 1980 (and 37% of the RN enrollment in baccalaureate programs in 1980). In addition there has been widespread acceptance of validation testing of prior knowledge and skill for placement in "generic" programs. Students typically test out of many of the sophomore and junior level courses, and "add" the senior year of nursing and required liberal education courses. This approach has been bolstered by societal pressures. For example, most community colleges are supported by public tax dollars. It has been difficult to explain to legislators why credit earned in "lower division" nursing education should not be directly applicable to "upper division" education.

No definitive research has been done to demonstrate that baccalaureate degree graduates from the "2+2 pattern" practice significantly differently from those who graduate from the "generic pattern." More controversial yet, data are mixed on whether or not associate degree graduates practice significantly differently than do baccalaureate graduates! Research is needed that will identify the significant variables in education and practice that produce practitioners whose differences can be clearly articulated. Then progress can be made toward appropriate educational and employment practices to ensure effective and cost-efficient nursing services.

Educational Mobility

Should educational mobility be encouraged? The opportunity for educational mobility has always characterized nursing education. However, in the past decade, this movement has assumed major proportions. In 1970, RNs comprised 13% of the enrollment in baccalaureate nursing programs. By 1980, RNs comprised 34% of the enrollment in baccalaureate nursing programs. Between 1971 and 1980, total enrollment in baccalaureate nursing programs nearly doubled (from 67,485 to 131,861), but enrollment of RN students in baccalaureate nursing programs increased 338%. It is projected that by 1990 about 100,000 of the 257,000 baccalaureate degree or higher prepared nurses will have earned the higher degree post-RN.

Several factors may have contributed to this phenomenon. The ANAs position in favor of baccalaureate education for entry to professional nursing has motivated a number of nurses to seek the credential in fear that lack of the baccalaureate degree in the future will either disenfranchise them, or limit job advancement opportunities. In addition, the 1970s were a decade of rapid growth in graduation of students from associate degree programs in nursing. These students already possess a significant number of academic credits that could be applied toward the higher degree. The early philosophy of the associate degree program as a "terminal" degree, began to change toward a conceptualization of associate degree education as an exit point for licensure, and part of a baccalaureate degree.

It is clear that societal influences in the 1980s will continue this trend. The population base for "generic" baccalaureate enrollment will continue to decrease. Thus, many baccalaureate programs that previously enrolled primarily high school graduates, now view the registered nurse population as a valuable source of students. As college costs continue to rise, many students seek associate degree education in community colleges close to home with the intention of working part-time while continuing their education toward the baccalaureate degree. All factors indicate that educational mobility will be an increasingly significant factor in baccalaureate nursing education.

DEVELOPMENT OF A SCIENCE OF NURSING

The purpose of a science has been described as "the discovery of new knowledge, the expansion of existing knowledge, and/or the reaffirming of previously held knowledge" (Andreoli and Thompson, 1977, p. 33), in order to "explain, understand, predict, and control natural events" (Kerlinger, 1973). Nursing needs a body of knowledge that will guide the practice of nursing and also provide a basis for the legitimacy and autonomy of the profession. It is fairly well accepted that nursing is in the beginning stages of developing a body of theoretical knowledge that will give clear direction to education, research, and practice (Feldman, 1980, p. 87). The development of nursing as a scientific discipline was discussed in Chapter 5, "Scientific Thought and Theory Development."

In developing the curriculum for the first school of nursing Florence Nightingale examined what nurses actually did in the hospital. As a consequence, the image of nursing became associated with the tasks and procedures that were the focus of the school curriculum. This "task orientation" persisted, eventually becoming associated with diseases of various body systems. According to Ellis (1982, p. 407), "rejection of the disease or body-systems perspective for nursing was forced by the identification of a burgeoning list of specific disease entities, the recognition of the import of psychologial and social factors in disease or in response to it, and by discovery or, at least, affirmation of the obvious: patients are people."

In the 1950s and 1960s a number of nurses presented definitions of nursing that changed the conceptualization of nursing. Currently most nursing curricula focus on concepts and on nursing process. This approach emphasized the knowledge needed for effective nursing planning, intervention, and evaluation, complementary to the nursing diagnosis and regimen. A number of models of nursing are presently being used to determine the selection and organization of nursing content. Some commonly used models were discussed in Chapter 8, "Models of Nursing."

In the past 10 years, in association with the development of models of nursing, there has been a radical increase in the interest in "nursing theory," in the growth of research training in masters and doctoral programs in nursing, and in the growing sense that a "science of nursing" is emerging. However, the development of nursing science is hindered by inadequate numbers of nurses who are prepared to conduct research, and by limited funding and visibility of nursing research.

Graduate Education

In 1980, 5% of all registered nurses held master's or doctoral degrees (IOM Study, 1983, p. 141). However, of the 80,000 master's prepared nurses, only two thirds or 55,055 had the master's degree in nursing. In 1980, 4,100 nurses had a doctoral degree. However, less than 850 (21% of those with doctoral degrees) had the degree in nursing. It is expected that by 1990, the deficit of master's and doctorally prepared nurses will become increasingly acute. WICHE projections of need (lower bound) are for 256,000 full-time equivalents (FTE) by 1990 for master's prepared nurses. The projected supply is less than half of that number. The need for nurses with doctorates by 1990 is projected at 14,000 FTE, almost three times the expected supply (IOM Study, 1983, p. 145). These data are shown in Table 17–2.

The lack of nurses with advanced education in nursing has particularly affected nursing administration and nursing research. Between 1971 and 1980 only about 7% of all graduates of master's programs in nursing had a concentration in administration (IOM Study, 1983, p. 135). Research in nursing has also been handicapped by inadequate levels of support. Between 1971 and 1981, $40 million was awarded for nursing research. During that same period, the National Institutes of Health received $1.7 billion for general biomedical research! The IOM Study concluded that "there is both a serious current and probable 1990 shortage of nurses educationally prepared for administration, teaching, research, and advanced clinical nursing specialties" (IOM Study, 1983, p. 149). Many of the recommendations of the IOM Study address the need for federal support for advanced education in nursing and nursing research (see Appendix).

TABLE 17–2. Comparison of Projected Supply of Nurses with Advanced Degrees in 1990 with WICHE Judgement of Need

Type of Degree	Total Employed November 1980	Projected FTE December 1990	Judgement of Need (WICHE)
Master's (all degrees)	65,200	112,400	256,000
Doctorate (all degrees)	3,000	5,600	14,000
Total	68,200	118,000	270,000

(Institute of Medicine: Nursing and Nursing Education: Policies and Private Actions, p 177. Washington, National Academy Press, 1983)

Funding and Visibility for Nursing Research

The IOM Study has already had several tangible results. For example, several recommendations addressed the need for financial support for nursing research. For fiscal year 1984, Congress has authorized $9 million for nursing research, up from a little more than $5 million the previous year. One specific recommendation was that "the federal government should establish an organizational entity to place nursing research in the mainstream of scientific investigation" (see Appendix). As of January 1984, a proposal to establish a National Institute of Nursing (NIN) had been approved by the United States House of Representatives and was to be debated in the United States Senate. The mission of the proposed National Institute of Nursing is:

> the conduct, support, and dissemination of basic and clinical research, training, and related programs in nursing. The programs of the Institute will be oriented primarily toward basic and applied scientific inquiry related to the promotion of health, prevention of illness, and understanding human responses of individuals and families to acute and chronic illnesses and disabilities. Included in the agenda for The Institute will be inquiry concerning health processes and related fundamental mechanisms as well as individual, family, and community behavioral processes underlying self-care and/or nursing care related to health, illness, disability, and recovery. In addition, The Institute will sponsor training of nursing research personnel, career development of new and established scientists, evaluation of specific nursing interventions, dissemination of new information about nursing and health, and demonstrations of alternative modes of delivery of nursing care.

These are positive signs that nursing research will receive increased visibility and more adequate funding. It is critical to the profession that graduate education *in nursing* (including research preparation) be expanded, and that nurses with appropriate training be encouraged and supported in their research efforts. There is nothing more critical to the future of the nursing profession than the development of its scientific base.

SUMMARY

The nursing profession has the potential to exert enormous power toward better health of consumers and a more responsive health care system to deliver health care. Progress is being made in a number of critical areas. For example:

1. For all practical purposes, nursing education has now moved into the mainstream of higher education. A number of national nursing organizations support the baccalaureate degree as preparation for professional nursing practice, including the NLN and the ANA. Graduations from associate degree, baccalaureate, master's, and doctoral programs continue to increase. There continues to be a need for clarification of the differences between technical and professional practice, and for facilitation of educational mobility for those who change career goals.

2. There is a growing recognition that the appropriate use of nurses in the work environment must be based on differences in educational preparation as well as experience. In addition, attention is being paid to the positive

factors that attract nurses to particular work settings, and help to maintain satisfaction and retention.

3. There is widespread agreement that public and private support is needed for graduate nursing education. The number of master's and doctoral programs in nursing is increasing. However, student financial support is critical if enrollments (especially fulltime) are to be maintained.

4. Scholarly work in nursing continues to expand. An increasing number of books and periodicals devoted to theory and research in nursing have appeared in recent years. Numerous workshops and conferences devoted to nursing research are now presented each year. The number of chapters of the National Honor Society (Sigma Theta Tau) is at an all time high and continuing to grow.

5. Nursing is clearly moving toward a scientific basis for practice and an organization of knowledge that identifies the unique contribution of the profession in the provision of health care to the public.

The ability of the nursing profession to come into its own will depend to a large measure on the self-confidence and professional self-image of its practitioners. As the rate of change accelerates, there is great potential for dynamic and profound development of the profession. This "self-actualization of the profession" is the goal toward which this book has been addressed.

APPENDIX

Recommendations of the Institute of Medicine Study

1. No specific federal support is needed to increase the overall supply of registered nurses, because estimates indicate that the aggregate supply and demand for generalist nurses will be in reasonable balance during this decade. However, federal, state, and private actions are recommended throughout this report to alleviate particular kinds of shortages and maldistributions of nurse supply.

2. The states have primary responsibility for analysis and planning of resource allocation for generalist nursing education. Their capabilities in this effort vary greatly. Assistance should be made available from the federal government, both in funds and in technical aid.

3. The federal government should maintain its general programs of financial aid to postsecondary students so that qualified prospective nursing students will continue to have the opportunity to enter generalist nursing education programs in numbers sufficient to maintain the necessary aggregate supply.

4. Institutional and student financial support should be maintained by state and local governments, higher education institutions, hospitals, and third-party payers to assure that generalist nursing education programs have capacity and enrollments sufficient to graduate the numbers and kinds of nurses commensurate with state and local goals for the nurse supply.

5. To assure a sufficient continuing supply of new applicants, nurse educators and national nursing organizations should adopt recruitment strategies that attract not only recent high school graduates but also nontraditional prospective students, such as those seeking late entry into a profession or seeking to change careers, and minorities.

6. Licensed nurses at all levels who wish to upgrade their education so as to en-

hance career opportunities should not encounter unwarranted barriers to admission. State education agencies, nursing education programs, and employers of nurses should assume a shared responsibility for developing policies and programs to minimize loss of time and money by students moving from one nursing education program level to another.

7. Closer collaboration between nurse educators and nurses who provide patient services is essential to give students an appropriate balance of academic and clinical practice perspectives and skills during their educational preparation. The federal government should offer grants to nursing education programs that, in association with the nursing services of hospitals and other health care providers, undertake to develop and implement collaborative educational, clinical, and/or research programs.

8. The federal government should expand its support of fellowships, loans and programs at the graduate level to assist in increasing the rate of growth in the number of nurses with master's and doctoral degrees in nursing and relevant disciplines. More such nurses are needed to fill positions in administration and management of clinical services and of health care institutions, in academic nursing (teaching, research, and practice), and in clinical specialty practice.

9. To alleviate nursing shortages in medically underserved areas, their residents need better access to all types of nursing education, including outreach and off-campus programs. The federal government should continue to cosponsor model demonstrations of programs with states, foundations, and educational institutions, and should support the dissemination of results.

10. To meet the nursing needs of specific population groups in medically underserved areas and to encourage better minority representation at all levels of nursing education, the federal government should institute a competitive program for state and private institutions that offer institutional and student support under the following principles:

    a. Programs must be developed in close collaboration with, and include commitments from, providers of health services in shortage areas.

    b. Scholarships and loans contingent on commitments to work in shortage areas should be targeted, though not limited, to members of minority and ethnic groups to the extent that they are likely to meet the needs of underserved populations, including non-English-speaking groups.

11. Differential allowances in payment should take into account the special burdens on inner-city hospitals that demonstrate legitimate difficulties in financing services because of disproportionate numbers of uninsured or Medicaid and Medicare patients. Federal, state, and local governments and third-party payers should pay their fair shares of amounts necessary to prevent insolvency and to support acceptable levels of service including nursing care.

12. The rapidly growing elderly population requires many kinds of nursing services for preventive, acute, and long-term care. To augment the supply of new nurses interested in caring for the elderly, nursing education programs should provide more formal instruction and clinical experiences in geriatric nursing. Federal support of such efforts is needed, as well as funding from states and private sources.

13. Nursing service staffs in nursing homes certified as "skilled nursing facilities" and other institutions and programs providing care to the elderly often lack necessary knowledge and skills to meet the clinical challenges presented by these patients. Such facilities, in collaboration with nursing education programs and other private and public organizations, should develop and support pro-

grams to upgrade the knowledge and skills of the aides, LPNs, and RNs who work with elderly patients. States should assist vocational and higher education programs to respond to these needs. Federal support of such programs should be maintained.

14. The federal government (and the states, where applicable) should restructure Medicare and Medicaid payments so as to encourage and support the delivery of long-term care nursing services provided to patients at home and in institutions. For skilled nursing facilities, such payment policies should encourage the continuing education of present staffs and the recruitment of more licensed nurses (LPNs and RNs), and should permit movement toward a goal of 24-hour RN coverage.

15. There is a need for the services of nurse practitioners, especially in medically underserved areas and in programs caring for the elderly. Federal support should be continued for their educational preparation. State laws that inhibit nurse practitioners and nurse midwives in the use of their special competencies should be modified. Medicare, Medicaid, and other public and private payment systems should pay for the services of these practitioners in organized settings of care, such as long-term care facilities, free-standing health centers and clinics, and health maintenance organizations, and in joint physician-nurse practices.

16. The proportion of nurses who choose to work in their profession is high, but examination of conventional management, organization, and salary structures indicate that employers could improve both supply and job tenure by the following:
    a. providing opportunities for career advancement in clinical nursing as well as in administration.
    b. ensuring that merit and experience in direct patient care are rewarded by salary increases.
    c. assessing the need to raise nurse salaries if vacancies remain unfilled.
    d. encouraging greater involvement of nurses in decisions about patient care, management, and governance of the institution.
    e. identifying the major deterrents to nurse labor force participation in their own localities and responding by adapting conditions of work, child-care, and compensation packages to encourage part-time nurses to increase their labor force participation and to attract inactive nurses back to work.

17. Lack of precise information about current costs and utilization of nursing service personnel makes it difficult for nursing service administrators and hospital managers to make the most appropriate and cost-effective decisions about assignment of nurses. Hospitals, working with federal and state governments and other third-party payers, should conduct studies and experiments to determine the feasibility and means of creating separate revenue and cost centers for direct nursing care units within the institution for case-mix costing and revenue setting, and for other fiscal management alternatives.

18. The federal government should establish an organizational entity to place nursing research in the mainstream of scientific investigation. An adequately funded focal point is needed at the national level to foster research that informs nursing and other health care practice and increases the potential for discovery and application of various means to improve patient outcomes.

19. Federal and private funds should support research that will provide scientifically valid measurements of the knowledge and performance competencies of nurses with various levels and types of educational preparation and experience.

20. As national and regional forums identify promising approaches to problems in the organization and delivery of nursing services, there will be a need for wider experimentation, demonstration, and evaluation. The federal government, in conjunction with private sector organizations, should participate in the critical assessment of new ideas and the broad dissemination of research results.
21. To ensure that federal and state policymakers have the information they need for future nurse manpower decisions, the federal government should continue to support the collection and analysis of compatible, unduplicated, and timely data on national nursing supply, education, and practice, with special attention to filling identified deficits in currently available information.

REFERENCES

Am Nurse 15:1, January 1983

American Nurses Association: Nursing: A Social Policy Statement, Kansas City, American Nurses Association (Pub. Code NP-63 35M), December 1980

Andreoli K, Thompson C: The nature of science in nursing. Image 9:2, 32–37, 1977

Bass BM: Stogdill's Handbook Of Leadership. New York, The Free Press, 1981

Burns JM: Leadership. New York, Harper Colophon Books, 1978

Claus KE, Bailey JT: Power and Influence in Health Care. St Louis, CV Mosby, 1977

Davis CK: Nursing and the health care debates. Image 15:67, Summer 1983

deSantis G: Power, tactics, and the professionalization process. Nurs Health Care 3:1, 14–24, January 1982

Eisenstein H: On the psychological barriers to professions for women. In Muff J (ed): Socialization, Sexism and Stereotyping. St Louis, CV Mosby, 1982

Ellis R: Conceptual issues in nursing. Nurs Outlook 30:406 410, July–August 1982

Fagin CM: Nursing as an alternative to high-cost care. Am J Nurs 82:56–60, January 1982

Feldman H: Nursing research in the 1980's: Issues and implications. Adv Nurs Sci 3:4, 85–92, 1980

French JRP Jr, Raven B: The bases of social power. In Cartwright D (ed): Studies in Social Power. Ann Arbor, University of Michigan, 1959

Griffith HM: Strategies for direct third-party reimbursement for nurses. Am J Nurs 82:408–414, March 1982

Henderson G: Nurses as risk-takers. In McCloskey JC, Grace HK (eds): Current Issues in Nursing, pp 593–597. Oxford, Blackwell Scientific Publications, 1981

Institute Of Medicine: Nursing and Nursing Education: Public Policies and Private Actions. Washington, National Academy Press, 1983

Johnson WL, Vaughn JC: Supply and Demand Relations and the Shortage of Nurses. Nurs Health Care:497–507, November 1982

Kalisch BJ, Kalisch PA: Politics of Nursing. Philadelphia, JB Lippincott, 1982

Kerlinger F: Foundations of Behavioral Research. New York, Holt, Rinehart & Winston, 1973

Knopf L: Registered nurses fifteen years after graduation: findings from the nurse career-pattern study. Nurs Health Care 4:2, 72–76, February 1983

Kramer M: Why does reality shock continue? In McClosky J, Grace HK (eds): Current Issues in Nursing, pp 644–653. Oxford, Blackwell Scientific Publications, 1981

Larsen J: Nurse power for the 1980's. Nurs Adm Quar 6:74–82, Summer 1982

Maraldo P: Reimbursement for nurses in the primary care arena: A cost saving for health care. National League for Nursing Public Policy Bulletin 1:5, November 1982

Mauksch I: Nurse–physician collaboration: A changing relationship. J Nurs Ad 11:35–38, June 1981

Moloney MM: Leadership in Nursing: Theories, Strategies, Action. St Louis, CV Mosby, 1979

Mundinger MO: Autonomy in Nursing. Germantown, Aspen Systems Corporation, 1980

NLN Nursing Data Book 1981. New York, National League for Nursing (Pub No 19-1882), 1982

Roberts SJ: Oppressed group behavior: Implications for nursing. Adv Nurs Sci 5:21–30, July 1983

Rogers JA: Toward professional adulthood. Nurs Outlook 29:478–81, August 1981

Stevens KR: Power and Influence: A Source Book for Nurses. New York, John Wiley & Sons, 1983

Tailor AR: Report of the Graduate Medical Education National Advisory Committee to the Secretary (Summary Report): Washington DC, US Department of Health and Human Services, Public Health Service. Health Resources Administration, April 1982

Weiss S, Remen N: Self limiting patterns of nursing behavior within a tripartite context involving consumers and physicians. West J Nurs Res 5:77–89, 1983

Yeaworth RC: Feminism and the nursing profession. *In* Chaska NL (ed): The Nursing Profession: Views Through the Mist. New York, McGraw-Hill, 1978

Yura H, Ozimek D, Walsh MB: Nursing Leadership: Theory and Process, New York, Appleton-Century-Crofts, 1981

.

Chapter 18

Future Perspectives

During the past 15 to 20 years, dramatic societal and professional changes have occurred that have influenced nursing education, service, and research. The forces that have influenced change have been detailed throughout preceding chapters. The intent of this chapter is to project current trends in order to gain a perspective on the nursing profession as it may appear at the turn of the century.

CHANGES IN HEALTH AND HEALTH CARE DELIVERY

Since 1950 there has been a demonstrable shift in the causes of mortality from the infectious diseases to chronic diseases and diseases associated with life stress. Although influenza and pneumonia continue to be the fifth largest cause of death in children aged 1 to 14, the mortality rate for these infectious diseases has decreased 84% since 1950. During the same time, death rates from homicide and suicide in adolescents (aged 15–24) have increased, and cirrhosis is the fifth largest cause of death among adults. Heart disease, while significantly decreased as a cause of mortality, is still the largest cause of deaths among adults and the elderly. Infant deaths are closely related to maternal smoking, alcohol, drug use, and poor nutrition. There is every indication that these trends will continue, if not accelerate, owing to people's increased life span and the rapid pace and increasingly technologic emphasis of modern life.

There has also been a demonstrable increase in people's interest in assuming responsibility for self-care, and in activities such as diet, exercise, and stress reduction that give promise of assisting in the promotion of health. This trend offers great potential for nursing to assume leadership in helping people to maintain health, promote well-being, and prevent illness.

Hospitalization has often been prescribed because of needed nursing care. Reasons for hospitalization, until fairly recently, have included diagnostic laboratory testing, routine care, or rehabilitation, in addition to restorative care. Increasingly, however, the high cost and highly specialized medical technology associated with hospitalization has led to use of hospitals primarily for diagnosis and attempted cure of serious acute illnesses and treatment of chronic disease. Minor illnesses and illness prevention have been provided through separately contracted ambulatory care in clinics, doctors' offices, and people's homes.

Central to the current organization of the health care delivery system is the concept that the client contracts with the physician for care, while nursing is supplied by the hospital as part of a package of services. The system is structured for the facilitation of medical cure. In the future, the system could move either toward increased centralization or decentralization of services. The decentralized model, consisting of a number of components separate from the hospital, could be facilitative of entrepreneurial nursing delivery systems. For example, nurses could form independent practices, or associate in partnerships with a variety of other health care professionals. With direct third-party reimbursement nurses could contract directly with the client for the provision of nursing services. With this model, nursing could assume responsibility for and control of nursing care delivery.

However, given the power, influence, and control of the medical-hospital industry, it is unlikely that the health care delivery system will be completely restructured in the forseeable future. It is highly possible that hospitals will move toward centralization of services in care centers that will include ambulatory services as well as inpatient care. This model could accentuate the current employee status of most nurses, and further consolidate the financial control of "health care" by hospitals and physicians. The challenge for nursing will be to gain autonomy within the system. For this, nurses will need equality with other health professionals that can only be accomplished through comparable educational qualifications and an equivalent allocation of authority.

The movement toward prospective payment is bound to become the standard for third-party reimbursement by private as well as public agencies, and for physicians and other professionals, as well as hospitals and other care institutions. Nursing must actively promote the cost and care benefits of well-educated, highly skilled professionals in the system, or run the very possible risk of replacement by less highly salaried workers. It is critical that the nursing profession emphasize the cost effectiveness of competent care, and assume initiative in documenting the unique contribution of nursing to the restoration of health and prevention of illness in clients. One positive aspect of prospective payment is the potential of clear labeling of the distinct contribution made by nursing to restoration of well-being, thus promoting the valuing of nursing services by the public.

CHANGES IN EDUCATION

The knowledge base and technology used in providing nursing care will continue to increase. With increasing need for skill in intensively acute aspects of care, as well as the necessity for diagnostic and decision-making ability, teaching, coordination of less skilled workers, and ability to collaborate with clients and health care professionals to improve the quality of health, nurses in the future will more than ever need a broad-based education, assertiveness skills, technical competence, and the ability to deal with rapid change.

In the past 20 years there has been an intensive national effort to promote the baccalaureate degree as the entry level for professional nursing. In that time, there has been an increase in the number of nurses prepared at the baccalaureate level, and a small increase in the percentage of nurses with that credential. However, in the same period of time there has been a dramatic increase in the percentage of nurses prepared at the associate degree level, so that about 70% of nurses are still being prepared at the technical level of nursing. Previously educated nurses comprise more than a third of baccalaureate enrollments.

Entry to nursing could conceivably occur at one of three levels, the associate degree, the baccalaureate degree, or the master's degree. Thus, there are at least three different patterns of education for nursing that might predominate in the future.

The current pattern, entry at the associate degree level, with professional education at the baccalaureate degree level might be perpetuated. Nursing is a profession that has been closely associated with upward mobility, especially for women. Most associate degree programs are located in community colleges, and thus are financially and geographically accessible. Demand can readily be met by an increased supply of licensed workers in a short period of time. Many students perceive the education at the baccalaureate level as additional and repetitive rather than different and enriching. Little incentive for professional education is provided by the delivery system, which lacks differential salary structures or clearly articulated differences in job expectations. Licensure as a registered nurse after associate degree education has served to reinforce this model.

There are some who propose that education for entry to professional nursing be moved to the master's level rather than the baccalaureate level. This level of education would prepare the student for a combination of specialized as well as generalized practice. All students would need a prior bachelor's degree for entry into nursing, which would strengthen the liberal arts and science base for practice, encourage recruitment of students from other fields, and raise the status and authority of the profession. This model for nursing education would probably include the associate degree for nursing assistants and the master's degree for licensed professional nurses.

A third and more feasible possibility is that the baccalaureate degree will become the entry level credential for professional practice, and be recognized as such with the appropriate licensure. Most major nursing organizations, including the American Nurses' Association (ANA) and the National League for Nursing (NLN) have now endorsed that goal. An increasing number of nurses are seeking baccalaureate education and the credential in order to practice at a professional level. The profession needs to better articulate and publicize the contribution to health promotion and restoration as well as illness prevention of a professionally educated practitioner. This book has identified the knowledge base and values that characterize the professional nurse in the hope that articulation will be a first step toward acceptance of scholarship and demonstration of professional competence in practice. If the baccalaureate degree does become the entry level for professional practice, the associate degree will probably become the accepted credential for practical nursing.

Regardless of which model is accepted by the year 2000, all educational programs must continue to modify their curricula to include changes in the theoretical and technical data base for nursing. For example, computer technology has begun to make an enormous impact on discovery, communication, and storage of knowledge. Yet few nurses are "computer literate," and only a few schools have included computer courses in their curricula. Little attention has yet been paid to the moral implications of a computerized society that engenders feelings of isolation associated with nonpersonal communication and invasion of privacy.

Other examples of developing knowledge include bioengineering, aerospace and underwater effects on man, and care of clients receiving artificial and human organ transplants (Leininger, 1978). The continuing development and testing of the theory base for nursing will lead to the development of knowledge that must be integrated into the educational curriculum.

NURSING RESEARCH

Such rapid development has occurred in nursing theory and research in the past 10 years that the promise for the next 15 years is very hopeful. What is most needed is the explication of theory that is predictive of nursing outcomes. It is possible that by 2000, there will be several accepted theories of nursing that will have been validated by research and be in use in practice as the basis for care. If such is the case, the promise for the future of professional nursing as described in this book will have become a reality.

REFERENCES

Leininger M: Futurology of nursing: Goals and challenges for tomorrow. In Chaska NL (ed): The Nursing Profession: Views Through the Mist. New York, McGraw-Hill, 1978

Schlesinger AM: Robert Kennedy and His Times. New York, Houghton Mifflin, 1978

Index

Numbers followed by an *f* indicate a figure; *t* following a page number indicates tabular material.

Age, well-being and, 160
Accountability, professional, 44, 198–202, 262, 304
  ANA Code on, 196
  to client, 199
  competence and, 202–203
  definition of, 195–198
  education and, 204–205
  to employing agency, 201–202
  ethics and, 203–204
  leadership skills and, 203
  positive aspects of, 205–208
  to self, 200–201
  theoretical basis for, 202
Adaptation, stressors and, 119
Adaptation model, 142–143
  concepts of, 142t
  terms of, 142
Adaptation theory, 119–122
  vs. other theories, 132t
Adolescence, stages of, 125
Advocacy
  coordination and, 286
  ethics of, 287–288
  facilitation and, 285–286
  meanings of, 284–286
  mutuality and, 285
  need for, 288–289
  protection and, 286
  theoretical basis for, 284
Ambulatory care, 178
The American Nurse, 14
American Nurses' Association, 9, 13, 14–15, 43
  agenda for health policy, 186
  Code for Nurses, 45, 46–47, 196, 198–199
  Commission on Nursing Services, 190
  Position Paper, 12
  and power for nurses, 301
  Social Policy Statement, 189, 297–298
  Standards of Nursing Practice, Service, and Education, 198, 212
  structure of, 270–271
Andragogy, 34
  comparison with pedagogy, 35t
Anxiety
  definition of, 241
  Freud on, 128
  interpersonal, 241

  nurses' role in controlling, 241
Associate degree, in nursing, 11
  minimal competencies for, 41
Association of Collegiate Schools of Nursing, 13
Authority
  formal, 258
  functional, 258
  leadership role and, 257–258
Autonomy
  in nursing practice, 303–304
  of patient, 287

Baccalaureate degree, in nursing
  accountability and, 204–205
  minimal competencies for, 41–42
  contributions of, to nursing research, 101
  enrollment in, 308
Behavior
  Freud on, 128
  preventive. *See* preventive behavior
Behavioral system model, 138–139
  subsystems of, 138–139
  terms of, 138
Being
  categories of, 23
  concepts of, 23–24
Biculturalism, 37
Blake and Moulton, leadership theory of, 251–252, 225t

Change
  capacity for, 268
  climate for, factors in, 275t
  definition of, 266
  developmental models of, 267
  implementation of, in nursing process, 278–280
  maintenance of, 270
  motivation and, 268, 269
  objectives for, 269
  organizational, 270–272
    classical theory of, 271
    systems theory of, 271–272
  phases of, 268–270
  resistance to, 272–274, 274t, 275t
    avoiding, 274
    cultural factors in, 272–273
    organizational factors in, 273
    psychological factors in, 273–274
    social factors in, 273
  systems model of, 267–270

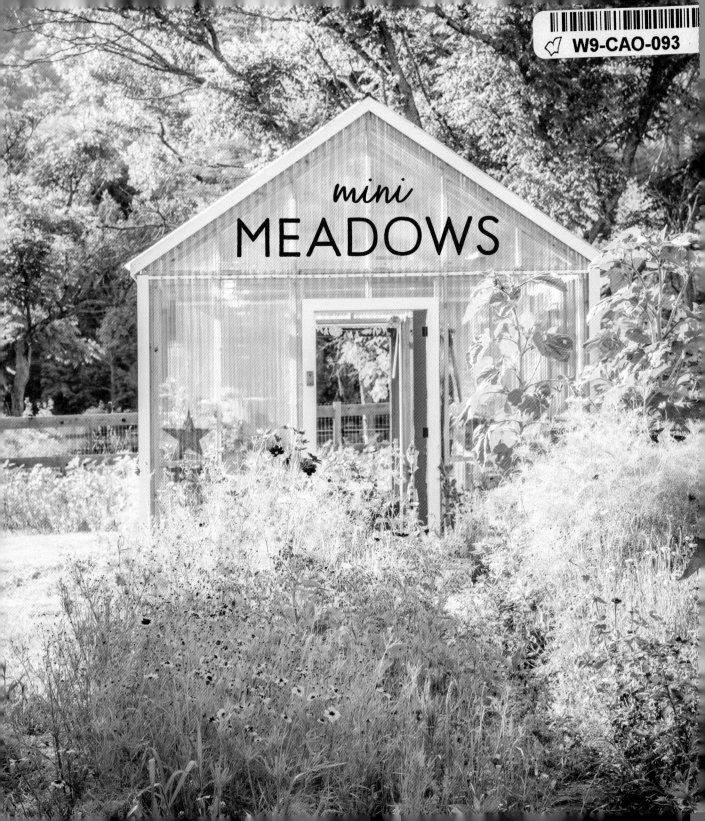

mini
MEADOWS

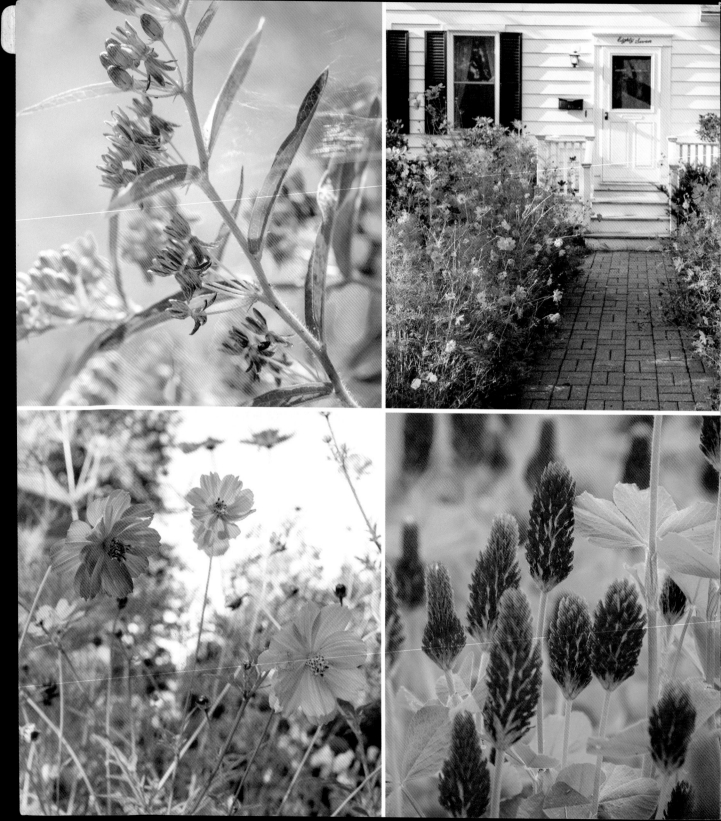

mini
MEADOWS

Grow a Little Patch *of* Colorful Flowers *Anywhere* around Your Yard

BY MIKE LIZOTTE

Photography by Rob Cardillo

Storey Publishing

*The mission of Storey Publishing is to serve our customers by
publishing practical information that encourages
personal independence in harmony with the environment.*

Edited by Carleen Madigan
Art direction and book design by Michaela Jebb
Text production by Erin Dawson
Indexed by Nancy D. Wood

Cover photography by © Rob Cardillo, front, back t.r. & b.l.; Mars Vilaubi, back t.l.; © Friedrich Strauss/GAP Photos, back b.r.; © emer1940/iStock.com, spine 2nd from b.; © joloei/iStock.com, spine 2nd from t.; © jumnong/iStock.com, spine t.; © khudoliy/iStock.com, spine 3rd from b.; © Snowbelle/Shutterstock, spine 3rd from t.; © Topaz777/iStock.com, spine b.; © VIDOK/iStock.com, spine 3rd from b.

Interior photography by © Rob Cardillo, with designs by Chanticleer, 20 r., 95 b.r.; Jonathan Alderson, 102, 118; Larry Weaner, 96; Northcreek Nurseries, 58

Additional photography credits on page 141

Storey Publishing
210 MASS MoCA Way
North Adams, MA 01247
storey.com

Printed in China by Printplus Ltd.
10 9 8 7 6 5 4 3 2 1

Library of Congress Cataloging-in-Publication Data
Names: Lizotte, Mike, author.
Title: Mini meadows : grow a little patch of colorful
    flowers anywhere around your yard / by Mike Lizotte.
Description: North Adams, MA : Storey Publishing, 2019. |
    Includes index.
Identifiers: LCCN 2018021754 (print) | LCCN
    2018027776 (ebook) | ISBN 9781612128368 (ebook) |
    ISBN 9781612128351 (pbk. : alk. paper)
Subjects: LCSH: Flower gardening. | Meadow gardening.
Classification: LCC SB404.9 (ebook) | LCC SB404.9 .L59
    2019 (print) | DDC 635.9—dc23
LC record available at https://lccn.loc.gov/2018021754

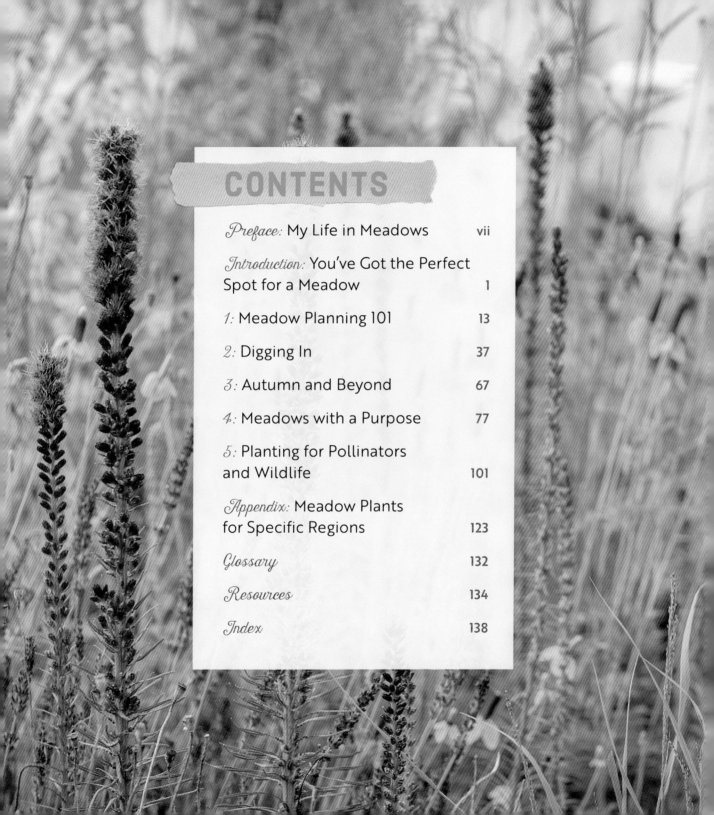

CONTENTS

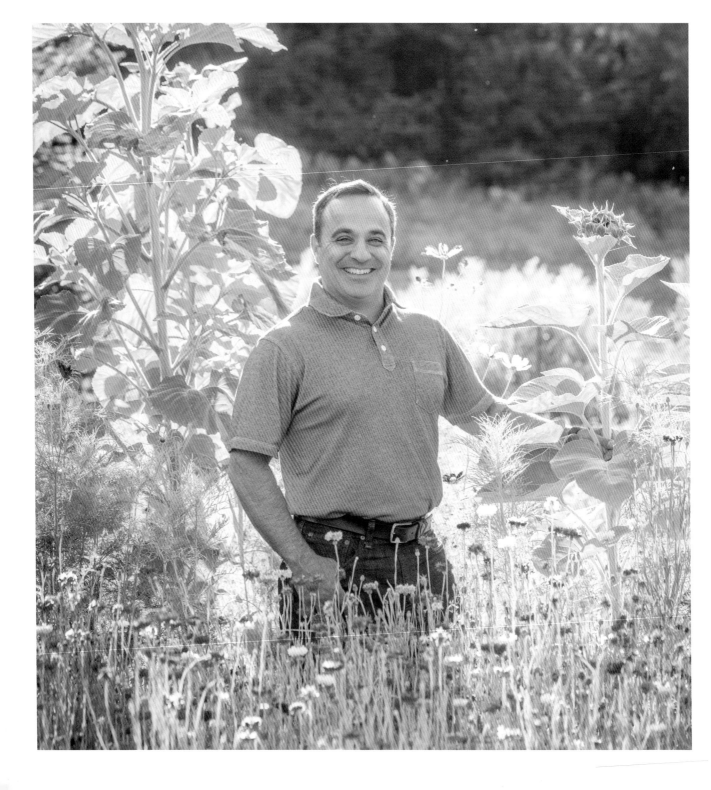

Preface
MY LIFE IN MEADOWS

It all started when I was 14 years old. A local seed company had a large shipment arriving, and a high school friend of mine who worked there recruited me to help out. Well, I must of have done something right, because they asked me to come back. I started mowing the display gardens and doing other outdoor maintenance on a regular basis. Shortly after that, I started packing seed on the weekends. And that's where my lifelong journey in meadow gardening began.

I must admit that I wasn't really into plants as a teenager. But as I began packing seed, I became familiar with hundreds of different flowers. You could lay the seeds of 50 different varieties on a table, and I could identify every single one. What I couldn't tell you, though, was what the flower looked like. So, unlike most people who learn about plants by gardening or looking at pictures of flowers, I learned the seed first and the plant and flower second. In the years that followed, I started working behind the counter at the company's retail location. I continued to learn about different plants, spending time in our display gardens and reading books on meadow gardening by authors such as Jim Wilson, Laura C. Martin, and Rick Imes.

As an 18-year-old, I got my fair share of doubter looks when people came to the retail counter to ask for meadow gardening advice. I used these looks as motivation to learn everything I could about the plants and how to grow them, so that I could prove to customers that I really did know what I was talking about.

It was also around this time that my nickname, "the Seed Man," came to be. As customers entered the seed shop, they'd see me behind the counter and say, "You must be the Seed Man." I loved it! I had T-shirts made with THE SEED MAN printed on the back in big letters.

Over the years, I developed relationships with customers from across the country. Many of them would come into the shop or call to tell me how their meadows were progressing and how much they were enjoying it. Knowing that I had helped them was rewarding and such a source of satisfaction for me. By the time I was 21 and out of college, I had been fortunate enough to engage with tens of thousands of enthusiastic gardeners.

In my job at the seed company, I wasn't just learning about plants and wildflowers. I was very much inspired by the owners of the company, Ray and Chy Allen, and their work ethic. They were the first ones in the office and the last ones to leave. They were so passionate about flowers and about their customers! They always smiled and treated everyone with the utmost respect. Even when an employee made a mistake, they never dwelled on it; rather, they encouraged people and helped them succeed. Their leadership, drive, and passion for the business motivated me. I wouldn't be where I am now without their inspiration.

In 2009 my business partner, Ethan, and I were fortunate enough to be able to take over the seed business from Ray and Chy. As a business owner, my responsibilities have changed through the years, but there's not much I enjoy more than talking to someone about planting meadows. I love sharing my knowledge and getting people excited about gardening! I hope I can inspire you to plant a meadow and experience the same joy and passion I've shared with people across the country for more than 27 years.

Mike Lizotte

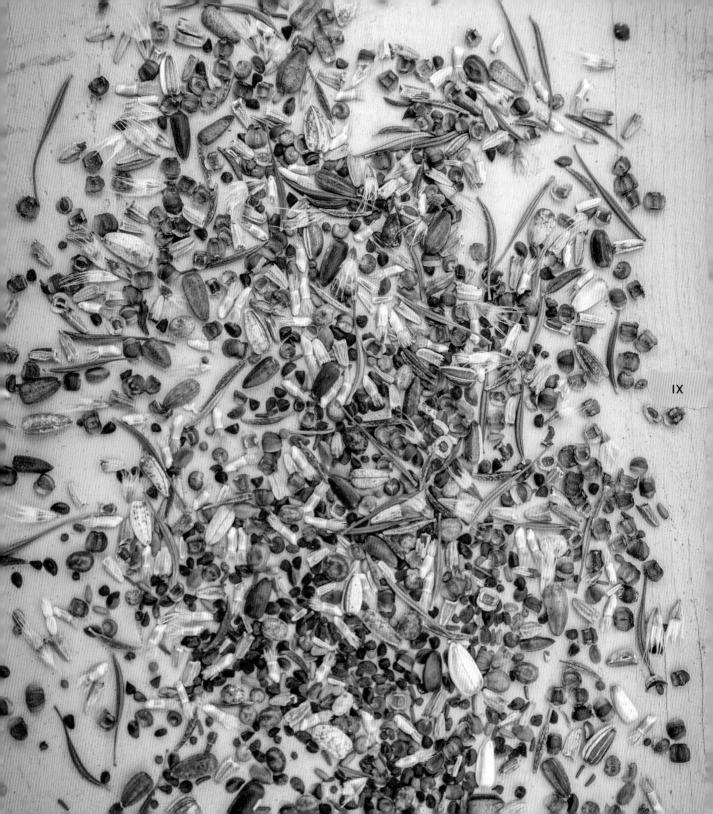

IX

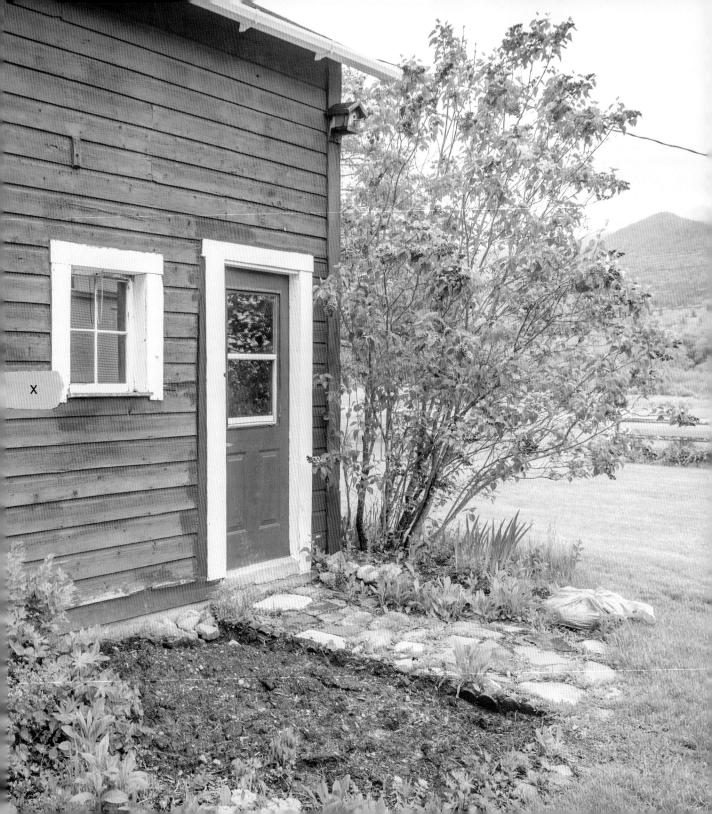

You've Got the Perfect Spot for a Meadow

What do you think of when you hear the word "meadow"? A wild, grassy expanse where birds nest and prairie dogs scurry? A hayfield? The dictionary defines a meadow as "land that is covered or mostly covered with grass." Maybe, in your vision, there are a few wild-flowers blooming among the grasses.

My definition of a meadow is slightly different. First off, I think of it as a place that isn't necessarily dominated by grasses but that includes all kinds of plants, both native and not, perennial and annual. A beautiful meadow should have flowers blooming from spring through the early frosts of fall. It most likely has a loose, naturalistic style and shouldn't be overly manicured. And because these plants typically offer food and habitat for insects and birds, there are butterflies and other pollinators flying around.

For the purposes of this book, a meadow can be any size — it can be in a planter box on your rooftop or it can occupy a few thousand square feet on the back edge of your property. It doesn't need to be big! The most important thing is to think of a meadow as a kind of garden that's loose and informal and that doesn't take a lot of time to maintain. It shouldn't be a burden. Allow it to develop and mature on its own, year after year, while you learn from and enjoy the process as you go.

For the past 25 years, I've been fortunate to have spoken and worked with gardeners of all levels, all over the world, walking them through the process of creating the meadow of their dreams. The fun and exciting part for me is that each meadow planting is unique and different — from a 300-acre commercial planting in Alabama to a rooftop garden in Dallas. Meadows can be defined in many ways, and each one carries its own unique stamp that reflects the aesthetics of the gardener as well as the conditions of the site; that's one of the great things about them.

In this book, I'm going to walk you through how to create your own meadow, step by step. Whether you have 10,000 square feet or 10, my instructions and planting tips will put you on the path to succeed and help you create a meadow that you can enjoy year after year. I'll also give you basic plant recommendations and hopefully leave you with ideas and tips to inspire you to create your very own mini meadow.

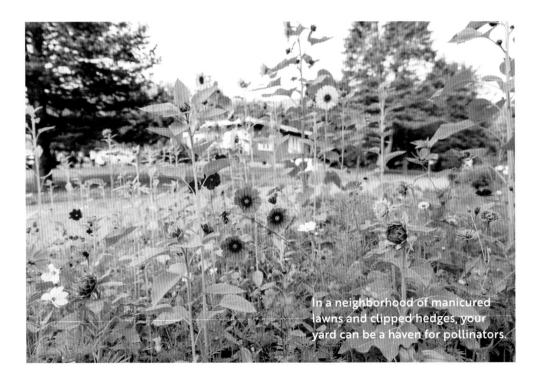

In a neighborhood of manicured lawns and clipped hedges, your yard can be a haven for pollinators.

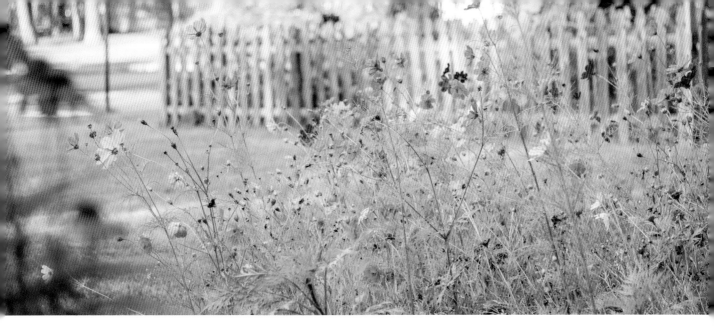

WHY PLANT *a* MEADOW?

I can't tell you how many times people call me after their first and second years with their meadow, raving about how much they've enjoyed it. They love the endless color, the ever-changing look, and the constant buzzing of pollinators. They also love not having to mow every week! Meadows require little maintenance once established and provide enjoyment for years to come. Here are just a few more reasons why you should consider converting part of your lawn into a beautiful meadow.

CULTIVATE BEAUTY

Who doesn't love flowers? Regardless of how big or small an area you may have, meadow gardening can bring color to your yard, year after year. The best part is that with a little planning, it's much easier than you might think. Want quick color? Incorporate some annuals into your meadow. If you want more lasting color, perennials are the perfect choice! You have hundreds of colors, heights, and sizes to choose from, allowing you to create a meadow that is specific to your growing area and conditions (see page 123). You'll be able to enjoy the meadow from afar while having fresh-cut flowers on your dining table all summer.

ENGAGE KIDS

There's nothing more satisfying to me than spending the summer exploring flower meadows with my six-year-old daughter, Sadie. Each year we sit down and plan our meadows, adding new flowers and Sadie's favorite colors or shapes. She also started a journal to identify all the different critters that visit each year. Whether you are sowing seeds or learning about pollinators, you'll find that meadow gardening is a great way to get kids involved in gardening at an early age. And thanks to the ever-changing blooms and colors, children will stay engaged. And I'm always surprised how quickly they absorb and understand the miniature world of the meadow.

"Why try to explain miracles to your kids when you can just have them plant a garden?"

Richard Brault

Guessing Bloom Time with Kids

My daughter and I like to play a game called "When will it bloom?" We go out to the meadow and identify different plants in bud, then try to guess how many days it will take the flower to open. It's a great way for both kids and adults to learn to identify flowers and figure out how long they take to bloom.

Guessing bloom time can also be a chance to learn how weather affects flowers. It's often surprising how bloom times can vary depending on the weather. In my own meadow, when we've had mild springs and hot summers, I've seen plants come into flower weeks earlier than in previous years. When we've had cold springs and damp summers, we usually see flowers bloom a little later.

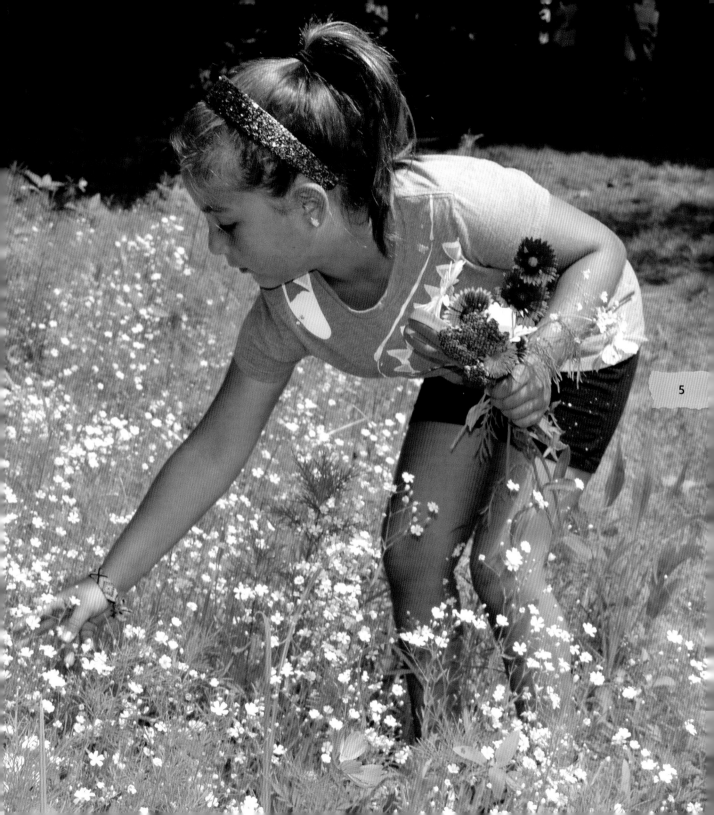

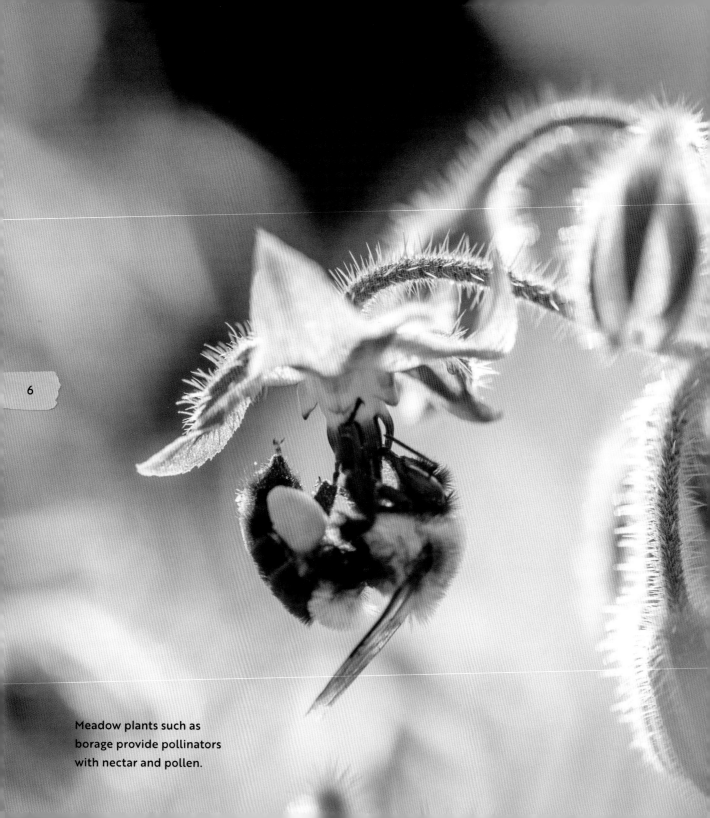

Meadow plants such as
borage provide pollinators
with nectar and pollen.

CONSERVE WATER

Did you know that landscape irrigation accounts for 9 billion gallons of water usage every day in the United States? The average American uses approximately 320 gallons of water a day, of which 30 percent is used on the lawn and gardening activities. That's a lot of H_2O! With proper planning, a meadow garden that includes drought-resistant and native varieties will help you cut back on watering and conserve thousands of gallons of water each year. Many meadow plant varieties require less moisture to thrive and can withstand longer periods of drought than varieties that you might find in a more formal garden setting.

HELP *the* POLLINATORS

Insects are critical to the pollination of crops that account for approximately 75 percent of food worldwide. In the United States, pollination plays a key role in producing crops such as almonds, apples, berries, and cucumbers — generating roughly 20 billion dollars' worth of food each year. And yet we are losing bees and other pollinators at concerning rates because of issues such as colony collapse disorder, pests and viruses, increased use of pesticides, and lack of genetic diversity. What better way to support pollinators than to create a meadow that includes nectar-rich meadow flowers, such as asters, butterfly weed, coneflower, joe-pye weed, zinnias, and cosmos?

ATTRACT BIRDS

A well-designed meadow will provide habitat and food for our winged friends. Flowers such as cosmos, daisies, and sunflowers produce seed that the birds will flock to for feeding. As the growing season winds down, the dead stalks and flower heads provide the perfect nesting material.

MOW LESS!

The U.S. Environmental Protection Agency estimates that more than 17 million gallons of gas are spilled each year by people fueling up lawn equipment. (Just so you know, that's more than the Exxon *Valdez* spill in Alaska.) The average gas lawnmower produces enough pollutants in one hour of use to equal 11 cars being driven for the same amount of time. When you replace your lawn with a beautiful meadow, you cut down on mowing and use (and spill!) less gas. Most meadow gardens are mowed only once or twice a year, which means you can spend more time enjoying your meadow and less time with the power equipment.

TACKLE HILLS and HELLSTRIPS

Do you have a hilly part of the yard that's a pain in the neck to mow every week? Or maybe a boggy area or a new septic field you'd like to plant over? How about beautifying that median or strip of grass along the sidewalk (also known as the "hellstrip")? Creating an eye-catching, low-maintenance, and tough-as-nails meadow is the perfect solution.

Most meadow gardens are mowed only once or twice a year, which means you can spend more time enjoying your meadow and less time with the power equipment.

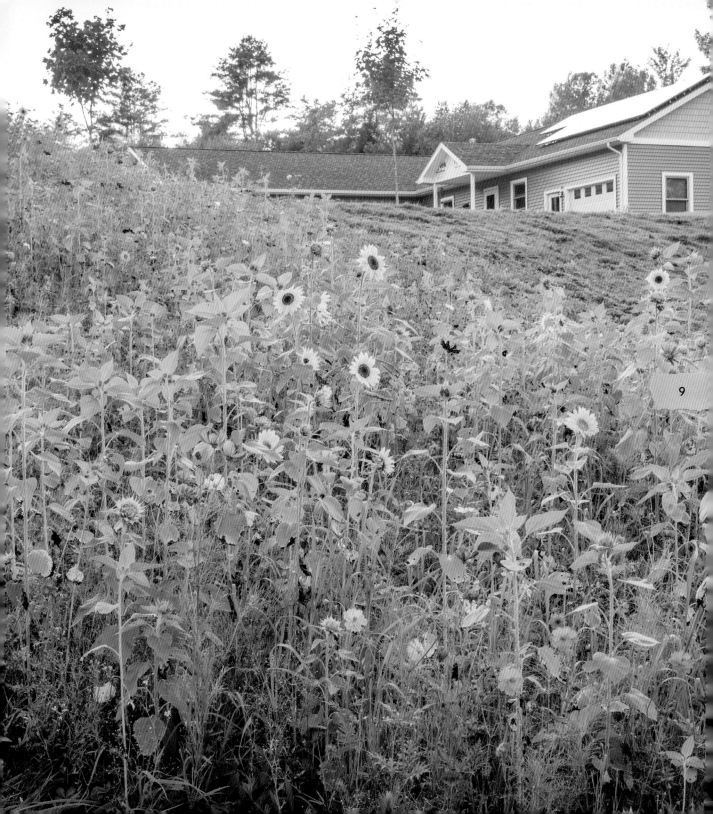

9

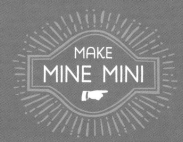

MAKE MINE MINI

a CUT-FLOWER MEADOW

Audrey planted up her walkway with a meadow mix designed to provide fresh-cut flowers all season long — a robust blend of annuals and perennials. There's nothing more satisfying than going out and cutting a fresh arrangement of flowers for the dinner table. A combination of annuals such as sunflowers, zinnias, cosmos, and cleomes can provide big color and beautiful cut flowers in year one. Perennials such as purple coneflower, bee balm, blanketflower, and blazing star will start bursting with flowers in the second year. To avoid creating bare spots in the meadow, it's best to avoid cutting too many flowers at a time. And adding grasses to a cut-flower meadow will contribute texture and beautiful contrast to any cut-flower bouquet.

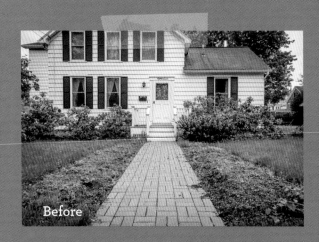

Before

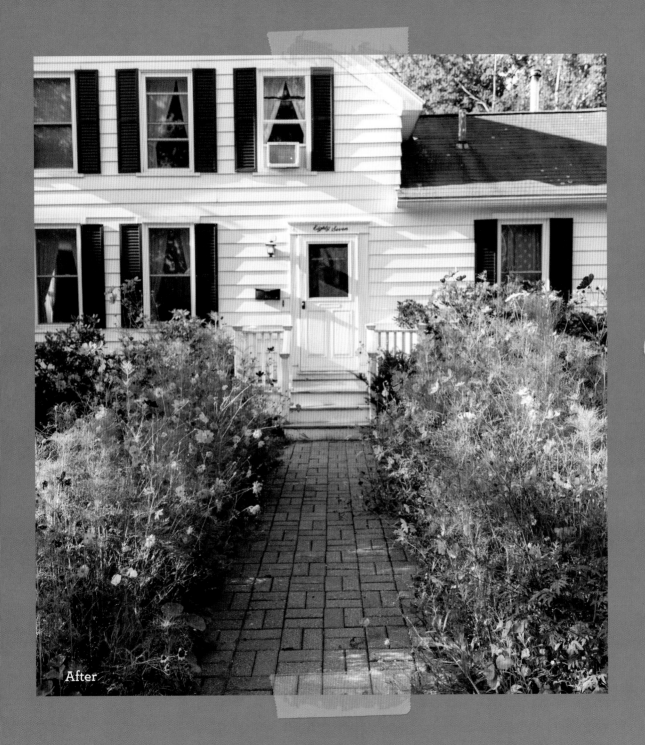

After

11

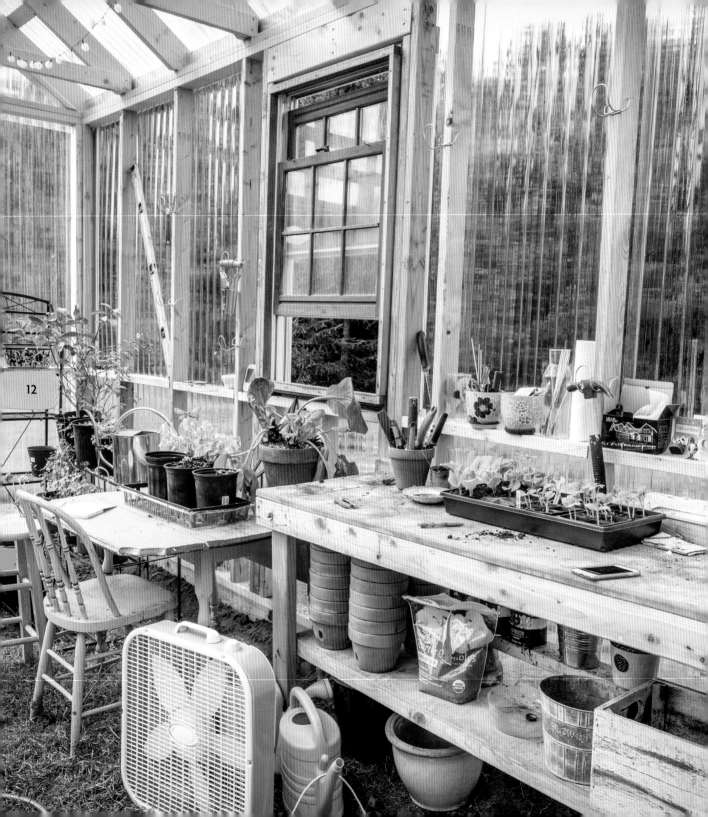

CHAPTER 1

Meadow Planning 101

Whether your meadow is big or small, it's important to set realistic expectations from the start, to avoid frustration and disappointment later on. After all, planting a meadow is much like planting any other kind of garden — good soil preparation and regular watering (especially early in the process, as the seeds are germinating) are very important.

To get the look you want, it's helpful if you identify the purpose, goal, or theme of your meadow planting. Let's say you're planning a wedding or other special event and you want a meadow as a backdrop for photography or to create some bouquets. The event is in the fall, and you want to plant this spring. You'll need to put in annuals, then — these will flower and complete their life cycle in one growing season. (Some popular annuals that you might already be familiar with are sunflowers, cosmos, zinnias, and marigolds.)

Or maybe you'd like to create a habitat to support pollinators. You're not in a rush, and you expect your meadow project to evolve over several years. There's no need for instant gratification in this scenario, so perennials — plants that come back year after year — can provide the perfect solution for creating a successful pollinator meadow. Knowing these details from the beginning will help you plan and better understand your meadow, how it may evolve, and the time and money it may take to achieve.

EVALUATE *Your* SITE

Now that you've done some thinking about what you want from your meadow, it's time to begin mapping out your plan of attack. There are a few keys to success that will apply to all planting scenarios, regardless of how big or small your meadow may be. What follows is a helpful meadow prep road map.

OBSERVE *and* TAKE NOTES

When I'm speaking with someone who wants to create a meadow, I usually recommend that we begin with a simple site analysis in the area they'd like to plant. You can learn a lot just by observing what's currently growing (or not growing) on your potential meadow site. Start by looking around and taking a few notes:

» Are there plants currently growing in the area you want to develop? How difficult will it be to remove them to prepare the site for your meadow?

» Are there any spots that are bare or have uneven growth? This could be an indicator of poor soil or lack of fertility; adding some compost will encourage better growth.

» Is the area boggy, or does it tend to be drier than other spots on your property? You'll want to select a plant mix that's suited to the site.

Fortunately, most meadow garden plants tend to be both hardy and tolerant of a range of soil conditions, so chances are you won't have to worry about getting a soil test or bringing in soil to establish your meadow. On pages 18 and 19, we'll learn more about how to evaluate your soil.

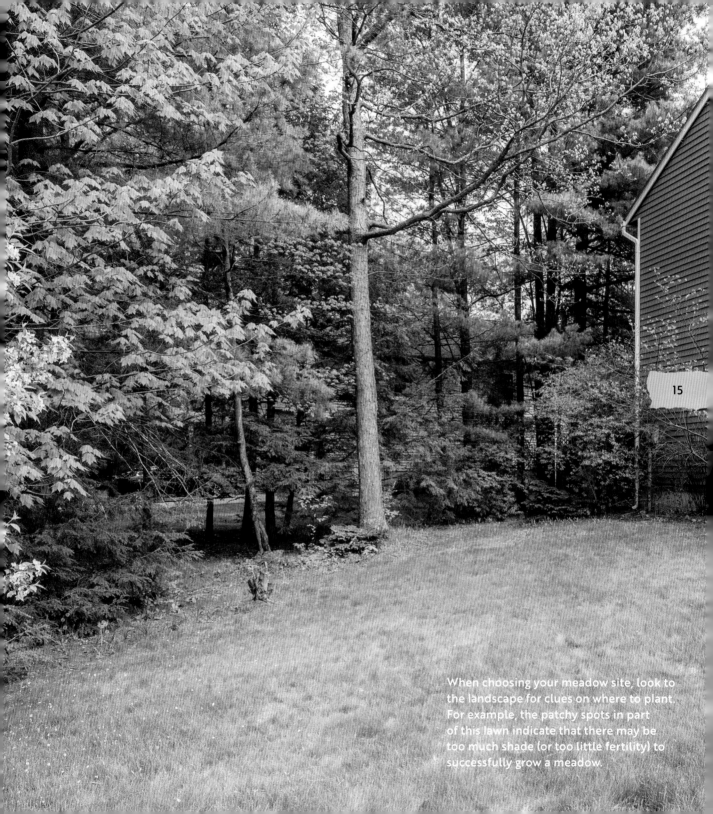

15

When choosing your meadow site, look to the landscape for clues on where to plant. For example, the patchy spots in part of this lawn indicate that there may be too much shade (or too little fertility) to successfully grow a meadow.

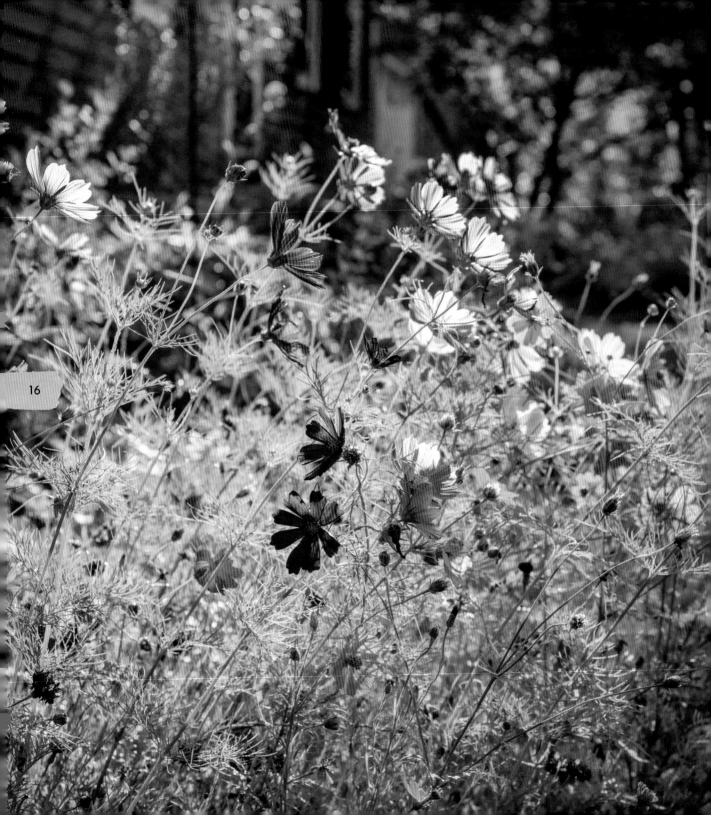

16

LET *the* SUN SHINE

Most meadow plant varieties are going to want some sun, so take note of how many hours a day the sun shines on your potential planting area. In addition, it's helpful to identify any trees that are on or near your site and where they cast their shade. Don't let a little shade get you down, though! In most cases, if the area receives five or six hours of direct sun a day, the meadow will thrive. And if you're getting only two or three hours of direct sun, or if the site only gets filtered sunlight, you should seek out varieties that grow well in partial shade. There are plenty of options to choose from, so don't feel discouraged if you don't have full sun.

Eight Plants for Partial Shade

If you're worried that you don't have enough sun to be successful with a meadow, try a few of these plants:

Wild columbine (*Aquilegia vulgaris*)

Johnny jump-up (*Viola cornuta*)

Forget-me-not (*Myosotis sylvatica*)

Siberian wallflower (*Cheiranthus allionii*)

Foxglove (*Digitalis purpurea*)

Drummond phlox (*Phlox drummondii*)

Sweet pea (*Lathyrus odoratus*)

Cornflower or bachelor's button (*Centaurea cyanus*)

GET TO KNOW *Your* SOIL

Even though most meadow plants are tough as nails, it's still a good idea to have a basic idea of what your soil conditions are, so that you can make adjustments as needed and so that you can choose the right seed mix for your site. A simple, fast, and free way to learn about your soil is to simply observe what's currently growing in your potential planting area. If the area supports lush growth of grasses and other plants, the soil is probably just fine for planting a meadow. If the area has spotty growth with lots of bare spots, or if you've tried to plant there in the past with little success, you'll probably have to amend the soil.

Meadow plants might be tough, but they aren't miracle workers; they still need nutrients from the soil to thrive and soil that isn't compacted. Sometimes adding compost or other organic matter is all that's needed, especially if you've planted seeds or plants in the past with mixed results (such as if the plants have lots of foliage but not many flowers, or if the plants don't grow quickly enough to outcompete the weeds). A soil test would be helpful for identifying how to best address the situation.

For a detailed analysis of your soil, take a soil sample and send it to your local branch of the Cooperative Extension Service (see Resources, page 134). There is usually a small fee, but the analysis will give you precise information about your soil composition and any deficiencies it might have.

The Importance of Soil Structure

There is one important aspect of your soil you can determine by simple observation: what type of soil you have. The three most common types are sandy, clay, or loamy. Knowing which of these components is most prevalent in your soil will help you choose plants for your particular conditions. For example, there are plants that actually thrive in clay soil and help break up compacted areas, for the benefit of other plants. (See page 20 for a list of these plants.)

Sandy. Sandy soil is very well drained, contains large particles, and is typically low in nutrients. It's usually very easy to work with when preparing a meadow. Plants that thrive in well-drained sites and can tolerate a lack of moisture are perfect for planting in sandy soil.

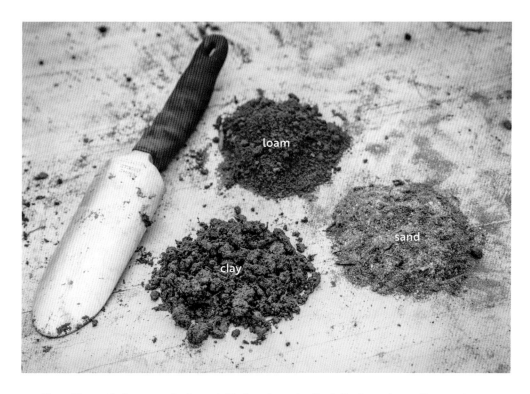

Clay. Clay soil does not drain quickly but is typically full of nutrients. It contains very small soil particles that stick together and is often compacted and challenging to work with. Choosing the rights plants is key, but you may also want to add organic matter to lighten the soil. If you have very heavy clay soil and you're going to use a tiller to prepare the area and mix in compost, it may take a few tillings for you to break up the soil. I recommend doing a test run to make sure your tiller can handle the density of the clay.

Loamy. Some might say a loamy soil is ideal, as it contains a nice balance of clay, sand, and organic matter. It usually the easiest to work, and most anything will grow in it. If you find yourself with a loamy soil, consider yourself lucky, as it's hard to come by in a natural setting. Most of us will be starting with a sandy or clay "base" and may have to amend by adding organic matter or compost to attain loamy conditions.

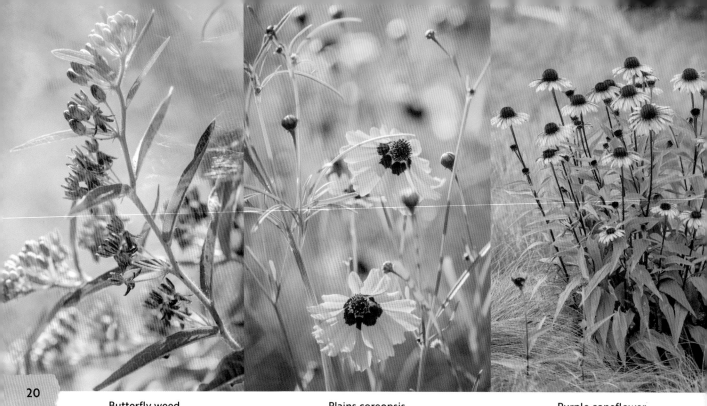

Butterfly weed
Asclepias tuberosa

Plains coreopsis
Coreopsis tinctoria

Purple coneflower
Echinacea purpurea

Eight Clay-Busting Plants

Some plants actually thrive in clay and can help break it down over time. A few of these claybusters are:

Purple milkweed (*Asclepias purpurascens*)

Butterfly weed (*Asclepias tuberosa*)

Plains coreopsis (*Coreopsis tinctoria*)

Purple coneflower (*Echinacea purpurea*)

Rough blazing star (*Liatris aspera*)

Black-eyed Susan (*Rudbeckia hirta*)

Mealycup sage (*Salvia farinacea*)

African marigold (*Tagetes erecta*)

The Ins and Outs of Fertilizer

Because most meadow plants are very hardy and can tolerate a range of growing conditions, you probably won't need additional fertilizer. If you decide you'd like to add fertilizer to give your plants a boost, here are a few tips to keep in mind:

Learn to read the labels. There are many different types of fertilizer, but they all usually include three numbers, separated by dashes — such as 10-10-10. These represent the three main nutrients plants need to survive: nitrogen (N), phosphorus (P), and potassium (K). The number is the percentage of each nutrient included. Nitrogen is primarily responsible for promoting vigorous green growth in plants. Phosphorus is critical in supporting healthy root growth and plays a role in flower production as well. Potassium supports the growth of the plants, from leaves to roots and flower production. It plays a key role in plant photosynthesis and respiration, activating enzymes that help the plant's overall growth and water use, which is critical in times of drought. Potassium also aids in cell production that strengthens and protects the plant from disease, heat, cold, and other extreme conditions.

Start with just a little. Regardless of the type of fertilizer you choose, it's important to remember that more isn't better. Adding fertilizer when it's not necessary can actually work against you, by making the soil just as inviting for weeds and grass as for your meadow plants. If you must add fertilizer, always read the instructions and start with a light application at first to see how the plants respond.

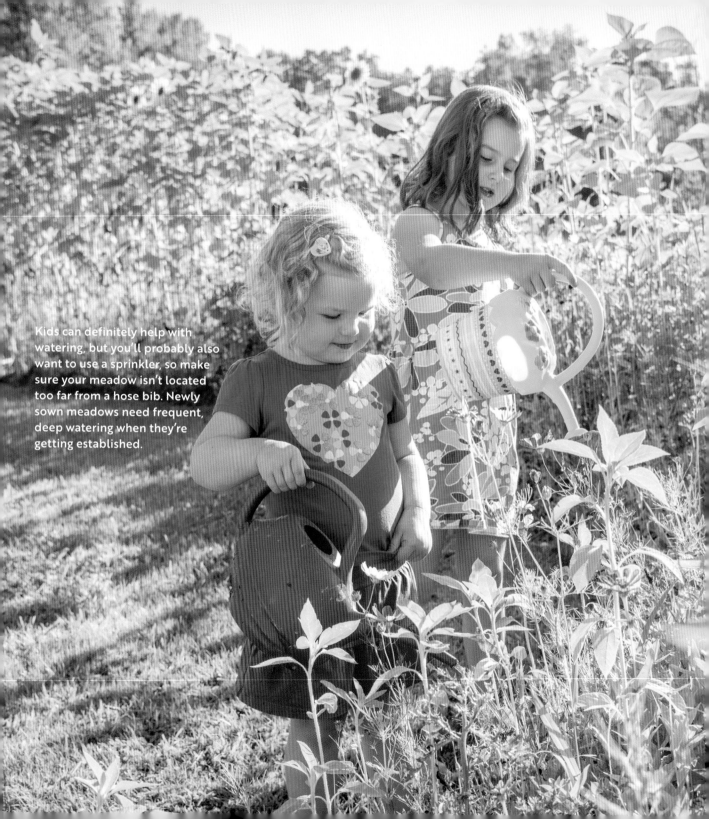

Kids can definitely help with watering, but you'll probably also want to use a sprinkler, so make sure your meadow isn't located too far from a hose bib. Newly sown meadows need frequent, deep watering when they're getting established.

PLAN for WATERING

Even though meadow plants can be remarkably drought tolerant once they're estab-lished, they benefit from regular watering early on — especially when the seeds are just starting to germinate. If seedlings don't have enough water at this stage, they may not be able to outcompete the weed seeds in the surrounding soil (which are better adapted to growing without much water). If you're able to set a sprinkler in your newly seeded patch, or if you schedule your planting to occur just before a stretch of rainy weather, you'll give your meadow a good start in life.

Decide how much you're willing to water after the meadow is established and make a plan for watering based on that. If you don't want to water your meadow, consider select-ing varieties that can grow with just the amount of rainfall your region receives. If you'd prefer to (or must) water, make sure to consider how far away your water source will be. This is important not only for a meadow in the ground but also for one in a raised bed or planter. How far will you have to carry your watering can or drag a hose?

Survival of the Fittest

What happens when you forget to water? One of our colleagues found out when she went away for a long weekend and the weather turned too hot and dry for her freshly germinated meadow. She watered and watered when she returned, but it was too late — most of the seedlings had died. She thought all was lost until she saw tiny sprouts of California poppy and marigold coming up. Although she didn't end up with the lush, multicolored meadow she was hoping for, she did have a lovely patch of orange flowers. And she learned a new appreciation for the most drought-tolerant plants in the meadow mix.

KNOW YOUR ZONE *and* REGION

Another important piece of gardening information to know is your USDA Hardiness Zone. These zones are based on the average minimum temperature in a given area, and they were created as a way to help consumers select plants that will survive the winter. Use the USDA Hardiness Zone Map (see page 135) to find your zone. When sourcing your plants, make sure they're all labeled with the proper growing zone.

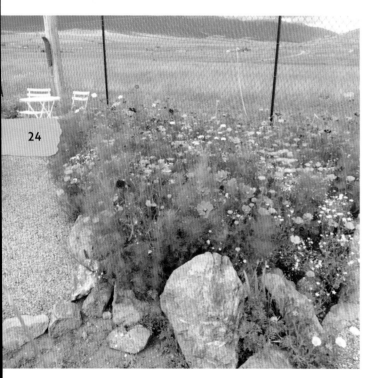

This mini meadow is a lush oasis in the dry Colorado landscape that surrounds it.

The good news is that a lot of plants do well in many different zones. Also keep in mind that every zone has micro-climates (areas that are cooler or warmer than the surrounding region). Because of that, you may well be able to grow plants that are not considered hardy for your area. You will learn over time how much wiggle room you have when selecting plants for your zone.

In some cases, meadow seed mixtures are marketed for particular regions rather than for zones. The reason for this is that most seed mixes contain a blend of flowering plants and/or grasses that can thrive in multiple zones. Also, gardeners (both novice and experienced) sometimes relate to the idea of regions a little more easily than to zones. See page 123 for some of my meadow mix recommendations for different regions.

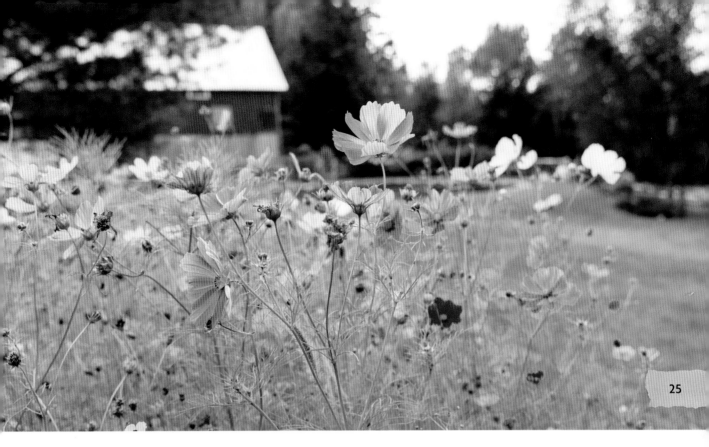

KNOW PLANT LIFE CYCLES *for* BETTER PLANNING

Whether you're a Master Gardener or you're planning your first meadow, it's important to understand the life cycles of the plants you'll be growing. This is key, both so that you have a sense of what to expect and so that you can create a successful planting plan. A good meadow mix should be properly marked with the species and life cycle information of each type of seed in the mix. Any plant you purchase should have a tag that indicates whether it is an annual, perennial, or biennial.

PLANT ANNUALS *for* QUICK *and* EASY COLOR

An annual is a plant that completes its life cycle in one growing season. The seed is planted, grows, produces a flower, develops and drops seed, and then dies. You'll only see that flower again next year if it produces seeds that overwinter in the soil and sprout the following spring.

If you're looking for quick color in the first growing season, plan on including some annuals in your meadow. Listed or shown below are some you might be familiar with:

» Spiderflower (*Cleome hassleriana*)
» Plains coreopsis (*Coreopsis tinctoria*)
» Cosmos (*Cosmos bipinnatus*)
» Rocket larkspur (*Delphinium ajacis*)
» California poppy (*Eschscholzia californica*)
» Indian blanket (*Gaillardia pulchella*)
» Baby's breath (*Gypsophila elegans*)
» Rose mallow or tree mallow (*Lavatera trimestris*)

» Scarlet flax (*Linum grandiflorum* var. *rubrum*)
» Sweet alyssum (*Lobularia maritima*)
» Lemon mint (*Monarda citriodora*)
» California bluebell (*Phacelia campanularia*)
» French marigold (*Tagetes patula*)
» Strawflower (*Xerochrysum bracteatum*)

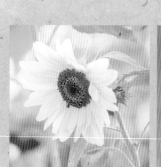

Sunflower
Helianthus annuus

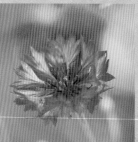

Cornflower or bachelor's button
Centaurea cyanus

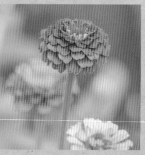

Zinnia
Zinnia species

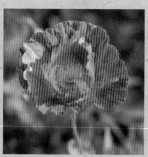

Red poppy, Shirley poppy, or corn poppy
Papaver rhoeas

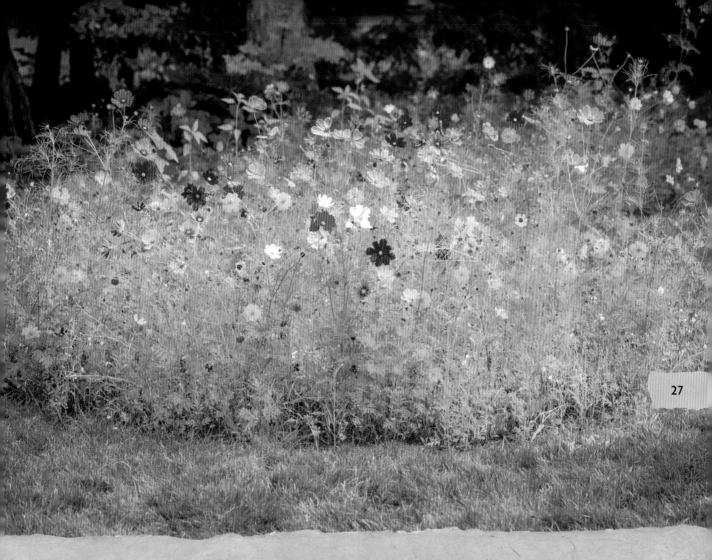

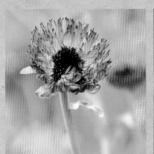

Calendula or pot marigold
Calendula officinalis

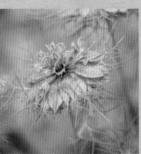

Love-in-a-mist
Nigella damascena

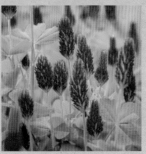

Crimson clover
Trifolium incarnatum

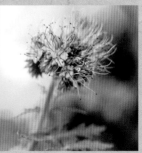

Lacy phacelia
Phacelia tanacetifolia

PLANT PERENNIALS *for* LONG-LASTING COLOR

For lasting color that comes back for several years, include a blend of perennial plants in your meadow. A plant with a perennial life cycle may not flower during its first year of growth from seed. The plant will go dormant during the winter and in the second growing season will put on growth and begin to flower. It will then continue to bloom every season thereafter, until the end of its life span (most perennials live for at least a few years).

If you are purchasing perennial plants or plugs and you notice they already have top growth and even flowers, it's always a good idea to ask how old the plants are. This will help you set the proper expectations for your meadow and better understand when your new perennials might bear blossoms. Most perennials come into bloom in the second growing season, but there are a few perennials that can produce a flower from seed in the first season.

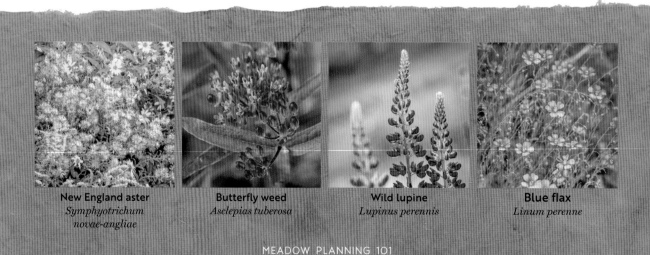

New England aster
Symphyotrichum novae-angliae

Butterfly weed
Asclepias tuberosa

Wild lupine
Lupinus perennis

Blue flax
Linum perenne

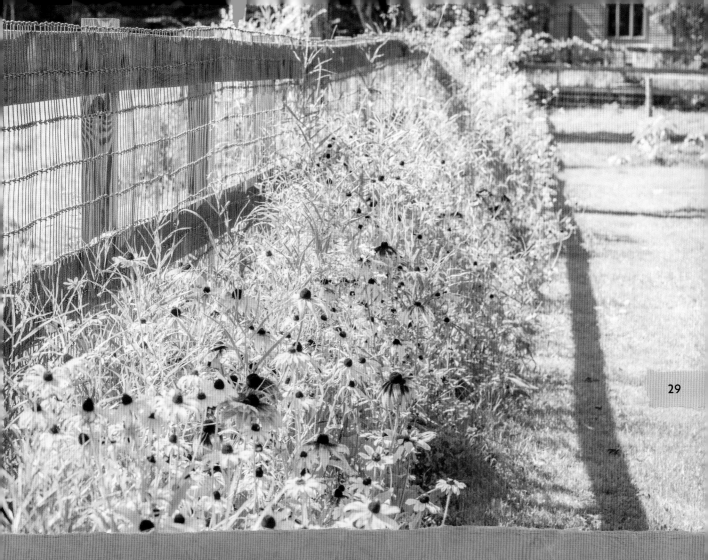

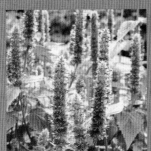

Anise hyssop
Agastache foeniculum

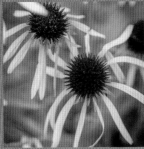

Pale purple coneflower
Echinacea pallida

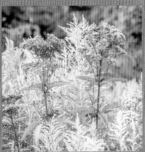

Spotted joe-pye weed
Eupatorium maculatum

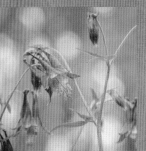

Eastern red columbine
Aquilegia canadensis

MEADOW PLANNING 101

DON'T FORGET BIENNIALS

A biennial plant completes its life cycle in two growing seasons. It will put on top growth in the first growing season from seed, then go dormant through the winter months and return the second year with flowers. After the flowers fade, they'll produce seed and the plant will then die; the only way it will reappear in your garden is if it reseeds. Although using biennials can present a challenge for planning, you may well count them among your favorite plants and want to include them in your meadow.

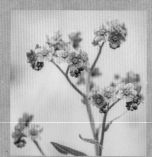

Sweet William
Dianthus barbatus

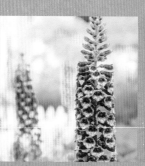

Hooker's evening primrose
Oenothera elata subsp. *hookeri*

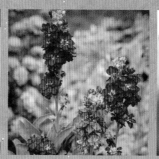

Stock
Matthiola incana

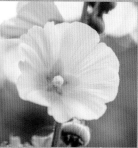

Hollyhock
Alcea rosea

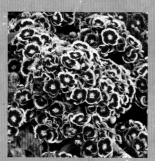

Forget-me-not
Myosotis sylvatica

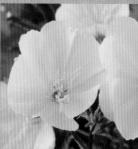

Foxglove
Digitalis purpurea

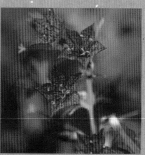

Standing cypress
Ipomopsis rubra

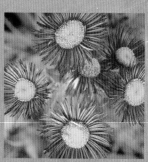

**Prairie aster or
tansy-leaf aster**
Machaeranthera tanacetifolia

NATIVE PLANTS

The term "native" generally refers to plants that are indigenous to a particular place. For example, purple coneflower (*Echinacea purpurea*) is a popular perennial that is native in much of North America. Some people have taken the designation a step further and try to determine what is native to their state or region in particular.

There are good reasons to include native plants in your meadow. Natives play a critical role in sustaining the biodiversity of our ecosystems. Most North American native varieties are very hardy and can withstand a wide range of growing conditions. They also tend to require less water and less maintenance overall. And last (but certainly not least!), they play a key role in feeding and providing habitat for native insects, pollinators, and other wildlife.

Native plants can be a little more expensive, but because native species tend to be much hardier and outlast many nonnative species, the cost will even out in the long run. If you're purchasing native seeds, check to make sure the origin is clearly marked, and always ask for the germination and purity information.

Here are some natives you might want to try:

» Eastern red columbine (*Aquilegia canadensis*)
» Common milkweed (*Asclepias syriaca*)
» Lanceleaf coreopsis (*Coreopsis lanceolata*)
» Purple coneflower (*Echinacea purpurea*)
» Spotted joe-pye weed (*Eupatorium maculatum*)
» Prairie blazing star (*Liatris pycnostachya*)
» Cardinal flower (*Lobelia cardinalis*)
» Wild bergamot (*Monarda fistulosa*)
» New England aster (*Symphyotrichum novae-angliae*)
» Prairie ironweed (*Vernonia fasciculata*)

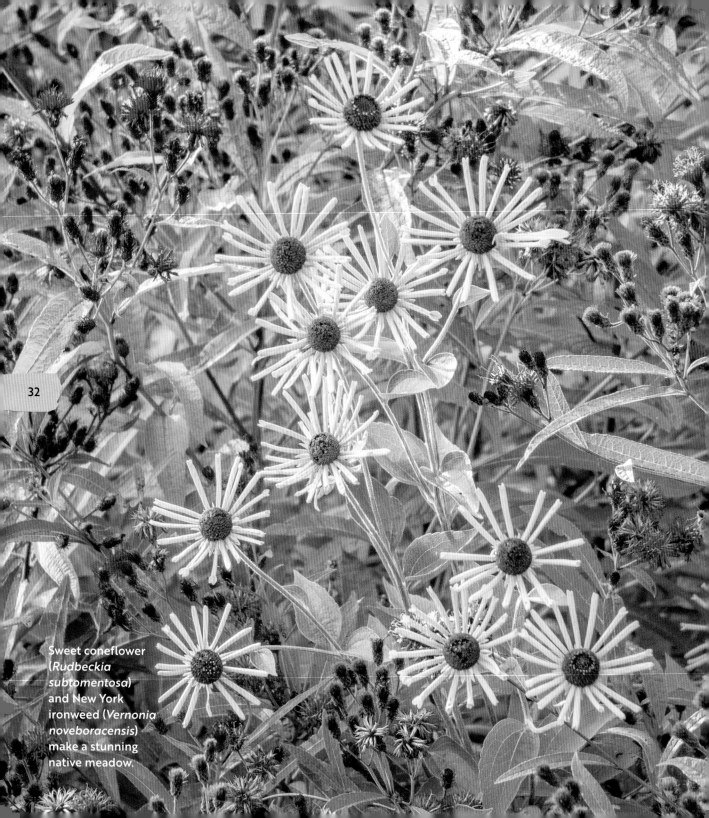

Sweet coneflower (*Rudbeckia subtomentosa*) and New York ironweed (*Vernonia noveboracensis*) make a stunning native meadow.

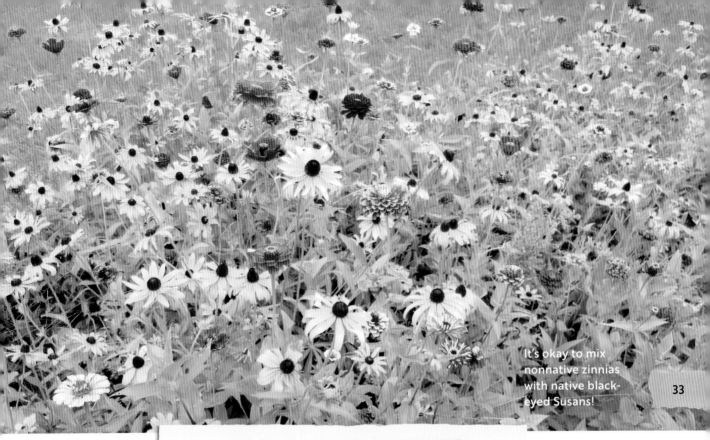

It's okay to mix nonnative zinnias with native black-eyed Susans!

MIXING IN NONNATIVES

Are you drawn to the idea of an all-native meadow but are secretly a fan of zinnias and poppies? That's okay! Nonnative annuals provide beautiful color in the first growing season, and they'll help suppress unwanted annual weeds that might be tempted to move in while your native perennials are establishing themselves.

Too often, when you mention the term "nonnative," people mistakenly interpret it as "invasive," or otherwise doing harm to the environment. This couldn't be further from the truth. Simply because a nonnative plant doesn't come from your region, or even from North America, doesn't mean that it won't be beneficial for the environment. You can definitely create a meadow with a nice variety of both native and nonnative varieties. Annual species such as zinnias, cosmos, and cleomes are popular meadow varieties that will add big, quick color to any meadow planting. They can also be very helpful to pollinators and wildlife.

HOW MUCH SEED WILL *You* NEED?

When planning your meadow, it's important to calculate the square footage of the area you'd like to plant. Having this measurement makes it easier to determine the amount of seed or plants to buy. It will also help you decide how best to go about preparing your site.

WHAT IF IT'S *not* SQUARE?

A meadow can take on any number of different shapes and sizes, which makes it difficult to figure an exact size. Here's how to calculate the square footage of different shapes:

Square or rectangle. These are the easiest! Simply multiply length times width.

Circle. If you're dealing with a circle, multiply pi (3.1416) by the radius of the circle squared.

Triangle. If your meadow is shaped more like a triangle, you'll multiply the base times the height and then divide by two.

HOW MUCH SEED *per* SQUARE FOOT?

How much seed to plant will vary depending on the look you'd like to achieve. If you're planting pure seed (see page 50), the package might suggest ¼ pound to cover an area of 500 square feet. If you wanted an especially lush stand of plants, you may choose to plant ½ pound of seed — and that's fine. But don't go overboard and plant 2 pounds of seed in your 500 square feet; if you put too much seed down, the plants will compete, choking each other out and not growing well.

How to Calculate Square Footage

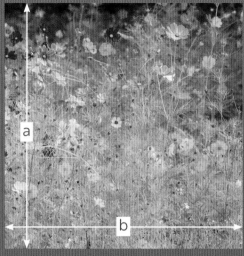

$$a \times b$$

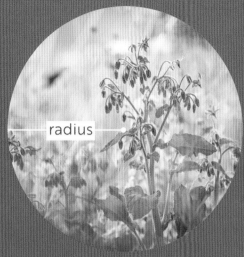

radius

$$radius \times 3.1416$$

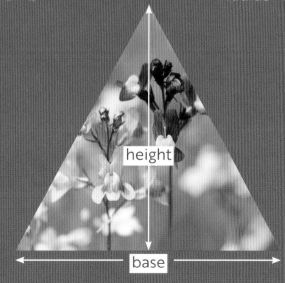

height

base

$$\frac{base \times height}{2}$$

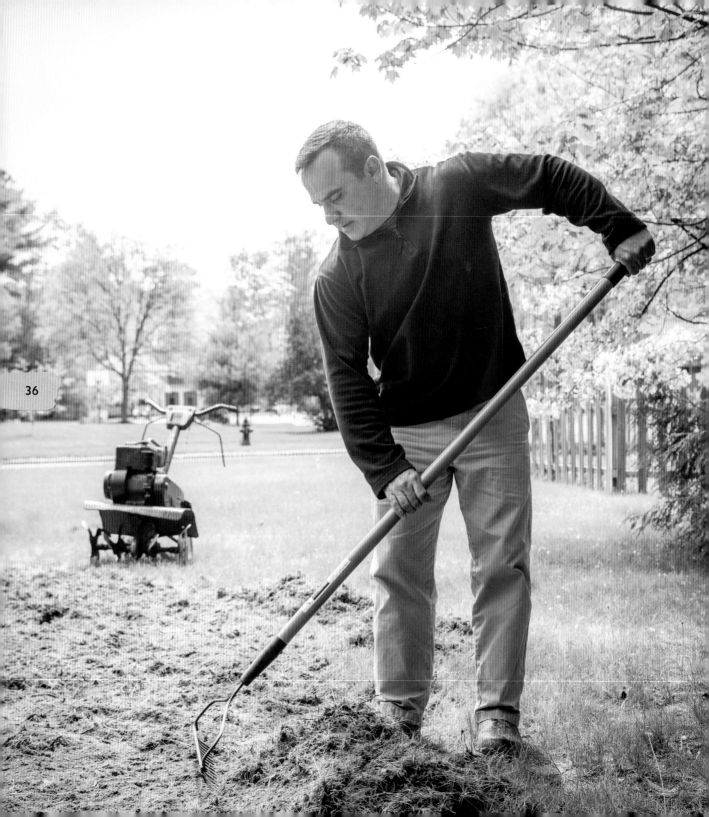

CHAPTER 2

Digging In

Now that you've learned the basics of meadow planning, it's time to dig in! Thorough site preparation, even seeding, regular watering after planting, and careful observation are keys to starting a successful meadow. Determining when to sow your seed may also be a consideration, depending on where you live.

If there's one step in the process that warrants spending a little more time to get right, it's site preparation. Meadow plants may be tough once they become established, but they still need help getting started — that means preparing a bed of loose, friable soil and giving them regular moisture once they've germinated. Just imagine if you tried to sow seeds for lettuce or carrots or any other crop into a bed of weedy, compacted soil! A meadow is still a garden and, like any other garden, the better you prepare your soil, the better results you'll have — both this year and in the future.

GETTING RID
of WHAT'S THERE

Listen up! This is the most important step in creating a successful meadow. The more time you spend clearing the area of unwanted grasses and weeds, the better your meadow will be. Through my 25 years of helping gardeners across the country establish meadows, I've seen firsthand that this is the one step that can make or break your meadow planting.

TILLING *up* TURF

One of the most common ways to prepare your meadow area is using a tiller. Tillers can be very effective in breaking up the soil while grinding up existing weeds and grasses. They vary in size, from a small walk-behind tiller to a three-point-hitch tiller that attaches to the back of a tractor. They can be rented at most hardware stores without breaking the bank.

You'll only need to till deeply enough to break up the surface layer of plants and their roots. There's usually no need to go any deeper than 6 to 8 inches. In most cases, you'll want to go over the area two or three times, to grind up all the surface growth and break apart any large clods of soil. Rake up any remaining clods of turf. You'll be left with a nice, fluffy bed of soil that will help your seed germinate easily and evenly.

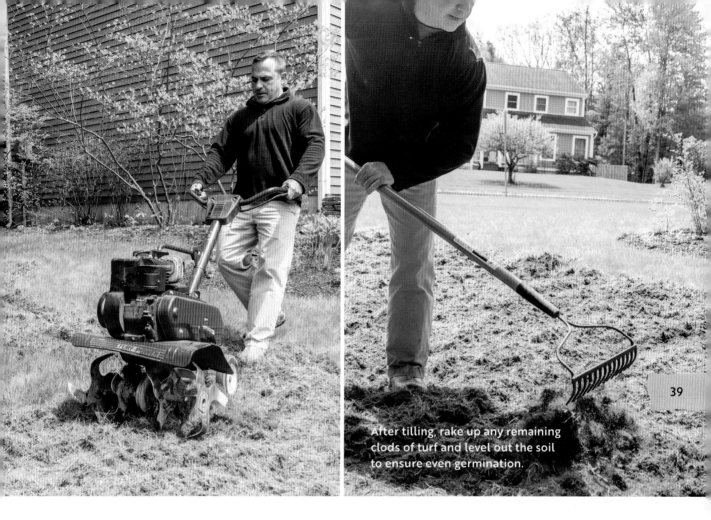

After tilling, rake up any remaining clods of turf and level out the soil to ensure even germination.

The Downside of Tilling

Any time you disturb the soil, you increase your chances of bringing dormant weed or grass seed to the surface, which isn't ideal when you're starting a meadow from scratch. Seeds can lay dormant in the soil for many years; when they're brought to the surface and exposed to sunlight and moisture, they germinate and create competition for your meadow seeds. When you're tilling your new garden, make sure you only go deep enough to break up the surface layer of growth. The deeper you till, the more seeds you'll bring up!

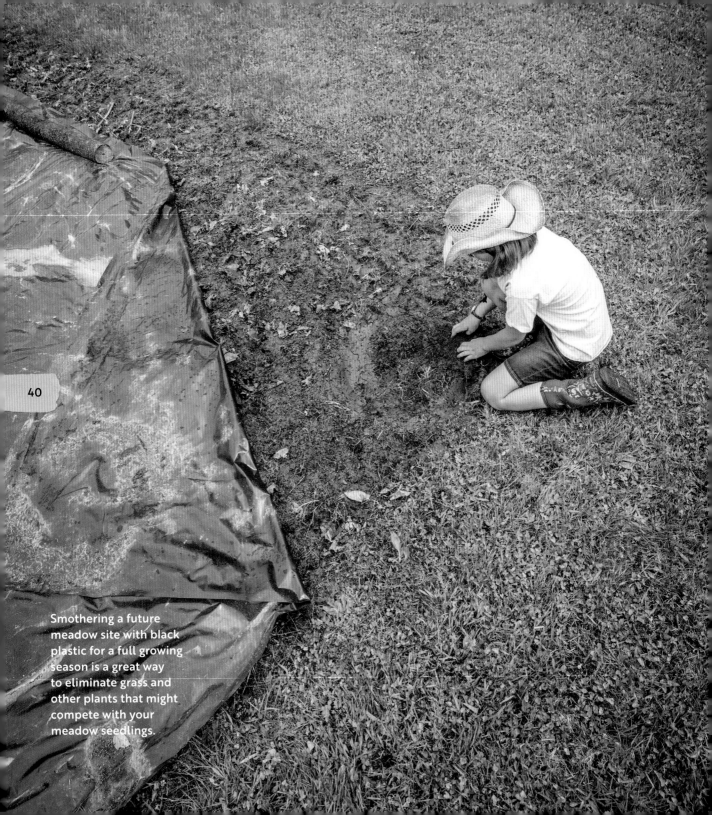

40

Smothering a future
meadow site with black
plastic for a full growing
season is a great way
to eliminate grass and
other plants that might
compete with your
meadow seedlings.

SMOTHER IT!

If you have a small meadow — let's say a few hundred square feet or less — you can eliminate existing plants by smothering them. Before smothering, it's helpful to mow the area well, both to outline where the meadow will be and to speed the process of breaking down the plants.

Plastic sheeting. A layer of black plastic, secured around the edges with boards or landscape staples, will kill the growth underneath by cutting off sunlight and air. Some advance planning is required for this; the plastic should be left in place for at least a month. After you remove the plastic, you'll want to loosen the soil with a garden fork before you sow seed.

Cardboard or newspaper. Instead of plastic, you might choose to use cardboard or layers of newspaper to smother existing plants. This method can take anywhere from four months to a full growing season to be effective, so make sure you plan ahead.

Cover the entire area with three to five layers of newspaper or a single layer of cardboard, dampen it with a hose to help hold it in place, then spread 2 to 4 inches of mulch on top. Check every couple of months to see if any plants are still alive, and only proceed to planting when all the vegetation has been killed.

If you're planting from seed, rake all the mulch and any bits of undecomposed newspaper or cardboard off to the side of the garden before you sow. Once your seedlings have sprouted, you may choose to add the mulch back around the base of the plants to help suppress weeds.

If you're starting a meadow from plants, your job is a little easier: You can simply scrape back a bit of the mulch, dig your hole right through the newspaper or cardboard (if it hasn't broken down all the way), and plant. Once you've gotten your plants in the ground, you can then add the mulch back at the base of the plants.

ORGANIC SPRAYS

There are organic sprays that can be quite effective in killing off the weeds when preparing your meadow. Regular white vinegar can be effective when sprayed directly on certain weeds; even more potent is the horticultural grade of vinegar, which has a higher level of acetic acid. As with any potentially dangerous product, always follow the instructions on the label.

SYNTHETIC HERBICIDES

Several types of synthetic herbicide are readily available at most hardware stores and garden centers. Whether or not to use them is obviously up to you. Are they effective in killing vegetation? Yes. Are some of them linked to various cancers, declines in pollinator populations, and other harmful environmental ramifications? Yes. If you are thinking of applying any of these chemicals, do your homework first.

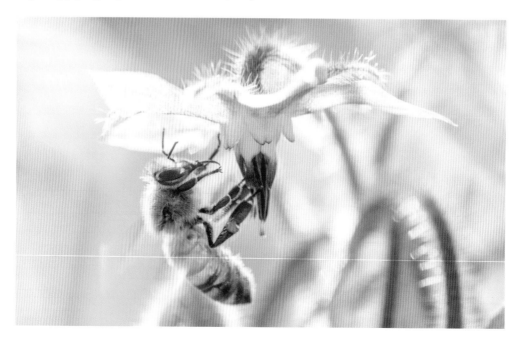

Preparing Soil for a Container Meadow

If you have a raised bed, window box, or other form of planter, preparation is also important but a lot easier. If you're planting in a raised bed, you could simply fill it with good, open-textured soil and a bit of compost. If you're planting in a container, make sure it has adequate drainage so that the plants' roots don't rot; containers should have enough holes in the bottom to allow water to flow through easily. Use potting mix rather than garden soil, which won't drain properly in a container.

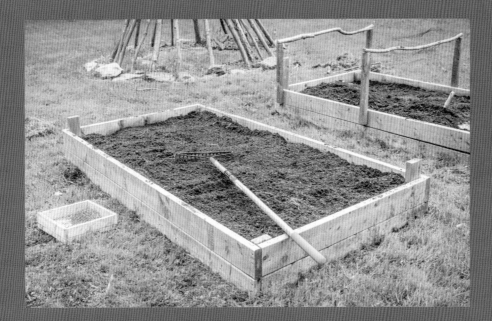

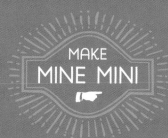

A MINI MEADOW *in* *a* RAISED BED

A meadow can be defined many ways and can take on any number of shapes and sizes. Some of us don't have a lot of space to work with — a small raised bed or container is all we can manage. Fortunately, planting a meadow garden in a constructed space like this offers some advantages, including greater control over soil and site, as well as better accessibility.

Whether you purchase a raised-bed kit or get creative and make your own, here are a couple of tips that will help you along the way:

Choose the right-sized kit. There are hundreds of raised-bed kits, plus different-sized whiskey barrels and containers that would all work for creating your meadow. Don't get overwhelmed or think you need to pick the biggest one. Choose the size that will work for your space and your level of commitment (bigger = more maintenance!). When in doubt, start small.

Plan your plants to fit your small space. Don't think just because you have limited space that means you have limited selection. There are lots of plants that will do just fine in a raised bed (see page 108).

Be vigilant about watering. With small-space gardening, the soil tends to warm up quickly. This is great for the plants that are getting established in your meadow, but it also means the soil could dry up just as fast. Be aware, keep a close eye on your plantings, and water when the soil feels dry when you plunge a finger into it.

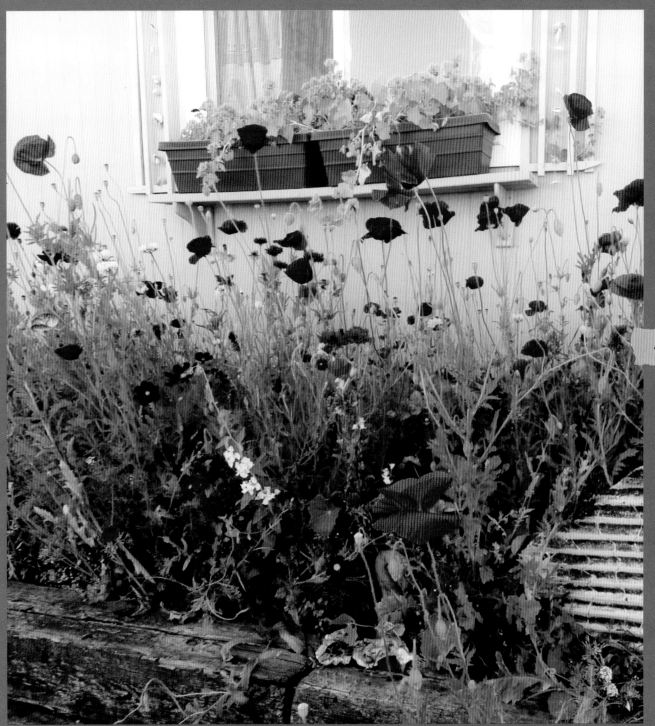

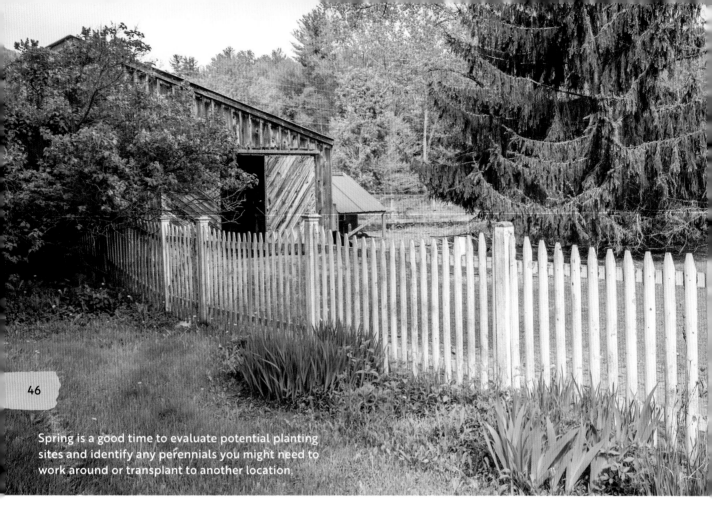

Spring is a good time to evaluate potential planting sites and identify any perennials you might need to work around or transplant to another location.

WHEN *to* PLANT

Both spring and fall can be good times to plant a meadow, depending on where you live and how much experience you have. For example, timing the fall planting of a cold-climate meadow can be a bit tricky. So if you're a northern gardener and this is your first time planting a meadow, I'd suggest sowing in spring. There's nothing wrong with a little experimenting, though, and you'll quickly learn which planting time is better for you.

PLANTING *in* SPRING

Spring is for gardening! We all get excited on that first mild day of spring after a long winter. We want to run outside and start planning our gardening projects for the season. Well, don't let that mild air fool you. The key to a successful spring planting is waiting until the *ground* temperature is warm enough, so that when you begin to plant, your seeds and plants will be ready to take off.

Wait for Warm Soil

Here's an analogy that I've been telling for years, which people seem to catch on to very quickly. I tell people that when you have that first warm day in spring, when it might get to be 65 or 75°F (18 or 24°C), you don't go jump into the Atlantic Ocean. Sure, the air temperature is nice, but the water is still 37°F (3°C). Ground temperature acts the same way: soil takes time to warm up in spring. So don't be fooled by warm *air* temperatures and plant too early. I can't tell you how many times the phone rings in early spring with customers panicking because they sowed their seed and nothing is happening after 20 days. We can usually trace their planting back to a warm day in March or April when the person planted, not realizing the ground temperatures were still very cold.

SEED MAN SAYS
Plant with Tomatoes

A good rule for planting your meadow in spring is to simply wait and sow seed at the same time you put your tomato plants out. That date will vary depending on where you live in the country, but it's usually a safe bet. It's always better to wait a little to plant than to sow too early.

What Happens if I Plant Too Early?

It's always best to be a little patient when planting in spring and let those ground temperatures warm up before you seed or plant your meadow. If you do make the mistake of planting too early, your seed will just sit on the cold ground until the soil warms up enough for germination to take place. If the seed actually does germinate and your garden is hit with a frost, your seedlings could be killed and you may have to sow more seed. If you've put plants in the ground, they'll act sluggish and may even wilt a bit until the ground warms up enough to stimulate the roots so they can begin growing. If a frost comes after they're in the ground, the plants should still be okay — they'll just need some time (and warmth!) to rebound.

FALL PLANTING MIGHT BE *for* YOU

Depending on where you live and what your growing season is like, fall may be a good time for planting. After all, in nature, seeds drop in fall, lay dormant through the winter months, and begin to germinate once the ground warms in spring. No matter where you live, fall is a great time to put plants in the ground; they won't be stressed from the summer heat, and the combination of warm soil and cool air means that roots will have time to settle in but the plants won't put energy into growing new foliage.

In Cold-Winter Regions

Fall seeding in regions that experience winters with freezing temperatures can be beneficial, allowing you get a jump-start on the following season and maximize your growing season. When planting your meadow from seed, you must wait until after you've had several frosts and the ground temperatures have cooled, so that the seed doesn't germinate. The seed will lay dormant through the winter months and begin to germinate once the ground warms in spring. I've seen fall-sown meadows bloom anywhere from 2 to 6 weeks earlier than spring-sown meadows.

If you're planting your meadow using container-grown plants or plugs, you'll want to get them in the ground up to a month before your first frost date. This will allow them enough time to set their roots in the warmer soil temperatures before the colder winter weather arrives.

In Warmer Regions

If you live in a region that experiences mild winters and hot summers, seeding or planting in fall works very well and gives your meadow the best chance to thrive. Cool temperatures and winter rains will help plants become established more easily and will get seeds off to a good start. A spring planting in warmer climates can be challenging and require constant watering, which isn't ideal.

If you live in a region that doesn't experience frosts or extended periods of cold weather, a fall planting can provide lasting color and flowers all through your winter, spring, and early-summer months. Once the extreme heat of summer arrives, your meadow will go dormant but will return come fall.

SEED MAN SAYS
Weed When Wet

Try to weed after a rainstorm, if you can. Pulling weeds when the soil is damp or wet is much easier. Also, if you do pull weeds, keep in mind it will create open pockets of soil. These are perfect for receiving more meadow seed, so be sure to have some extra on hand.

PLANTING *from* SEED

Now that you've prepared your meadow, it's time to sow. As with anything, you should always follow the instructions on your package of seed. Planting a package of 100 percent pure seed is different from planting a mix that is mostly filler.

When you open your seed packets, start by just noticing all the different seed sizes and shapes. They're amazing! Spend some time sifting them through your hands and observing. How many different varieties are you able to identify?

MIX SEED *with* SAND

When using 100 percent pure seed, you'll want to mix it with builders' or sandbox sand, at a ratio of five parts sand to one part seed, to make sure the seed is distributed evenly. If you were to spread your seed without adding a dispersing agent like sand, the lighter seed would fall in some areas and the heavier seed would fall in other areas. Mixing with sand also makes it easier to see exactly where the seed has been spread; the light color of the seed-and-sand mix is easy to identify as it lands on your dark soil. Be sure the sand is dry; otherwise, it won't mix evenly and will clog your spreader.

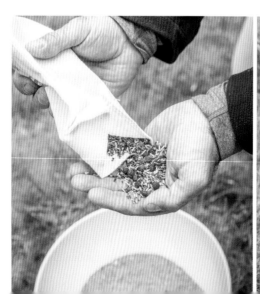
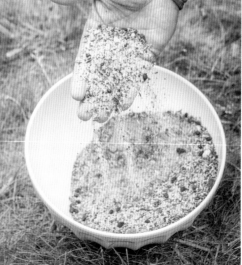

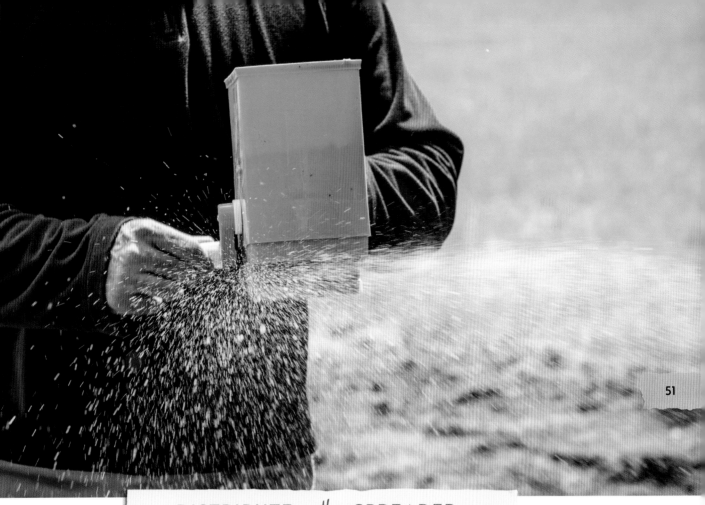

DISTRIBUTE *with a* SPREADER . . .

There are several ways you can go about sowing your seed, depending on the size of your meadow. A simple shoulder spreader can be very effective and a little faster than hand spreading. There are many handheld spreaders that will also do the trick. If you have a larger area that may have required a tractor to prepare, you can rent a steel seed spreader that fits on the back of the tractor.

Most spreaders allow you to adjust the settings based on the size of the seed you're sowing. I always recommend using the finest or smallest setting when spreading your meadow mix, though it may take a little experimenting with just sand to find the proper setting on your particular spreader.

. . . OR SPREAD *by* HAND

My preference is to forgo the spreader and do it by hand. I mix my seed and sand in a 5-gallon pail or wheelbarrow and then divide the mix into four equal parts. Then I fill a smaller bucket with a quarter of the seed-and-sand mix and walk around the meadow area, tossing handfuls of the mix with an underhand motion and a little flick of the wrist. After I've made one pass, I'll fill my bucket with another quarter of the mix and go over the entire area again in a different direction, then repeat until I've spread all the mix. By going over the entire area several times, I ensure a nice, evenly sown meadow.

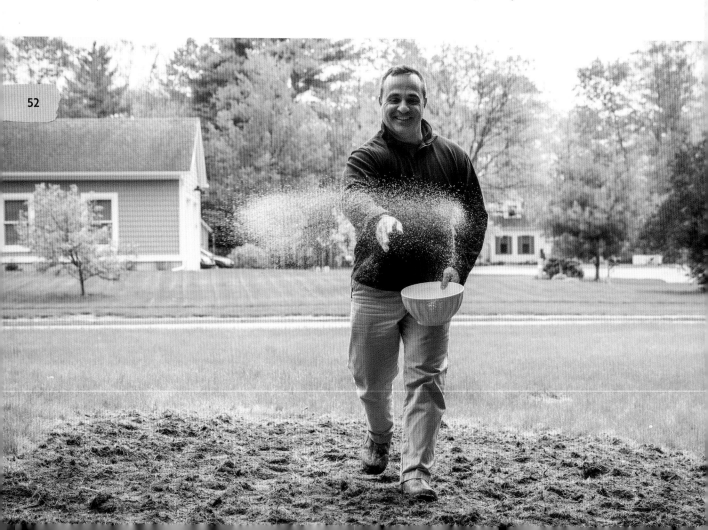

Look for Quality Seed

When you're shopping for a meadow mix, you'll want the best-quality product you can find. Here's what to look for:

- A good meadow mix should have a balance of species that bloom all season long, with a nice blend of different heights and textures.

- Any product you buy should be 100 percent pure seed; many of the lower-quality products are mostly filler.

- The seed should be lab tested with germination and purity information provided on the label.

- The meadow mix should be from a reputable seed company, as they will be able to answer any questions you might have and provide additional information.

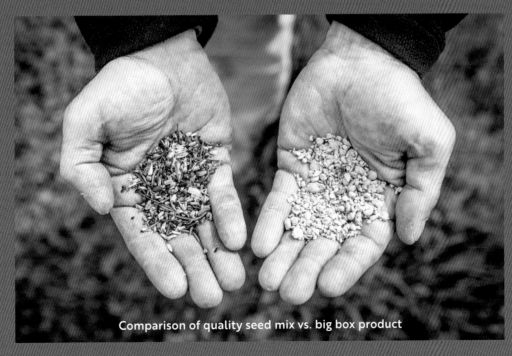

Comparison of quality seed mix vs. big box product

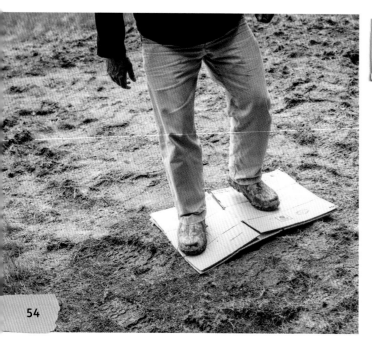

PRESS THE SEED *into the* SOIL

Once you've sown your seed, lightly press it into the soil. With smaller plantings, this can be done by simply laying a piece of cardboard over the planting area and walking over it. For larger meadow plantings, you can use a water-fill roller (which is usually available for rent if you don't own one). There's no need to add much water, as you don't need a lot of weight — just a little pressure to push the seeds down to ensure good seed-to-soil contact and better germination.

DO *Not* COVER

People often ask if they need to rake their seeds into the soil or cover them with soil. In most cases, the answer is no. Most wildflower or meadow mix seeds are small enough that if you rake them or cover them, some of them may end up planted too deep in the soil, and this would affect the germination rate of the mix.

The only time I recommend covering your seed is if you're planting on a slope. A light cover of chopped straw (not hay, as this may contain weed seeds) would help hold the seed. If the area is exposed to a lot of wind, you might also cover the seeds to keep them from being blown away. Be careful not to cover seeds too thickly; you still want water and sunlight to be able to penetrate. You also want your seedlings to be able to come up through the straw once they begin to germinate.

In the first day or two after seeding, don't be surprised if birds or other critters visit your soon-to-be meadow and munch on some seeds. Don't worry — they can snack on seeds without affecting the outcome of your meadow. When planting 100 percent pure seed, there could be between 200,000 and 300,000 seeds per pound (depending on your mix formulation). So if the birds eat a few, don't panic — there's plenty to go around.

WATER and WATCH for GERMINATION

Once you've planted your meadow, watch for the first signs of germination. Watering the area right after sowing will certainly help speed up the germination process. If you're not able or willing to water, you might consider scheduling your planting around a forecast period of rainy weather. In most cases, a high-quality meadow mix should germinate in 10 to 20 days. I've had seed sprout in as little as 5 days over a stretch of sunny weather when I kept the meadow well watered.

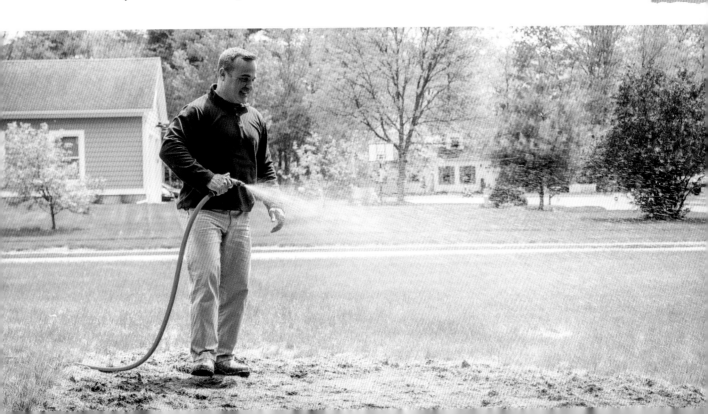

STORING SEEDS

If you have leftover seed after you've planted your meadow, you can store it for up to two years. Any container you choose — a mason jar or a plastic food container with a lid — should be securely sealed after it has been filled with seeds, so that no moisture can enter. Be sure to label the containers and store them in a cool, dry place. A refrigerator, kitchen cupboard, or a dry basement would work fine.

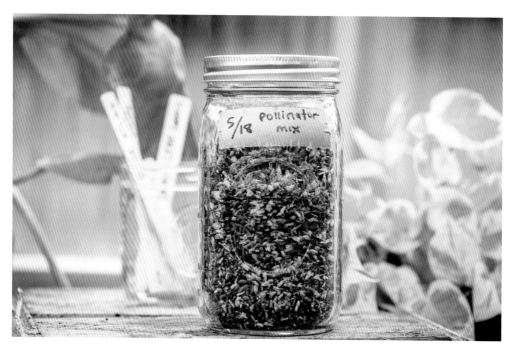

Buy a Blend or Mix Your Own?

Rather than purchase a premixed blend of seeds, you may choose to design your own mix or plant individual species from seed. This does take a little more understanding of the heights and bloom times of each flower, but it can be very rewarding and allows you to plant species exactly where you want them in your meadow.

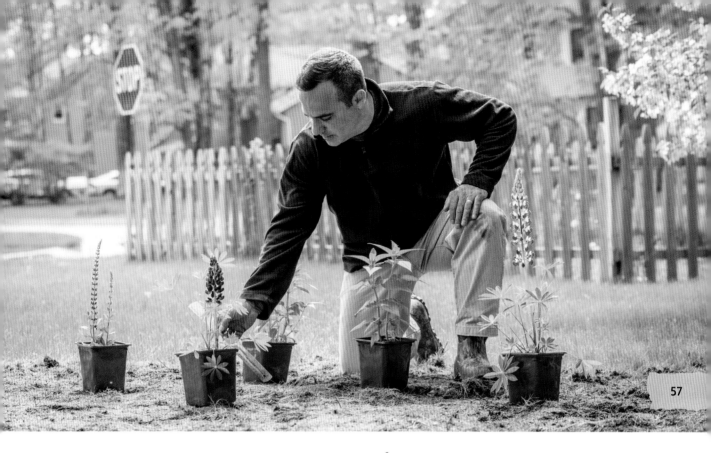

STARTING *with* PLANTS *or* PLUGS

If you're looking for faster results, consider starting a meadow with both seed and plants.
Most garden centers or nurseries offer a nice selection of both annuals and perennials
in all sorts of colors, heights, and bloom times so you can plan your garden accordingly.
Don't be afraid to ask for help at the garden center when choosing plants or mapping
out your meadow garden. There are a lot of little details to consider, such as how tall and
wide the plants will eventually be, as well as when they'll bloom. A good garden center or
landscape designer can help put you on a path to succeed.

CHOOSING PLANTS

You will find meadow plants offered in a variety of different sizes. Bigger is not better when it comes to plants in pots, though. A 2- to 4-inch potted perennial will grow and become established more quickly than a plant that's in a 1-gallon or larger pot. After a year or two, the smaller plant will have become just as big as the larger plant, and most people wouldn't be able to tell the difference between the two. But where you *will* be able to tell is in your savings of money! The smaller plants are usually a fraction of the cost of the larger plants.

Once you've prepared your list of plants, I suggest that you make a planting plan, so that you know how many plants you'll need. Take into consideration how tall the plants will get and how much they'll spread. This will allow you to get a more accurate count on the quantity needed and calculate your costs properly.

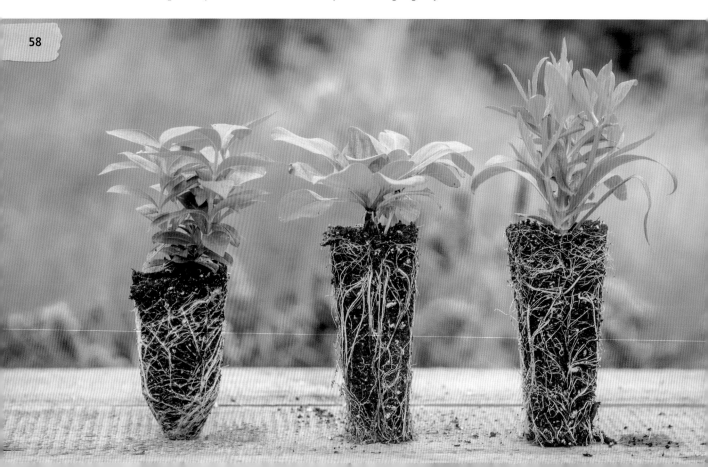

GET PLANTING!

Having a planting plan will help you space plants appropriately, so they have room to grow. A common mistake people make is putting their plants too close together; the plants may look small in the beginning (especially if you're planting plugs), but in just a few short months, those plants will grow quickly.

Once you know the spread of your plants, you can mark the soil where you're going to dig your holes. Dig your holes so that they're twice the size of the pot that your plant is currently in; the extra space will encourage the roots to expand quickly in their new site. Tuck the plant into the hole, backfill with compost or topsoil, water it well, and cover the root zone (but not the foliage) with an organic mulch to help keep the soil moist.

It's not unusual to see some plants droop a little shortly after they go into the ground. This is natural as the plants adjust to their new environment and will usually last only 24 to 48 hours; then you should see them bounce right back.

A big benefit to using plugs or plants from containers is that most of the plants will be ready to flower that growing season. If you're putting in annuals, they could be ready to bloom in a matter of weeks. Perennials might also be ready to bloom quickly, depending on how old they were when you purchased them.

SEED MAN SAYS
Know Your Bloom Time

Know the bloom times of the plants and plugs you've selected, and don't choose too many that bloom at the same time as this could leave other times of the year with limited color. A landscape designer or nursery should be able to help you with this planning. Bloom time information should be found on all the plant tags as well.

Your MEADOW IS ALIVE!

As those first few weeks go by, continue to take notice of the weather, as this will play a big part in the development of your meadow. It's ideal to have some rain in the forecast or to water your meadow to stimulate growth during those first few weeks after sowing or planting. If it's been sunny and you've been watering or getting rain and things *still* seem slow to progress, it's a good time to troubleshoot.

TROUBLESHOOTING *Your* MEADOW

No germination at all. If a few weeks have passed and the area has been receiving lots of sun and regular moisture, yet the ground still looks pretty bare, this raises some concern. A high-quality meadow mix should germinate in 10 to 20 days with proper sun and moisture. If it's been 30 days and there's very little growth, the problem may be a lack of soil fertility. You might consider doing a soil test to help pinpoint the possible areas of concern.

It looks like there are just grasses and weeds growing. This may be the result of sowing seed too sparsely. Did you calculate the area or square footage properly to ensure you purchased the right amount of seed? If you sowed too little in relation to the actual size, this could allow weeds to gain the upper hand.

There's growth in some areas but not others. This suggests that the seeds weren't evenly sown. Keep a close eye on the areas that seem to be slow to develop; another possibility is that those areas are just a little slower to develop than the others because of a difference in the soil, but they will fill in soon. If a few more weeks go by, there's been sun and rain, and you still have bare spots, you may want to add compost or fertilizer to those areas. The good news here is that if the problem is detected early enough, you can address it and add more seed if needed.

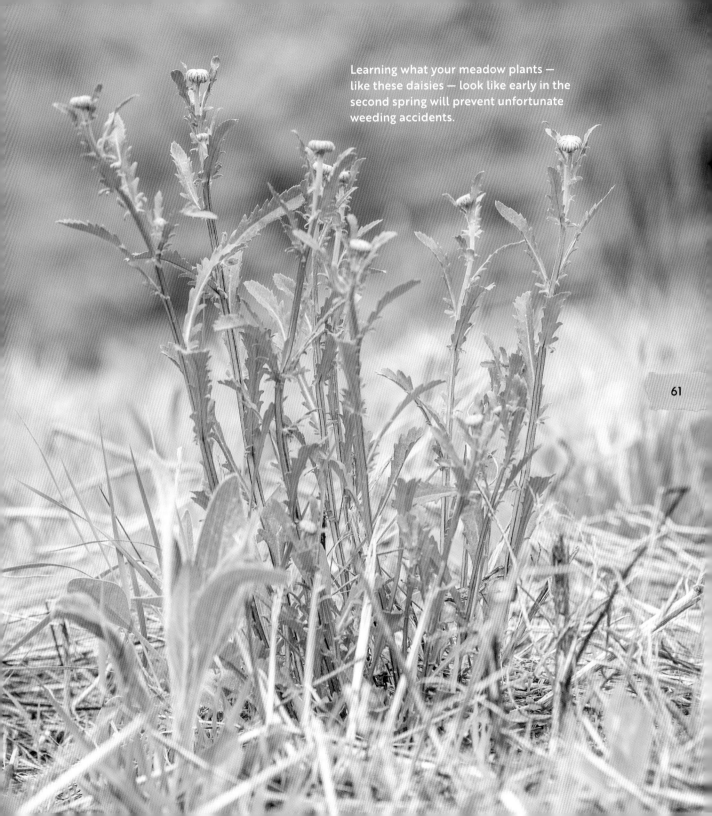

Learning what your meadow plants — like these daisies — look like early in the second spring will prevent unfortunate weeding accidents.

How Many Pollinators Can You Find?

As a new growing season arrives and my meadow begins bursting with color, I look forward to seeing all the different pollinators that may visit during the year (we also get the occasional deer, moose, or black bear, too, but I don't count them!). My daughter, Sadie, and I keep a journal and spend many days waiting patiently to see who might come flying in for a visit. This is a great way to learn about our winged friends and teach myself and the next generation of gardeners how critical pollinators are and the role they play in our ecosystem. We have different categories in our journal, such as Butterflies, Hummingbirds, Bees, and Insects, and we jot down the different species that come to visit. We try to take photos and videos to document as well, just adding to the fun. We'll usually share on social media with other gardening enthusiasts.

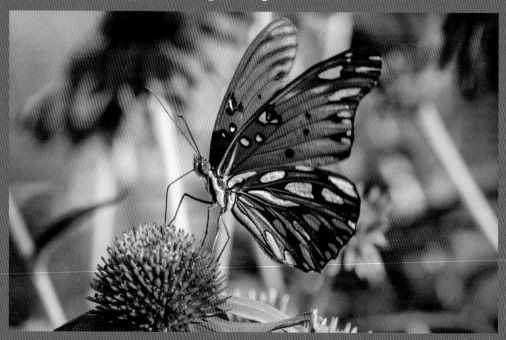

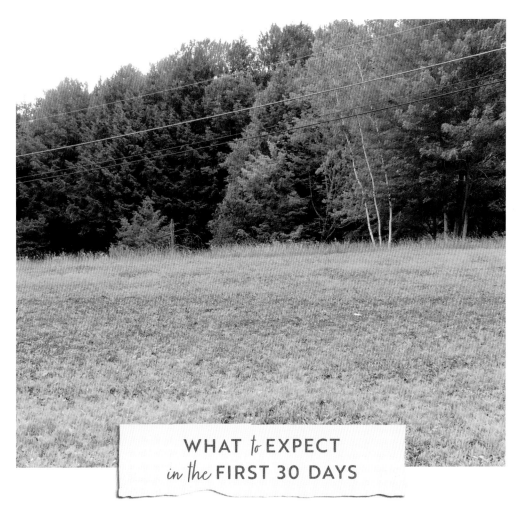

WHAT *to* EXPECT *in the* FIRST 30 DAYS

At this point, your meadow should be coming in nicely. You should see similar-looking seedlings scattered evenly throughout your meadow. Your plants or plugs should show noticeable signs of growth as their roots settle in and get acclimated to their new growing conditions.

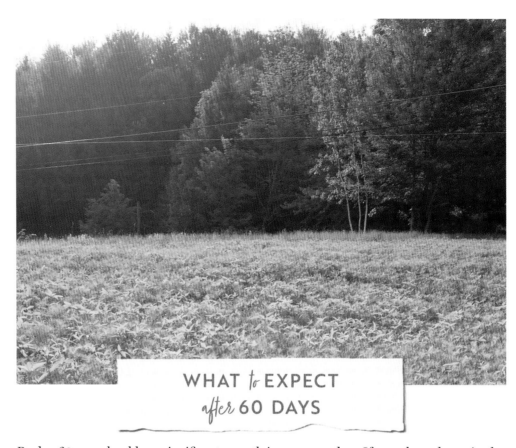

WHAT *to* EXPECT *after* 60 DAYS

By day 60, you should see significant growth in your meadow. If you planted or mixed some annuals from seed into your meadow mix, you may even be noticing the first flowers. If you planted perennial plants or plugs, they, too, may be showing buds or be in bloom. The perennials and biennials you planted from seed will show top growth, while belowground their root structures continue to develop and mature.

This is a great time to identify and pull any unwanted grasses or weeds. If you've planted a large area and you're not willing or able to pull weeds, don't worry too much; most meadow varieties should be able to hold their own against most weeds. If you're not able to identify a weed from a wildflower, don't pull anything just yet and let your meadow continue to develop.

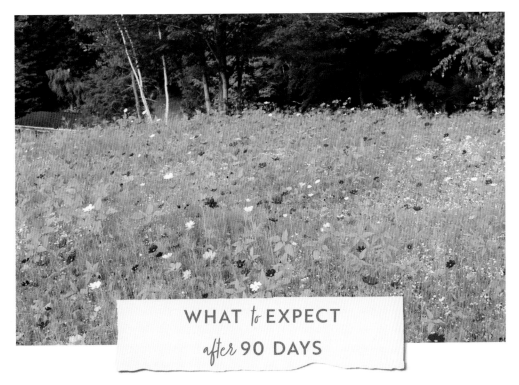

WHAT *to* EXPECT *after* 90 DAYS

Hopefully by now you're enjoying the fruits of your labor. Perennial plants and plugs should be blooming. Perennials that you planted from seed should show lots of green top growth as their roots continue to develop, but probably not a lot of (if any) flowers. Annuals planted from seed should be showing lots of color. Hopefully you're seeing bees, birds, and butterflies visit your garden each day. Your meadow should require very little maintenance at this stage. If you're seeing weeds and grasses at this stage, either pull them or snip the tops off (to prevent them from going to seed).

This is a great time to get to know your flowers. Observe all the different colors, heights, and bloom times of plants throughout the summer. Take lots of pictures and notes. This will help you learn the different bloom times and record the color combinations you prefer.

As the weather cools and the fall season approaches, it's time to think about the second season of your meadow!

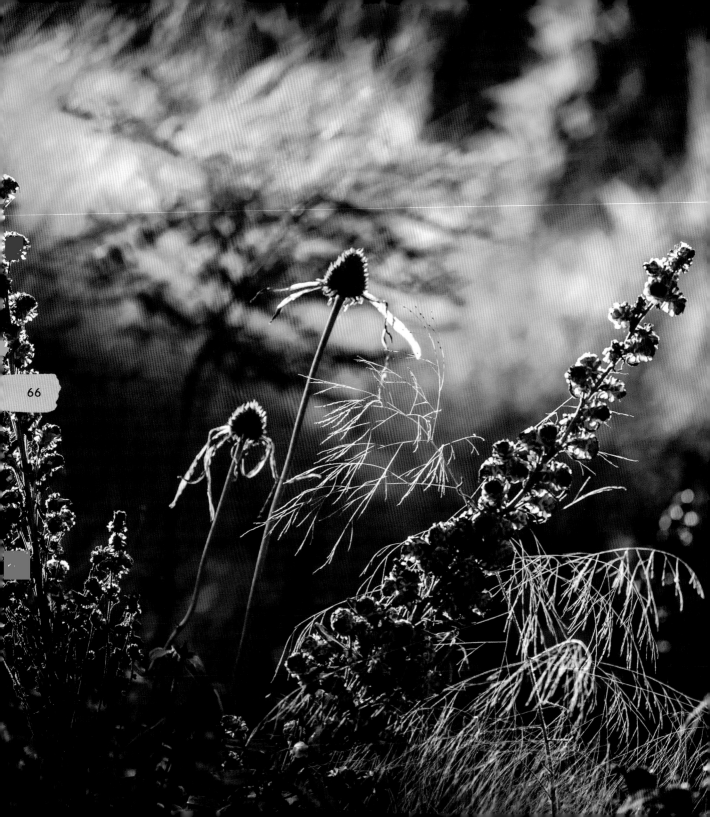

CHAPTER 3

Autumn and Beyond

As the cool temperatures of fall set in and your meadow flowers fade, your plants will produce and drop seed for next year's flowers. Following the garden's lead, now is the ideal time to evaluate your meadow and add more seed where it's needed.

Fall is also a great time to try your hand at collecting seeds. You first need to identify the flowers and where the seed is developing. Seeds can take on many shapes and sizes and can develop in pods or nestle in seed heads on the plant. If you've never collected before, start with seeds that are easy to identify and collect, such as lupine, zinnia, or baptisia. You'll need to wait for the seed to mature fully before you begin collecting.

Keep in mind that flowers mature and produce seeds at different times throughout the growing season. If there's a plant you want to collect seed from, note when it flowers, then wait 30 to 45 days from flowering for the seeds to ripen. For most plants, the seed is ready to harvest when the case or pod is brown and dry. Although you may gather lots of seed, not all of it will be viable.

SOWING SEED *for* NEXT YEAR

Fall is a good time to evaluate your meadow and sow additional seed. Maybe your meadow had a bare spot or you want to add more of the annuals you especially liked this year. Your favorite annuals can help fill out the planting, and join the perennials that have already established themselves, in next year's riot of color.

When adding seed in fall, you won't dig up the whole meadow again and prep the soil as you did in spring; you don't want to disturb any perennials that have taken root. Instead, take a hard rake and rough up small pockets in the meadow. This will expose some bare soil for seed sowing while minimizing damage to surrounding growth. Simply sprinkle your seed and press it into the disturbed soil with your foot.

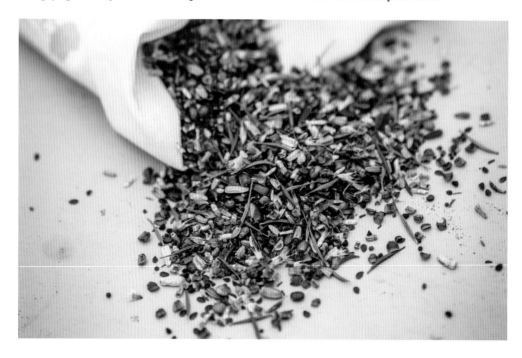

Collecting Seed with Kids

Collecting seed with kids is a fun way to show them where the seed develops on a plant, to appreciate all the different sizes and shapes of seeds and pods, and to engage in creative play (baptisia pods make great rattles!). It's also a chance to teach kids about the importance of the garden for supporting wildlife.

Milkweed is a good example of this. It's critical to the survival of monarch butterflies, which feed on its flowers and whose larvae eat the foliage. Whether you're growing them in your meadow or just hunting for them along the side of the road, it's fun to look for these pickle-shaped seedpods when they burst open in fall, sending their fluffy, seed-laden floss into the air. You can blow into the pods to help spread the seed, or you can pick the pods, bring the seeds indoors to germinate (after a month or so of cold storage in the fridge), then plant the seedlings outside.

My daughter and I keep a journal to identify all the different birds and insects that visit our meadow each year, including which flowers they prefer and which seeds they eat. Monarchs, fritillaries, swallowtails, luna moths, honeybees, and Japanese beetles are just a few of the critters that we're fortunate enough to have visit us each year. Some of these are not exactly welcome (Japanese beetles), but as long as they're not causing major damage, we let them hang around.

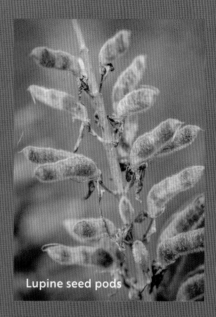

Lupine seed pods

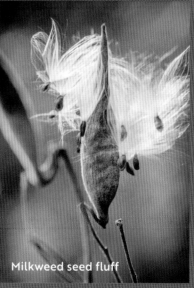

Milkweed seed fluff

WHEN *to* MOW

Cutting your meadow back once a year is a good idea to help new growth, and fall is one time to consider mowing. If you decide to add more seed to your meadow (see page 68), cutting back the meadow prior to seeding can make this process a lot easier; removing dead foliage and stems provides better access to ensure good seed-to-soil contact.

If you're not adding seed in fall, I suggest waiting to cut your meadow until the following spring. The stems from this year's growth can provide valuable habitat and food for birds and beneficial insects through the winter months. Just a few short weeks after being cut back in spring, the new growth will be coming on and the cuttings will begin to decompose into the soil.

A brush hog or weed whacker works just fine to cut down the growth. And keep in mind that there's no need to scalp your meadow; it's perfectly fine to cut it back to 4 to 6 inches high. You can also chop up the stems you've cut, so that they break down more quickly.

WHAT ABOUT BURNING?

People ask me whether they should burn their meadow once a year. Burning can be effective in stimulating the growth of some types of native plants and help some kinds of seeds break dormancy. But it can also be very dangerous and is not allowed in some regions of the country or at certain times of the year. It also seems overkill for a very small meadow! Before you burn, check your local ordinances and speak with someone from your local fire station. He or she should also be able to confirm if it's legal in your area to perform a controlled burn.

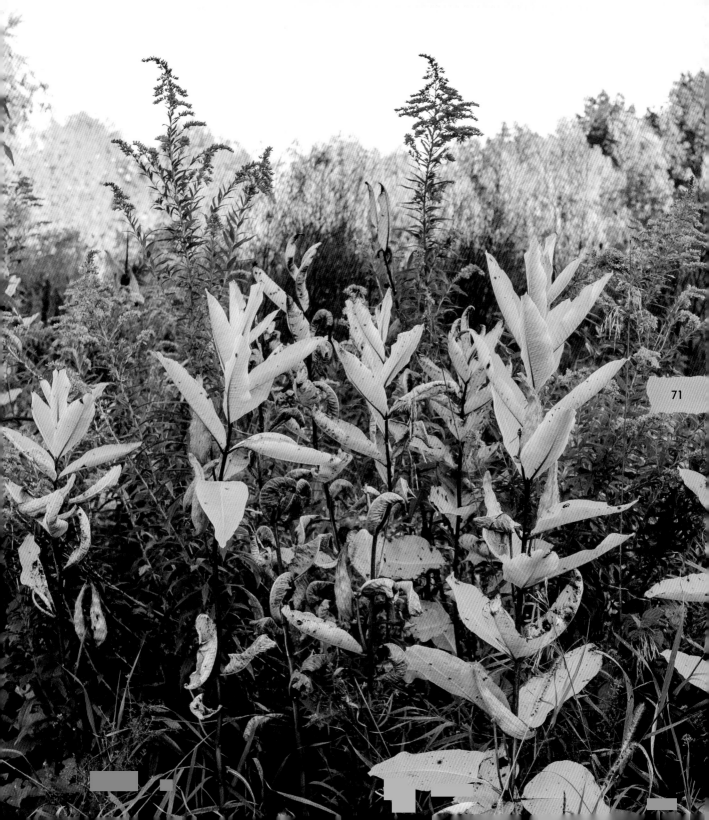

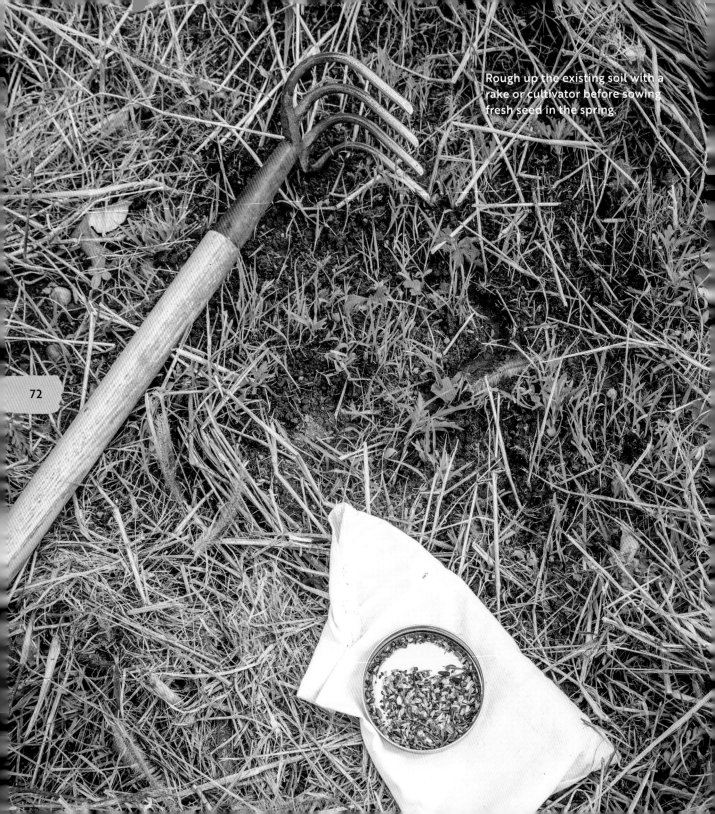

Rough up the existing soil with a rake or cultivator before sowing fresh seed in the spring.

YOUR MEADOW *in* YEAR TWO *and* BEYOND

As spring arrives, it's time to get excited for another year of meadow magic. If you didn't mow last fall, this would be a good time to knock down the dead stalks and other debris before significant spring growth starts. Cutting now will allow for better sun exposure on the returning plants. You can leave the cuttings right in the meadow, where they will break down and enrich the soil.

Spring is also a good time to revisit the list of plants in your meadow mix, so you can be on the lookout for second-year perennials that might be starting to bloom. Don't get discouraged if a few of your perennials don't flower in the second year. Regardless of whether you planted them from seed, plants, or plugs, some varieties are just slow to develop; some may not flower until their third or fourth year in the meadow. But once they do begin to flower, they should return with flowers for years to come.

If you'd like to see more of your favorite annuals this season, now is the time to sow seed for them (assuming you didn't sow in fall; see page 68). Remember to rough up the soil surface with a hard rake first to ensure good seed-to-soil contact, and to press the seed firmly into the soil to speed up germination.

Cutting back dead stalks in spring will allow the sun to reach perennials growing for their second season.

ONCE YOUR MEADOW
Is ESTABLISHED

Your meadow will continue to evolve as it matures, offering you a chance to play with your plantings. As varieties grow and fill out, you might think about thinning some of them to make room for other plants. You can divide and move plants around your meadow or, even better, share them with friends. You might find yourself adding a new variety or two each year as you learn about different plants. A variety might fade, or a plant just doesn't take; that simply means there's room to try something new!

Gardeners often ask me what kind of maintenance they should do at this point. Here's one of the attractions of this kind of gardening: once a meadow is established, it should require only minimal maintenance — especially if you've chosen the right plants for your growing conditions. Your meadow shouldn't require constant watering or fertilizing or constant weeding.

Rather than worrying about maintenance, consider other ways to enhance your enjoyment of the space. Maybe put out a bird feeder to invite more winged friends, or add a bench or chair so that you can sit and observe the comings and goings in your meadow. Maybe mow a new path through your meadow to add visual definition and provide different access points. These are all things you might include or expand on as the years go by.

Maybe put out a bird feeder to invite more winged friends, or add a bench or chair so that you can sit and observe the comings and goings in your meadow.

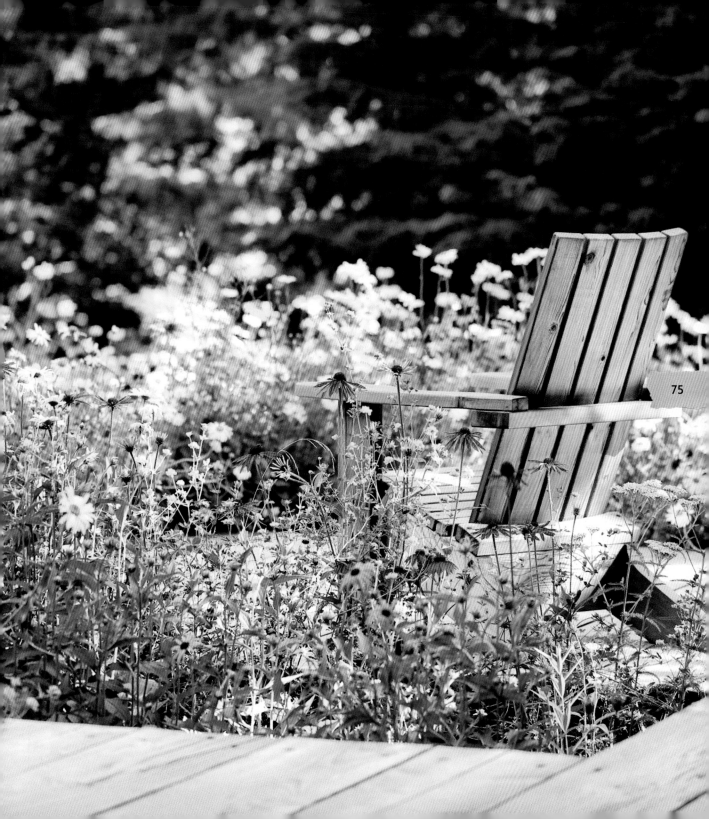

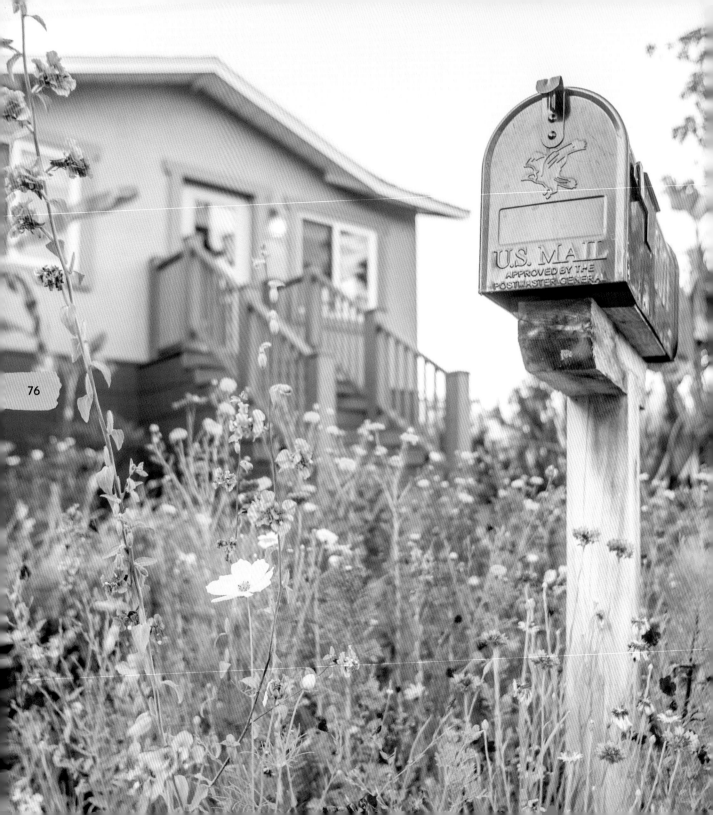

CHAPTER 4

Meadows with a Purpose

If you have a challenging landscape to work with — such as a sloped hillside, hard-to-reach area, or leach field — a meadow can act as a problem solver for you. Many wildflowers, in particular, adapt to extreme growing conditions and require little maintenance, meaning they'll not only look beautiful but also serve a purpose on your property.

The first step is to determine your purpose, then find the right plants for the job. For example, if you're trying to stabilize soil on a hill, you'll want plants that establish quickly and require little supplemental water once they've grown in. If you're filling a marshy spot, you'll want plants that tolerate a lot of moisture. If you're trying to make your urban plot more nature-friendly, you might want plants that attract pollinators.

Meadow plants can solve all kinds of problems. One spot that's perfect for planting a meadow is over the leach field for a septic system. In addition to adding color and visual interest, the plants soften the look of the area and do a good job of helping a constructed "mound" leach field blend into the surrounding landscape. The reduced mowing is also a benefit. And unlike trees and shrubs, which send their roots farther underground and can infiltrate leach pipes, meadow plants pose no risk to the septic system.

MEADOW PLANTS *for* EROSION CONTROL

Do you have a pesky hill that's a pain to mow each week or one that's losing soil to erosion? Converting it to a meadow might be the answer. With careful soil preparation and plant selection, your hillside can become a place of enjoyment rather than a weekly chore.

It can be challenging to prepare the soil for a hillside planting. Sometimes the area is too steep to till or to break up the soil. You might have to get creative; instead of

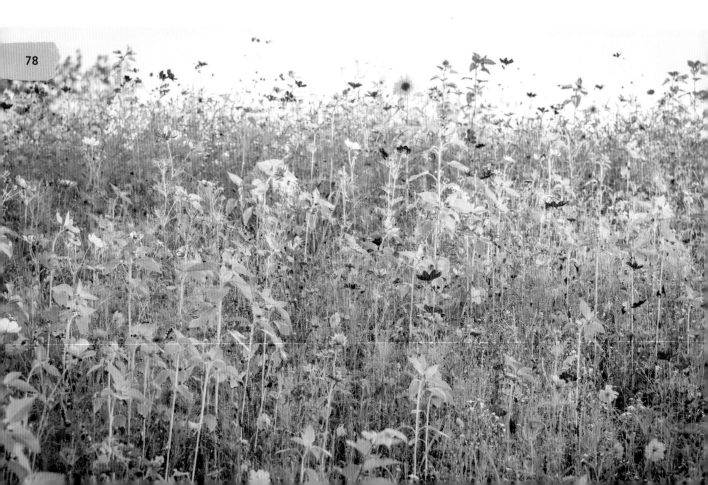

trying to prepare the entire area at once, you might divide it up and tackle smaller areas at a time. This can mitigate soil erosion by not exposing the entire slope all at once. If the area is just *too steep* to seed even a little at a time, you may try terracing the area by creating retaining walls using wood, stone, or concrete blocks to prevent water runoff. Another option for an extremely steep slope is to use plugs in the area instead of seed.

Choosing the right plants will play a big part in whether your meadow is successful. When planting on a slope, include a combination of perennials and annuals. Annuals germinate quickly and help keep the weeds down and the soil secured while your perennials are being established. As perennials send their roots deep into the soil, they'll provide long-term stability and erosion control year after year.

Seeding the slope. It's important to account for the slope itself when determining the proper amount of seed for a hillside. I recommend adding 25 to 50 percent more seed when seeding a slope or hill. For example, let's say you have a flat and level 1,000-square-foot area to sow; I might recommend ¼ to ½ pound of meadow mix for this area. If the same 1,000 square feet was sloped, I would recommend 1 full pound of seed. This is to make sure we have enough seed and account for any runoff that you might experience in those first few weeks after seeding. Many times I find that people aren't spreading enough seed to account for the runoff common when planting a slope.

Seeding a slope is one case when I do recommend covering the seed, simply to help hold it on the slope and to prevent the seed washing away. A few bales of straw — not hay, which contains seed — will usually do the trick. Cover the area lightly, so that newly germinated seedlings are able to grow up through it.

Hydroseeding large areas. If you're planting an area that's more than 10,000 square feet, you may want to consider getting a quote for having the meadow hydroseeded by a landscape professional. This can be an affordable, time-saving solution for seeding larger meadows, and the mix of seed and tackifier holds very well on a slope.

Plugs or plants. Another option for establishing a meadow on a slope is to start with plugs or plants, or to use a mix of plants and seed. The plants will set roots quickly and can help with erosion while your seedlings are beginning to grow.

Stabilizing Plants for Hillsides

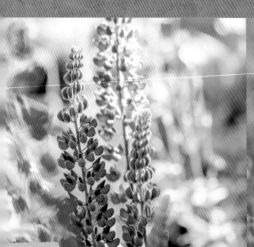

Wild lupine
Lupinus perennis

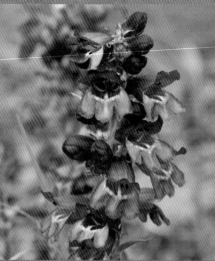

Rocky Mountain penstemon
Penstemon strictus

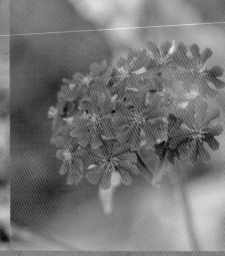

Maltese cross
Lychnis chalcedonica

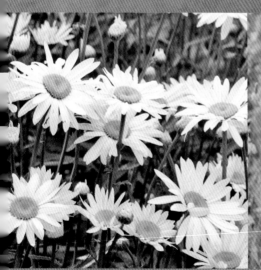

Shasta daisy
Leucanthemum × superbum

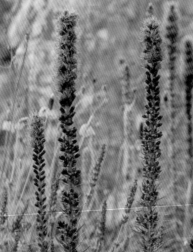

Blazing star or gayfeather
Liatris spicata

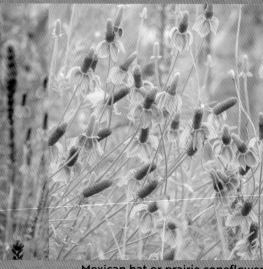

Mexican hat or prairie coneflower
Ratibida columnifera

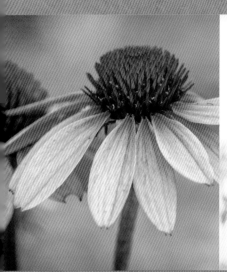

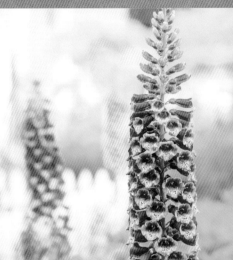

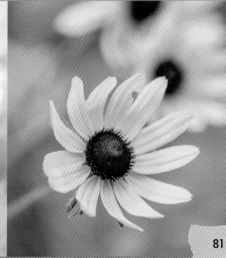

Purple coneflower
Echinacea purpurea

Foxglove
Digitalis purpurea

Black-eyed Susan
Rudbeckia hirta

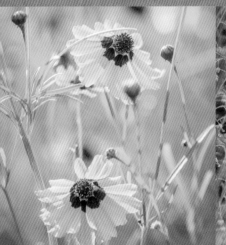

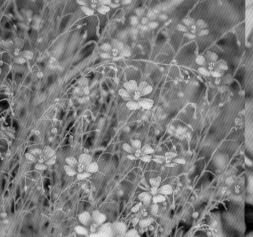

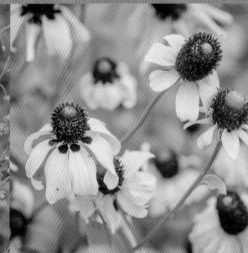

Plains coreopsis
Coreopsis tinctoria

Blue flax
Linum perenne

Clasping coneflower
Rudbeckia amplexicaulis

MEADOWS WITH A PURPOSE

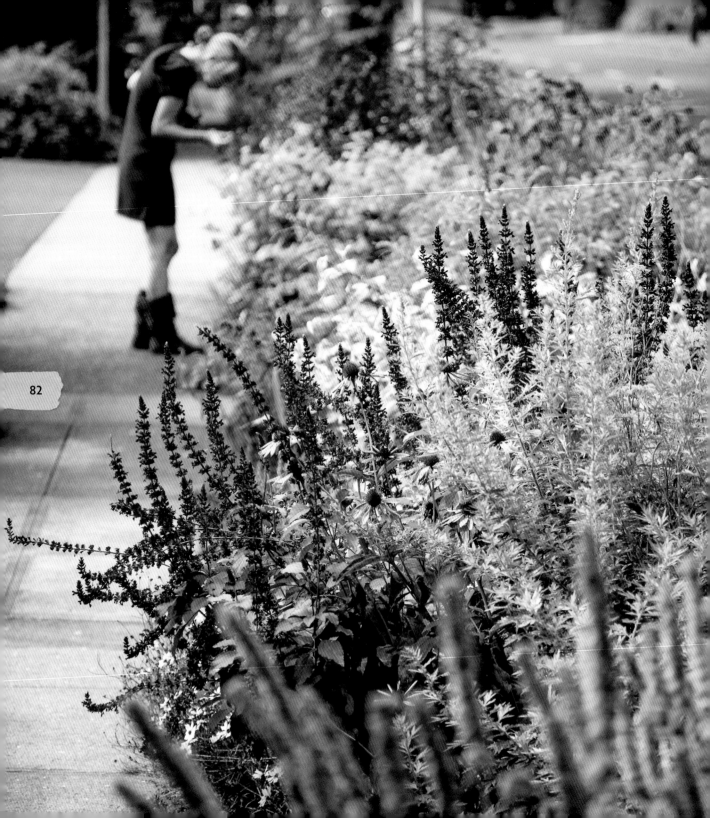

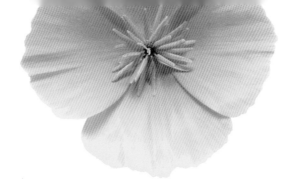

A HELLSTRIP MEADOW

Okay, so you might be wondering what the heck a hellstrip is. It's that area between the street and a sidewalk that is usually planted with grass or inundated with weeds, and you're never sure if *you* should mow it or if the city takes care of it. Why not replace the grass and weeds with a meadow planting? These meridians or sidewalk planting strips are the perfect spot for some tough meadow plants: they're usually in full sun, have poor soil, and aren't highly maintained.

Once you've confirmed that you're responsible for this area (check with your local department of public works), ask whether there are any height restrictions for plants in the hellstrip. Some towns place restrictions on hellstrips so they don't impede visibility of buildings or roads. Tough plants such as coreopsis, asters, penstemons, and baptisia are good choices. Adding grasses such as little bluestem and blue grama would complement the flowers and add texture.

Tough Plants for the Hellstrip

Common yarrow
Achillea millefolium

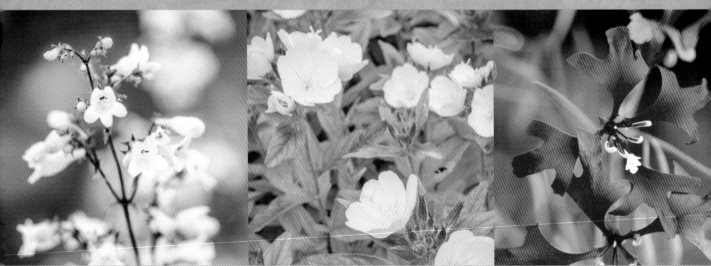

Little bluestem
Schizachyrium scoparium

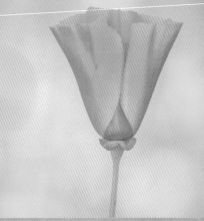

California poppy
Eschscholzia californica

Beardtongue
Penstemon digitalis

Evening primrose
Oenothera species

Deerhorn clarkia
Clarkia pulchella

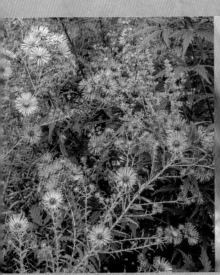

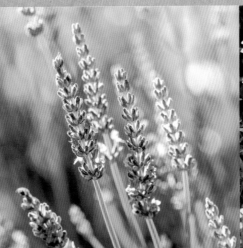

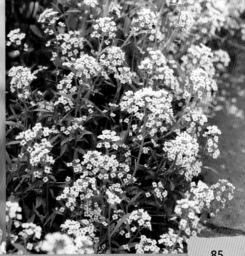

New England Aster
Symphyotrichum novae-angliae

Lavender
Lavandula angustifolia

Sweet alyssum
Lobularia maritima

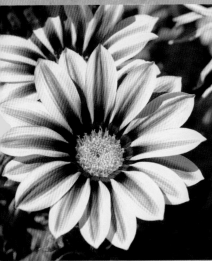

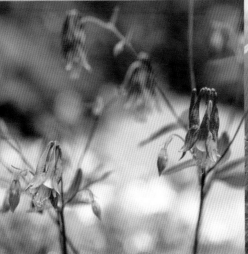

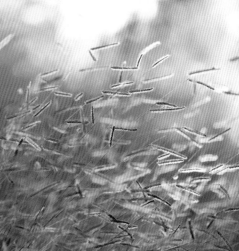

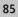

Gazania
Gazania splendens

Eastern red columbine
Aquilegia canadensis

Blue grama
Bouteloua gracilis

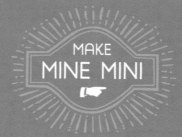

MAKE
MINE MINI

A YARDFUL
of MINI MEADOWS

The Velázquez family was growing tired of their large expanse of lawn in the front yard and wanted to bring a bit of color to the neighborhood. They decided to till up patches to plant with different meadow mixes that would offer a variety of blooms throughout the summer. The neighbors were intrigued by all the activity at first — and very impressed at bloom time!

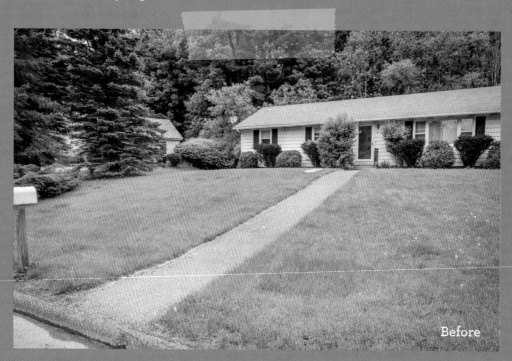

Before

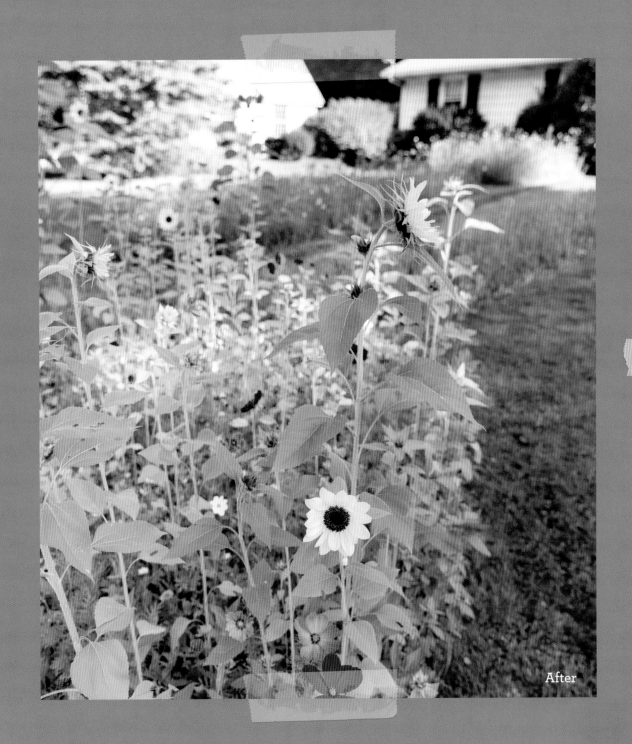

After

A DROUGHT-TOLERANT MEADOW

Increasingly warmer summers with inconsistent rainfall can make for some very stressful growing conditions for a lot of plants. In recent years, we've seen an increase in drought conditions across the country, from Connecticut to California. As a result, there has been a big increase in demand for drought-tolerant plants in home gardens. A meadow planting of drought-tolerant plants can actually thrive and provide years of color in these less-than-ideal conditions. Just keep in mind that whether you're planting seeds or plants, they'll need watering at the early stages to get them established. All young plants need regular water, especially seedlings, so think about how you will get some water to them in the first few weeks after planting.

Drought-tolerant plants can actually thrive and provide years of color in less-than-ideal conditions.

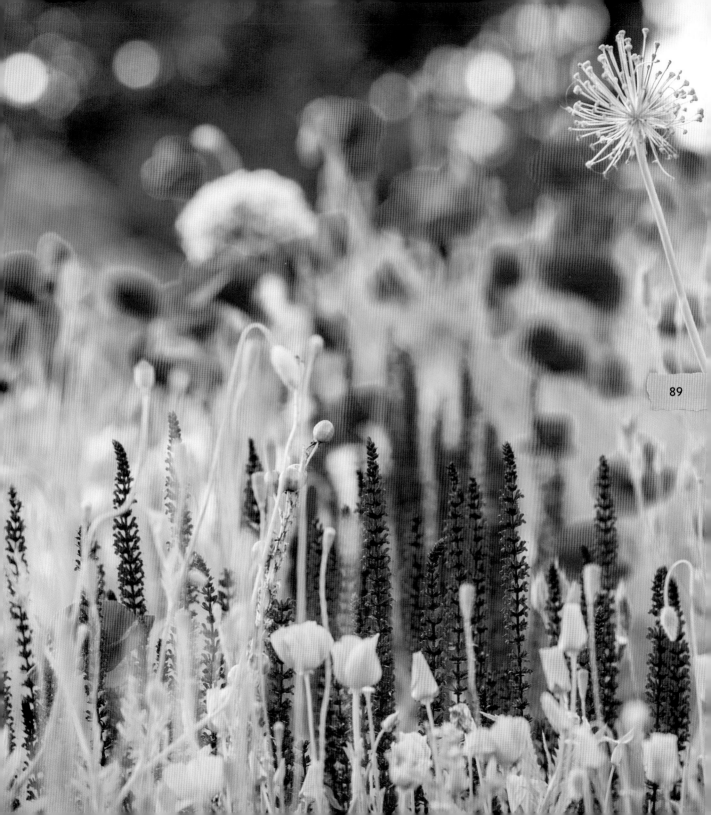

Drought-Tolerant Meadow Plants

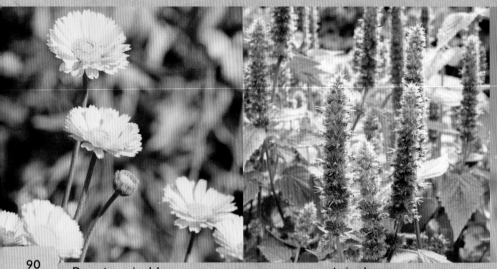

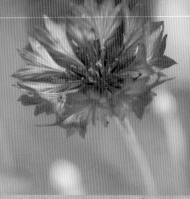

Desert marigold
Baileya multiradiata

Anise hyssop
Agastache foeniculum

Cornflower or bachelor's button
Centaurea cyanus

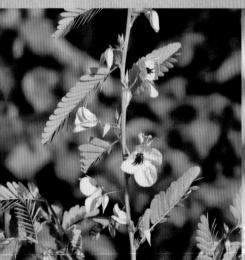

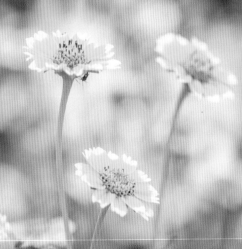

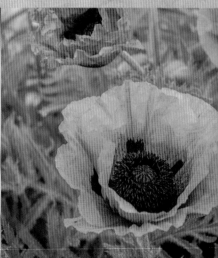

Partridge pea
Chamaecrista fasciculata

Tidy tips
Layia platyglossa

Oriental poppy
Papaver orientale

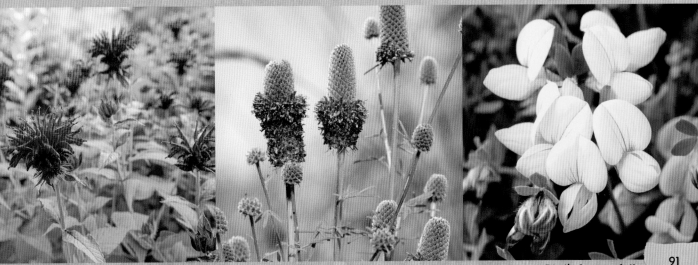

Bee balm
Monarda didyma

Purple prairie clover
Dalea purpurea

Bird's foot trefoil
Lotus corniculatus

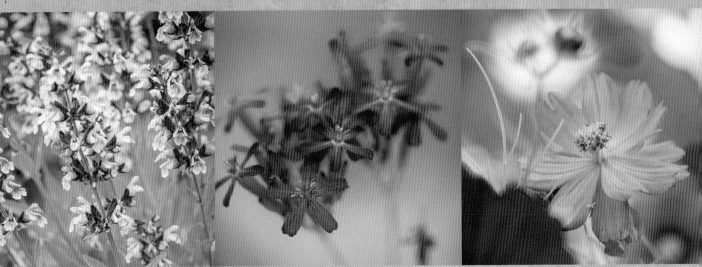

Sage
Salvia officinalis

None-so-pretty or catchfly
Silene armeria

Sulphur cosmos
Cosmos sulphureus

DEER-RESISTANT MEADOW PLANTS

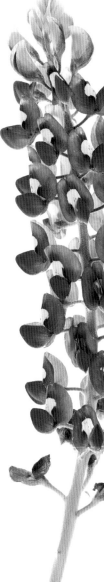

How can I create a meadow that the deer will not eat? This is certainly one of the top ten questions I've gotten from customers over the past 25 years. So let me be honest and realistic: this can be a difficult task. If the deer are starving, they will eat just about anything to survive; the success of your garden depends on just how hungry the deer are.

Here in Vermont we have lots of deer, but we also have plenty of rural land for them to graze, so they aren't interested in the meadows I've planted. Not far away in New Jersey and Pennsylvania, gardeners also have high deer populations, but they also have high human populations and residential areas have impinged on deer territory. The lack of wild food sources has caused Bambi to become quite a pest in residential gardens.

If you'd like to try a "deerproof" meadow, start by choosing plants that aren't especially appetizing, which includes varieties that are usually fragrant and taste bitter to them. Low-interest plants for deer include asclepias, marjoram, foxglove, monkshood, and catnip. On the following pages, I've included a list of additional plants that will hopefully work for you. Also be sure to pay a visit to your local nursery and ask them for deer-resistant selections for your region.

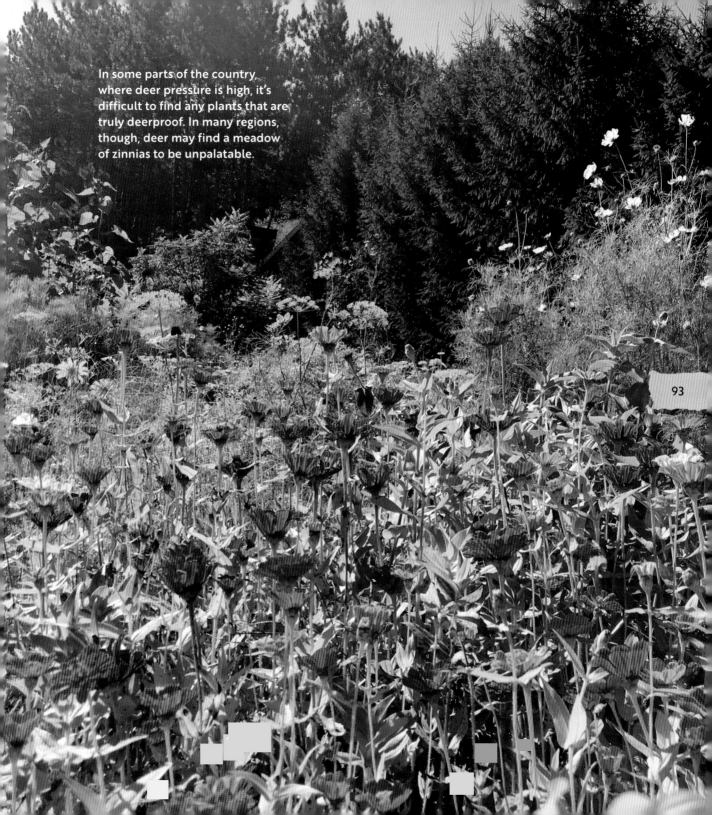

In some parts of the country, where deer pressure is high, it's difficult to find any plants that are truly deerproof. In many regions, though, deer may find a meadow of zinnias to be unpalatable.

Deer-Resistant Plants

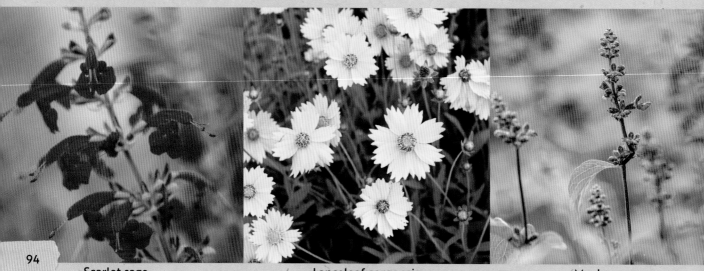

Scarlet sage
Salvia coccinea

Lanceleaf coreopsis
Coreopsis lanceolata

Mealycup sage
Salvia farinacea

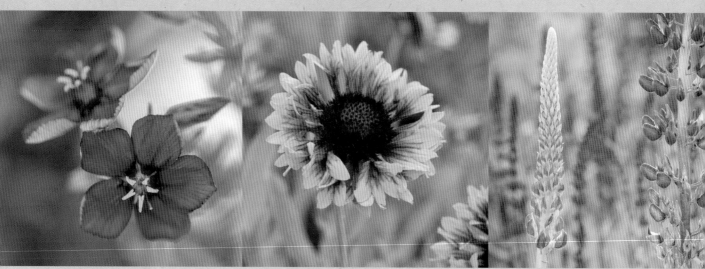

Blue pimpernel
Anagallis monelli

Blanketflower
Gaillardia aristata

Wild lupine
Lupinus perennis

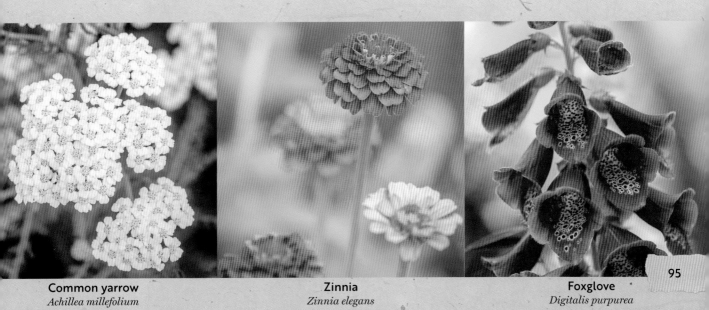

Common yarrow
Achillea millefolium

Zinnia
Zinnia elegans

Foxglove
Digitalis purpurea

95

Sweet alyssum
Lobularia maritima

Black-eyed Susan
Rudbeckia hirta

**Red poppy, Shirley poppy,
or corn poppy**
Papaver rhoeas

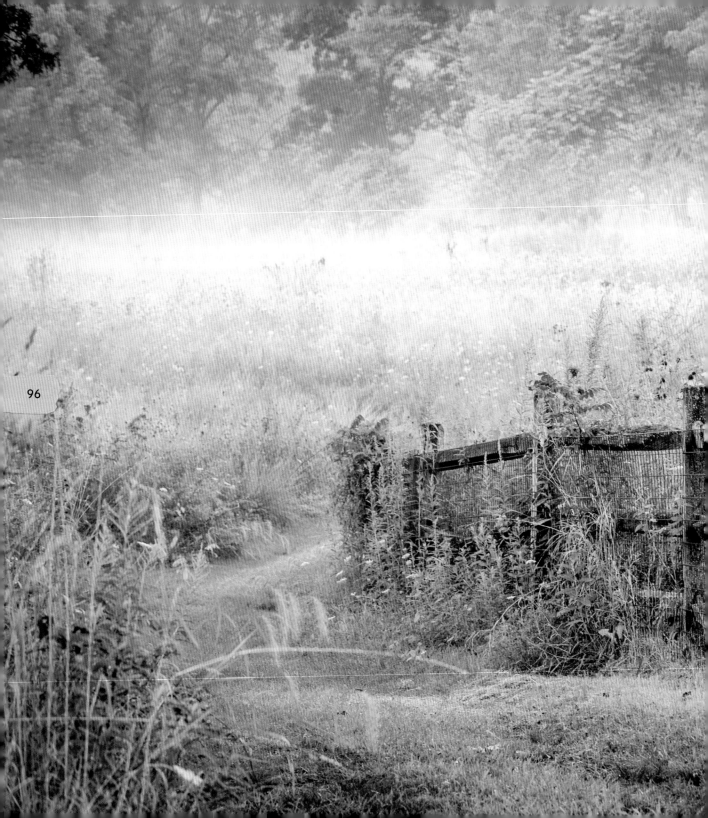

A BOGGY MEADOW

If you have an area on your landscape with poorly draining soil that collects water — especially in the spring — you may try your hand at planting wildflowers to create a boggy meadow. Typically these boggy spots are found at the bottom of slopes where water collects or in newly cleared wooded areas.

Before you get started, it's important to first survey the area. Is there actual standing water in this area and if so, how often? Most meadow plants won't thrive in constant standing water, so if this is the case with your area, you may want to create drainage to give the water a place to go.

There are plenty of meadow plants that thrive in damp soil. This area of your property may quickly become one of your favorite colorful spots to enjoy throughout the season.

Some plants thrive in spots that tend to be boggy, but not in areas with permanent standing water.

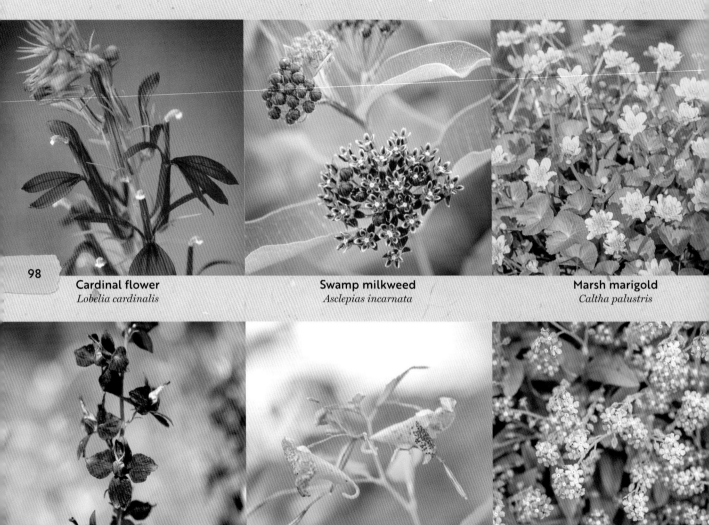

98

Cardinal flower
Lobelia cardinalis

Swamp milkweed
Asclepias incarnata

Marsh marigold
Caltha palustris

Rocket larkspur
Delphinium ajacis

Jewelweed
Impatiens capensis

Forget-me-not
Myosotis sylvatica

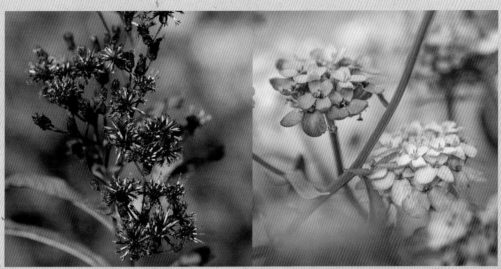

Giant ironweed
Vernonia gigantea

Globe candytuft
Iberis umbellata

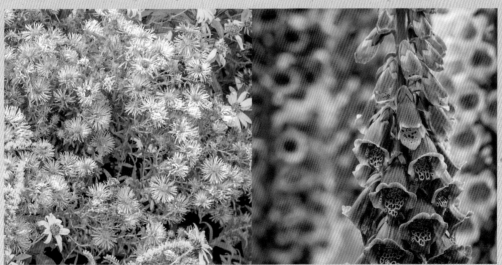

New England aster
Symphyotrichum novae-angliae

Foxglove
Digitalis purpurea

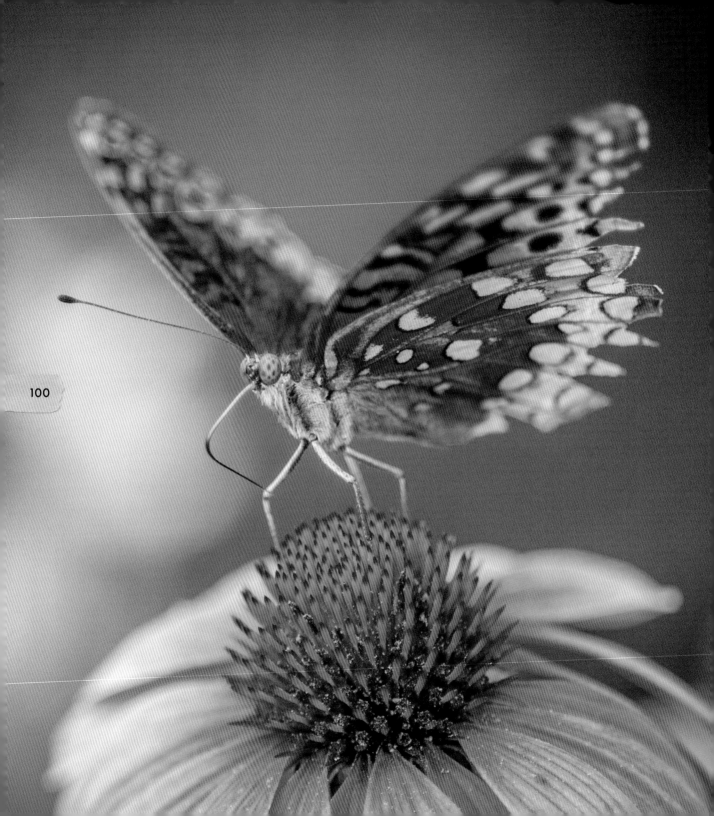

100

CHAPTER 5

Planting for Pollinators and Wildlife

Many people have become aware of the huge problem facing pollinators — those insects that move pollen from flower to flower, helping to produce most of our food crops. They are disappearing at an alarming rate, which affects not only the natural ecosystem but also our food supply.

The good news is that there is a lot we can all do to help solve the problem. As home gardeners, we can make a big difference by avoiding the use of pesticides, by providing a source of water for insects and birds, and by growing a meadow that's full of plants to attract pollinators and other beneficial insects. Pollinators include many different species of bees, butterflies, moths, flies, beetles, and even bats. Depending on your region, you will see a variety of these pollinators native to your area around your garden.

Planting a combination of annual and perennial flowers allows for early flowers in the first growing season — which pollinators depend on — and provides long-lasting habi-tat that insects can come back to year after year: another key to their survival. Planting a "near-native" landscape (one with both native and nonnative species) usually results in longer bloom time and more nectar and pollen sources throughout the season, which benefits a wider range of pollinators.

PROVIDE HABITAT

To provide habitat for beneficial insects, it's best to leave dead stems and flower heads standing through the winter, then cut them back in early spring. Pollinators need these natural settings in your garden or property to stay protected from predators and to lay their eggs. If you absolutely must mow (perhaps because of homeowners' association rules), consider putting out a nesting box. Nesting areas and boxes are easy to make yourself and provide shelter for bees, butterflies, and hummingbirds.

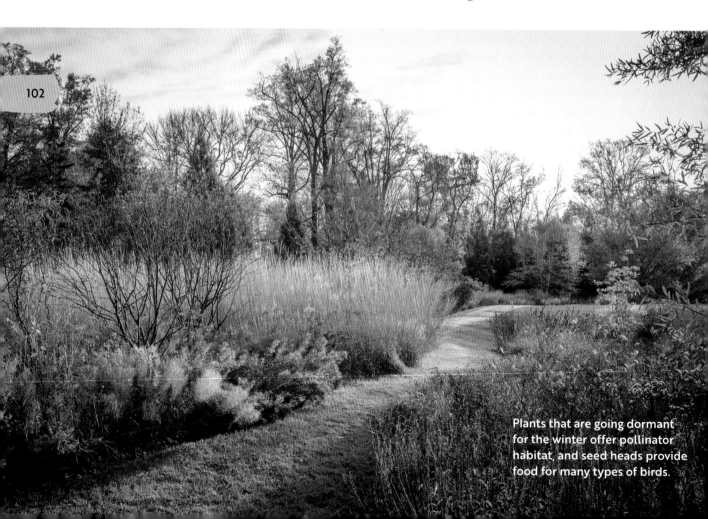

Plants that are going dormant for the winter offer pollinator habitat, and seed heads provide food for many types of birds.

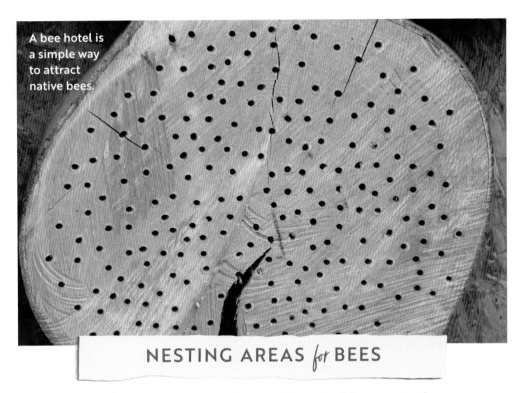

A bee hotel is a simple way to attract native bees.

NESTING AREAS *for* BEES

There are more than 20,000 species of bees, and not all of them nest in the same way. Many native bees nest in the ground and need easy access to bare soil. Come spring, clear away plant debris to expose a 2-square-foot (or smaller) area of bare soil near your garden. This area should get as much sun as possible. If you have space restrictions, you can fill a planter with a mixture of sand and loam to help these native bees nest.

Other native bees nest aboveground. Online, you'll find many intricate examples of "bee hotels" you can build. Though they do add style to the garden, a bee nest doesn't have to be that complicated. Simply take a log, old stump, or block of lumber (that hasn't been pressure treated) and drill ¼- to ⅜-inch holes along one side. The holes should only be about 3 to 5 inches deep and not go through the entire piece of wood. Depending on the size of your stump or log, you can drill anywhere from 50 to 100 holes in one nest. Place your nest at least 3 feet above the ground on a stake, another stump, a fence, or any other secure area. Make sure the side with the holes is facing south and has full morning sun.

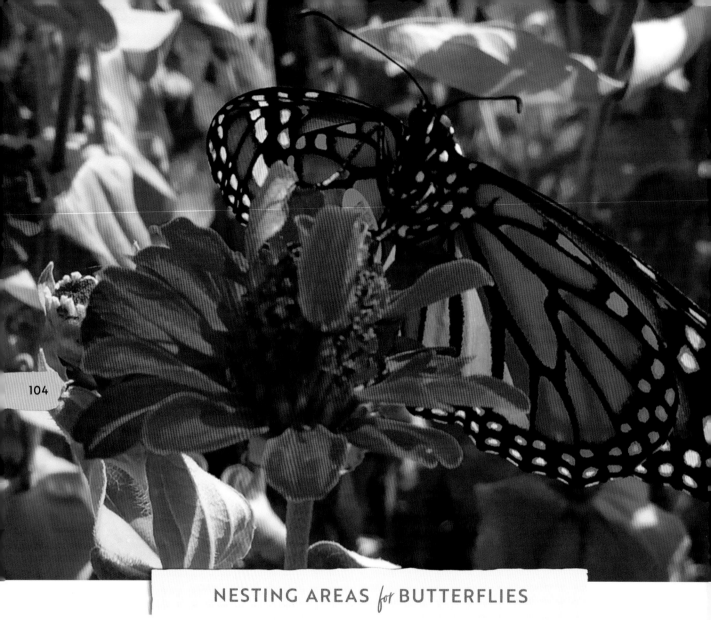

NESTING AREAS *for* BUTTERFLIES

Butterflies lay their eggs on the host plant for their species. It's important to provide plenty of nectar-rich meadow plants as well as these host plants in your garden. With a diverse offering of both, butterflies will have a safe spot to lay their eggs, and the caterpillars will have plenty of food when they emerge.

Common Butterflies and Their Host Plants

Try to offer as many host plants in your landscape as possible to help the different species of butterflies in your area. If you have limited space (or growing conditions), milkweed is always a great choice. Even though it only serves as a host plant for monarchs, it provides extremely important nectar for all butterflies and for other pollinators.

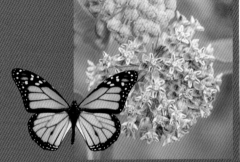

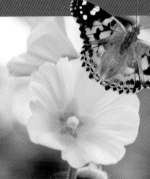

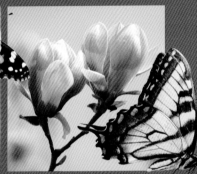

Monarch butterfly
Milkweed

Painted lady butterfly
Thistle, hollyhocks, sunflowers

Eastern tiger swallowtail butterfly
Magnolia, mountain ash, willow

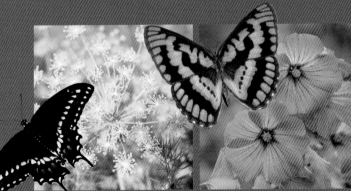

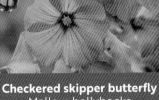

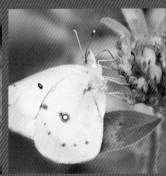

Black swallowtail butterfly
Dill, parsley, fennel, carrots

Checkered skipper butterfly
Mallow, hollyhocks

Dogface butterfly
Prairie clover, baptisia

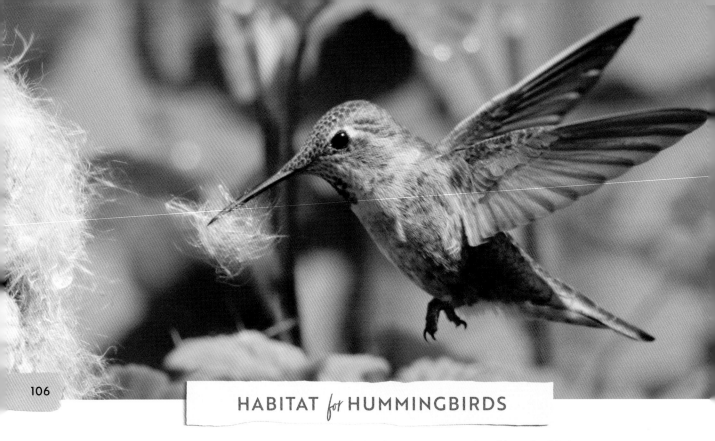

HABITAT *for* HUMMINGBIRDS

Hummingbirds nest high up in trees and shrubs, so you won't be able to build them a nesting area, but you can encourage them to nest on your property by providing them with the materials they need to build their nests:

» Leafy trees and shrubs

» Ornamental grasses

» Plants with soft, fuzzy foliage (like lamb's ears)

» Plants with soft seedpods and fiber (like milkweed, blanketflower, and honeysuckle)

In addition to offering nesting material, be sure to plant plenty of nectar-rich plants for them to feed on! Hummingbirds are most attracted to plants with long, tubular blooms in shades of red, orange, blue, and yellow. Favorite meadow plants include cardinal flower, golden aster, bee balm, and zinnias. Hummingbird feeders help provide these busy birds with plenty of energy and are a great addition to your property.

Citizen Science: Track Your Pollinators

Once you've taken the time to help pollinators in your own garden, you can take your efforts to the next level. Look online at the variety of great citizen science projects that you can be involved with. Many of these track different species of pollinators throughout the country. One of my favorite initiatives is the Million Pollinator Garden Challenge organized by the Pollinator Partnership, an organization with a mission to promote the health of pollinators through conservation, education, and research. The goal of the challenge is to register a million public and private gardens that support pollinators. Once you've planted your pollinator meadow or garden, you can register it on their site (see page 137) and learn all about how you can help raise awareness for their cause.

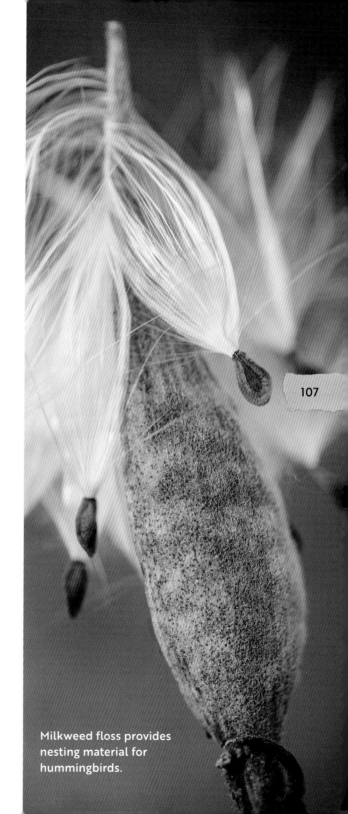

107

Milkweed floss provides nesting material for hummingbirds.

Every SMALL SPACE COUNTS!

Even if you're gardening in a tiny plot, such as in a raised bed or on a balcony in the city, you can still do your part to help pollinators by providing just a window box or other container with pollinator-friendly plants like the ones listed below. Pair these easy-to-grow container plants with a hummingbird feeder, some type of water feature (a birdbath is perfect), and a nesting box or nesting supplies, if you have the space. These three elements — food, water, and shelter — can help pollinators in a big way, even in your small space. Here are a few plants you might consider for your small plot:

» Calendula or pot marigold (*Calendula officinalis*)
» Plains coreopsis (*Coreopsis tinctoria*)
» Dwarf cosmos (*Cosmos bipinnatus*)
» Chinese forget-me-not (*Cynoglossum amabile*)
» Baby's breath (*Gypsophila elegans*)
» Dwarf sunflower 'Sunspot' (*Helianthus annuus* 'Sunspot')

» Sweet alyssum (*Lobularia maritima*)
» Dwarf lupine 'Pixie Delight' (*Lupinus hartwegii* 'Pixie Delight')
» Baby blue eyes (*Nemophila menziesii*)
» French marigold (*Tagetes patula*)
» Mexican sunflower (*Tithonia rotundifolia*)
» Zinnia (*Zinnia elegans*)

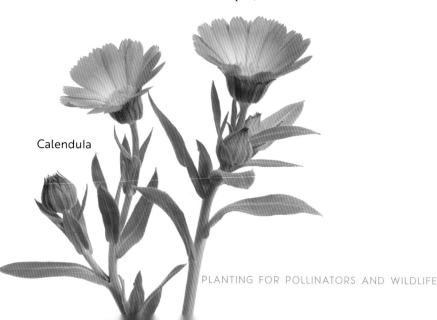

Calendula

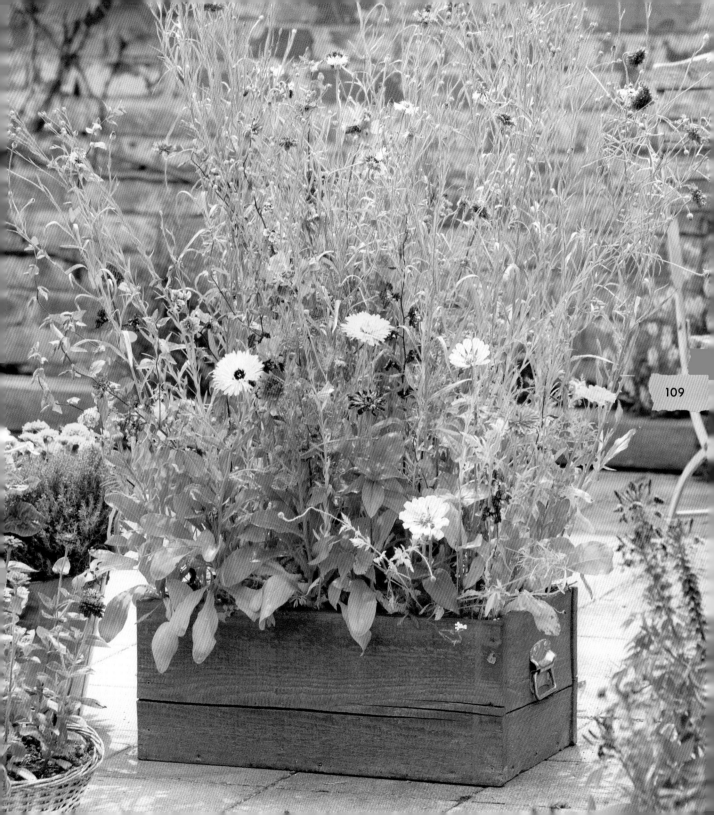

109

Toadflax

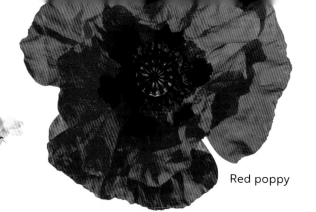

Red poppy

Zinnia

Plains coreopsis

ANNUAL WILDFLOWERS *for* POLLINATORS

Annual wildflowers are extremely beneficial to pollinators: they serve as a quick food source for bees, butterflies, and hummingbirds while your perennials continue to develop. Even if your plan is to create a low-maintenance perennial meadow for pollinators, planting some annuals each year — even after your perennials are established — is extremely helpful. Many annual wildflowers, like those on the list below, are extremely nectar-rich, providing essential nutrition for a variety of different pollinators.

- » Partridge pea (*Chamaecrista fasciculata*)
- » Plains coreopsis (*Coreopsis tinctoria*)
- » Rocket larkspur (*Delphinium ajacis*)
- » California poppy (*Eschscholzia californica*)
- » Toadflax or baby snapdragon (*Linaria maroccana*)
- » Arroyo lupine (*Lupinus succulentus*)
- » Red poppy, Shirley poppy, or corn poppy (*Papaver rhoeas*)
- » Lacy phacelia (*Phacelia tanacetifolia*)
- » Zinnia (*Zinnia elegans*)

Lacy phacelia

Quick-Blooming Annual Wildflowers for Pollinators

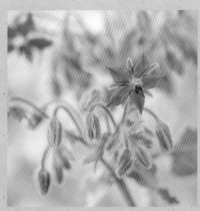

Borage
Borago officinalis

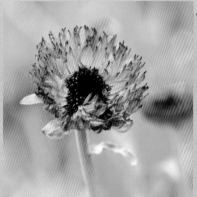

Calendula or pot marigold
Calendula officinalis

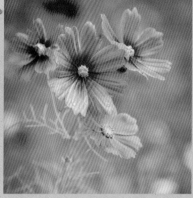

Cosmos
Cosmos bipinnatus

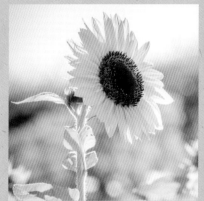

Common sunflower
Helianthus annuus

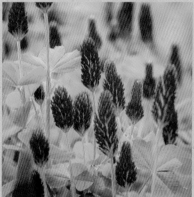

Crimson clover
Trifolium incarnatum

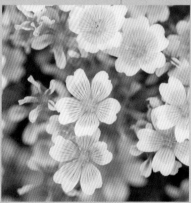

Meadow foam
Limnanthes douglasii

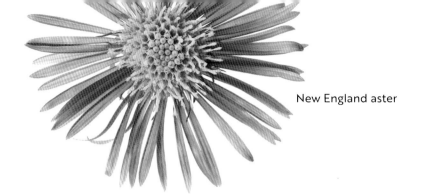

New England aster

PERENNIAL WILDFLOWERS *for* POLLINATORS

Many perennial wildflowers not only act as a dependable food source for pollinators but also provide shelter and serve as host plants. Additionally, perennials are a great way for gardeners to provide a variety of wildflowers for pollinators and not have to worry about planting each year. Here are a few perennials to plant for the pollinators:

» Common yarrow (*Achillea millefolium*)
» Plains coreopsis (*Coreopsis tinctoria*)
» Blanketflower (*Gaillardia aristata*)
» Wild lupine (*Lupinus perennis*)

» Mexican hat or prairie coneflower (*Ratibida columnifera*)
» New England aster (*Symphyotrichum novae-angliae*)
» Thyme (*Thymus vulgaris*)

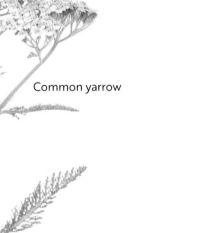

Common yarrow

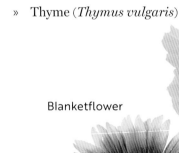

Blanketflower

Plains coreopsi

Long-Lasting Perennial
Wildflowers for Pollinators

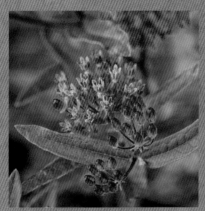

Butterfly weed
Asclepias tuberosa

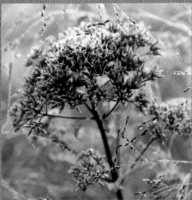

Joe-pye weed
Eupatorium maculatum

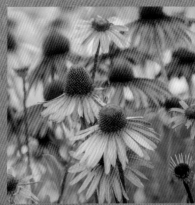

Purple coneflower
Echinacea purpurea

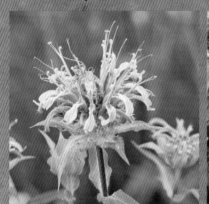

Wild bergamot
Monarda fistulosa

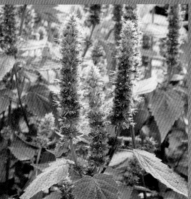

Anise hyssop
Agastache foeniculum

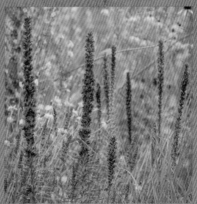

Blazing star or gayfeather
Liatris spicata

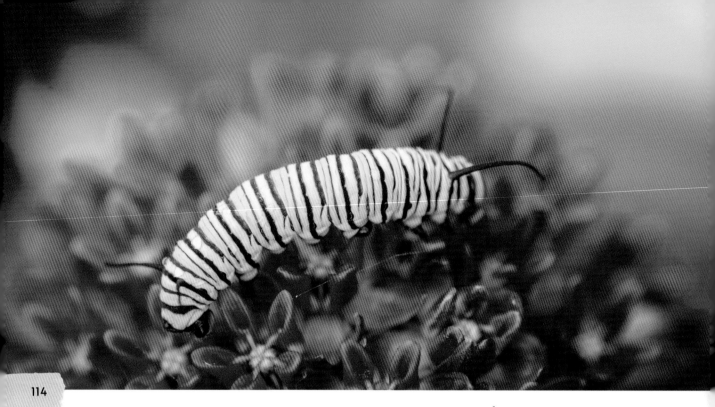

HOST PLANTS *for* POLLINATORS

Host plants play another important function for pollinators: they provide optimal egg-laying sites. One of the most well-known and critical host plants is milkweed (any of a number of species of *Asclepias*), which is the only plant monarch butterflies will deposit their eggs onto. Milkweed and many of these other plants play a key role in helping a wide range of pollinator species, so plant them with abandon:

- » Butterfly weed (*Asclepias tuberosa*)
- » Swamp milkweed (*Asclepias incarnata*)
- » Purple coneflower (*Echinacea purpurea*)
- » Common sunflower (*Helianthus annuus*)
- » Shasta daisy (*Leucanthemum × superbum*)
- » Black-eyed Susan (*Rudbeckia hirta*)
- » New England aster (*Symphyotrichum novae-angliae*)

Easy-to-Grow Host Plants
for Pollinators

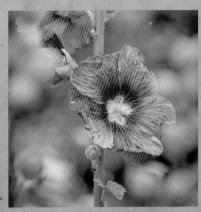

Hollyhock
Alcea rosea

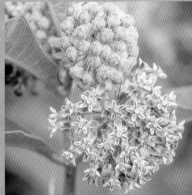

Common milkweed
Asclepias syriaca

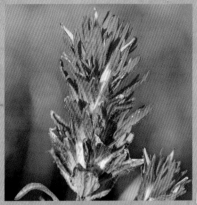

Indian paintbrush
Castilleja coccinea

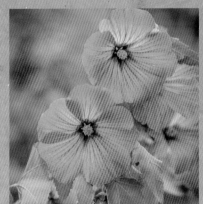

Rose mallow or tree mallow
Lavatera trimestris

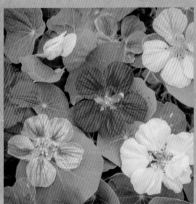

Nasturtium
Tropaeolum majus

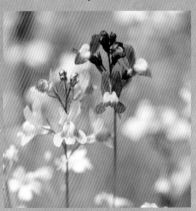

Toadflax or baby snapdragon
Linaria maroccana

Baby blue eyes

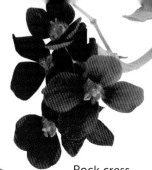

Rock cress

PLANTS *to* ATTRACT BENEFICIAL INSECTS

Cosmos

116

One of my favorite ways to control unwanted insect pests such as aphids, thrips, and mites is to choose plant varieties that attract beneficial bugs to the garden — including lacewings, ladybugs, hoverflies, and parasitic wasps. These insects help keep pest populations in check. Many of the same plants that are attractive to pollinators also attract beneficial insects. Here are a few to consider for your garden:

» Dill (*Anethum graveolens*)
» Lanceleaf coreopsis (*Coreopsis lanceolata*)
» Cosmos (*Cosmos bipinnatus*)
» Purple prairie clover (*Dalea purpurea*)
» Siberian wallflower (*Erysimum × marshallii*)

» California poppy (*Eschscholzia californica*)
» Globe candytuft (*Iberis umbellata*)
» Rock cress (*Aubrieta deltoidea*)
» Wild bergamot (*Monarda fistulosa*)
» Baby blue eyes (*Nemophila menziesii*)

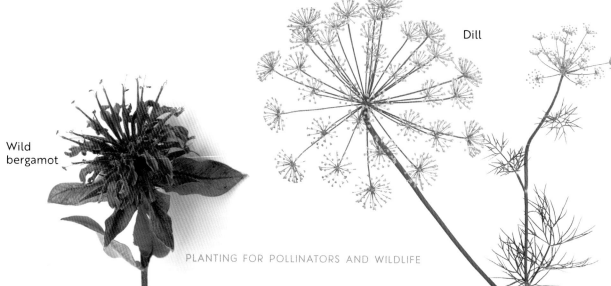

Dill

Wild bergamot

Easy-to-Grow Plants
to Attract Beneficial Insects

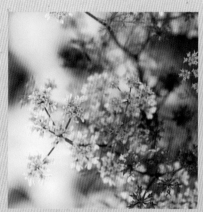

Cilantro
Coriandrum sativum

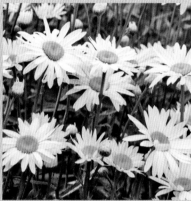

Shasta daisy
Leucanthemum × superbum

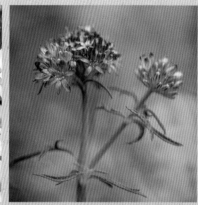

Globe gilia
Gilia capitata

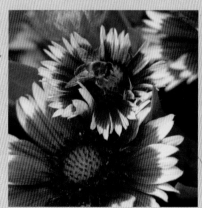

Indian blanket
Gaillardia pulchella

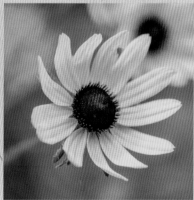

Black-eyed Susan
Rudbeckia hirta

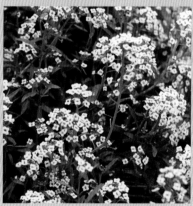

Sweet alyssum
Lobularia maritima

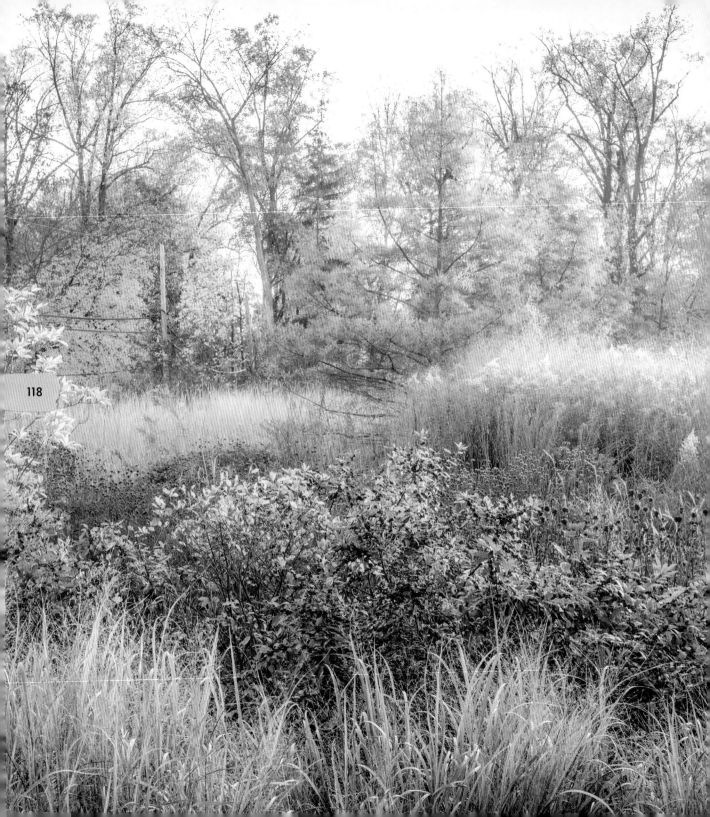

A NATIVE GRASS MEADOW *for* WILDLIFE HABITAT

We've been talking about the different ways meadows can serve a purpose in your landscape, and a native grass meadow provides year-round interest and habitat for local wildlife. One of my favorite winter sights is a native grass meadow dusted in snow. As an added bonus, you'll often spot birds coming to and from your native grass meadow for food and shelter throughout the colder months.

When planning your meadow, consider adding some grasses into the mix along with flowers. No matter what you do, Mother Nature will always toss some unwanted grasses and weeds into your meadow. The more varieties of flowers and grasses that you deliberately include in your meadow mix, the smaller the chance of "unwanted" varieties showing up.

Grasses complement meadow flowers. Their different textures, heights, and colors offer lasting color throughout the growing season, and their seed heads provide food for the birds and offer shelter during winter months. Native grasses are also low maintenance and very adaptable, requiring little water and tolerating poor soils — just like meadow flowers. They have identical traits that make them a nice fit together. Ideally you want to select clump-forming grasses, as they are less aggressive and will thrive well together with your flowers.

Some popular varieties include little bluestem (*Schizachyrium scoparium*), sheep fescue (*Festuca ovina*), sideoats grama (*Bouteloua curtipendula*), and switchgrass (*Panicum virgatum*). These can be purchased in both seed form and as plants or plugs and will adapt nicely whichever way you choose to plant.

If you are going to add grasses into your meadow, the ratio I generally recommend is 25 percent grasses and 75 percent flowers. This usually strikes a nice balance, regardless of the varieties you choose. Of course, you can certainly adjust this depending on your preferences. If you want more flowers, plant more flowers; if you want more grasses, plant a higher ratio of grasses. Whomever you purchase your plants or seeds from should be able to give you some professional advice and make the proper recommendations for your meadow. Below are some common meadow grasses.

» Broom sedge (*Andropogon virginicus*)

» Sideoats grama (*Bouteloua curtipendula*)

» Prairie brome (*Bromus kalmii*)

» Canada wild rye (*Elymus canadensis*)

» Virginia wild rye (*Elymus virginicus*)

» Purpletop (*Tridens flavus*)

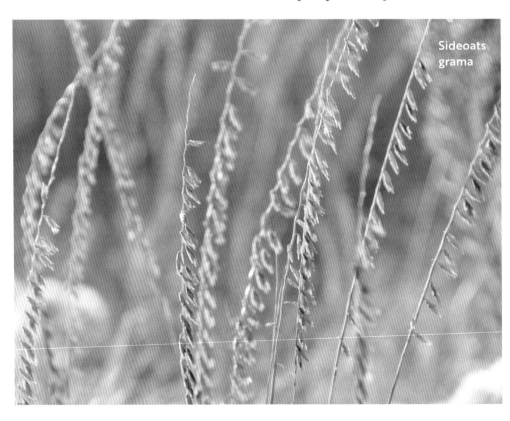

Sideoats grama

Plants for a Native Grass Meadow

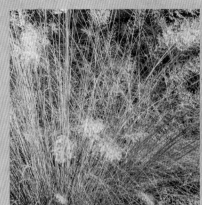

Prairie dropseed
Sporobolus heterolepis

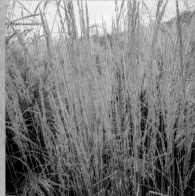

Switchgrass
Panicum virgatum

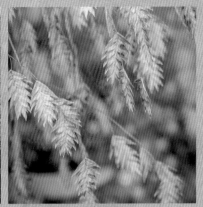

Northern sea oats
Chasmanthium latifolium

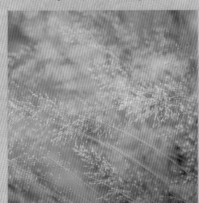

Big bluestem
Andropogon gerardii

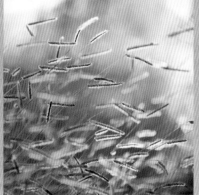

Blue grama
Bouteloua gracilis

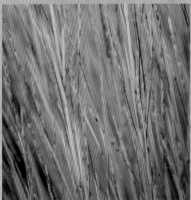

Little bluestem
Schizachyrium scoparium

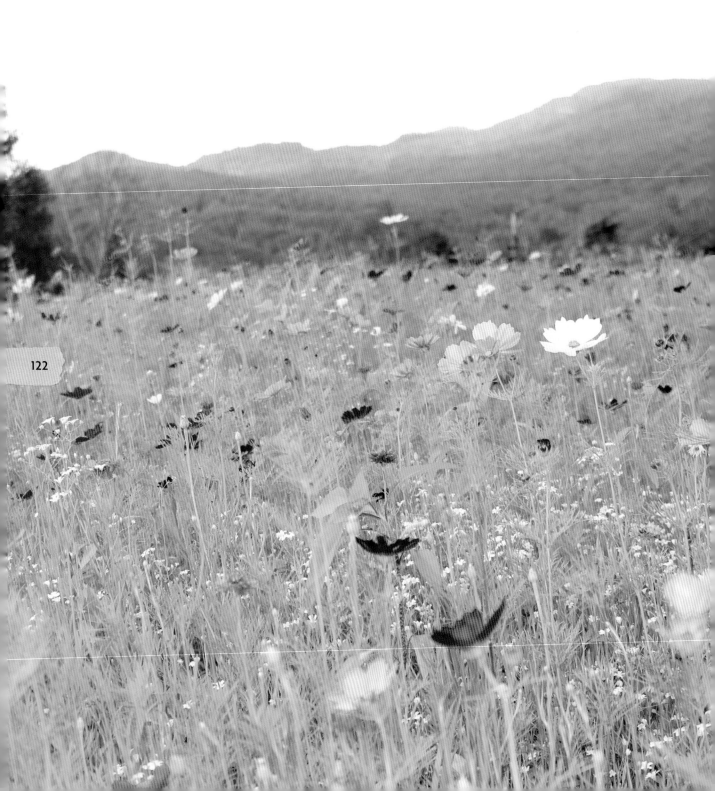

APPENDIX
Meadow Plants for Specific Regions

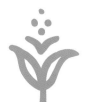

When you visit a garden center, you'll notice that many of the plant labels indicate particular growing zones. These are the USDA Hardiness Zones, and they refer to the average annual low temperatures experienced in each region across the United States and Canada. This information can be helpful when you're selecting perennial plants, particularly when taken into consideration with local site conditions (dry or rainy climate, rich or poor soil, etc.) and microclimate (warm or cold pockets on a site or weather patterns in a region that can affect plant hardiness).

I've found that instead of getting bogged down by figuring out growing zones, many people relate better to the concept of growing *region*. Many common meadow plants are hardy across several different zones, anyway: butterfly weed, lupine, purple coneflower, and daisy are all examples of perennial meadow plants that will provide years of lasting color in a wide variety of conditions. So for the sake of simplicity, I've identified six different growing regions and have made recommendations for hardy and easy-to-grow meadow species. These lists represent just a small sampling of the many options available. You'll certainly find more when you begin researching.

NORTHEAST REGION

This region includes: Connecticut, Delaware, Maine, Maryland, Massachusetts, New Hampshire, New Jersey, New York, Pennsylvania, Rhode Island, Vermont, West Virginia, as well as Quebec and the Eastern Provinces. A short growing season with cold winters, unpredictable weather, and four distinct seasons are synonymous with Northeast weather. But don't let that deter you. You can still grow many annual and perennial meadow flowers and some unique ones, too. A meadow can provide big impact with lots of color and maximize the growing season.

» Eastern red columbine (*Aquilegia canadensis*)

» Swamp milkweed (*Asclepias incarnata*)

» Butterfly weed (*Asclepias tuberosa*)

» Calendula or pot marigold (*Calendula officinalis*)

» Cornflower or bachelor's button (*Centaurea cyanus*)

» Partridge pea (*Chamaecrista fasciculata*)

» Lanceleaf coreopsis (*Coreopsis lanceolata*)

» Plains coreopsis (*Coreopsis tinctoria*)

» Larkspur Giant Imperial Mixed (*Consolida ajacis*)

» Cosmos (*Cosmos bipinnatus*)

» Sulphur cosmos (*Cosmos sulphureus*)

» Sweet William (*Dianthus barbatus*)

» Purple coneflower (*Echinacea purpurea*)

» Siberian wallflower (*Erysimum × marshallii*)

» California poppy (*Eschscholzia californica*)

» Spotted joe-pye weed (*Eupatorium maculatum*)

» Blanketflower (*Gaillardia aristata*)

» Indian blanket (*Gaillardia pulchella*)

» Baby's breath (*Gypsophila elegans*)

» Dwarf sunflower 'Sunspot' (*Helianthus annuus* 'Sunspot')

» Oxeye sunflower (*Heliopsis helianthoides*)

» Globe candytuft (*Iberis umbellata*)

» Rose mallow or tree mallow (*Lavatera trimestris*)

Wild lupine

- » Shasta daisy (*Leucanthemum × superbum*)
- » Blazing star or gayfeather (*Liatris spicata*)
- » Scarlet flax (*Linum grandiflorum* var. *rubrum*)
- » Blue flax (*Linum perenne*)
- » Wild lupine (*Lupinus perennis*)
- » Wild bergamot (*Monarda fistulosa*)
- » Baby blue eyes (*Nemophila menziesii*)
- » Love-in-a-mist (*Nigella damascena*)
- » Common evening primrose (*Oenothera biennis*)
- » Red poppy, Shirley poppy, or corn poppy (*Papaver rhoeas*)
- » Beardtongue (*Penstemon digitalis*)
- » Mexican hat or prairie coneflower (*Ratibida columnifera*)
- » Brown-eyed Susan (*Rudbeckia triloba*)
- » Black-eyed Susan (*Rudbeckia hirta*)
- » Sweet coneflower (*Rudbeckia subtomentosa*)
- » None-so-pretty or catchfly (*Silene armeria*)
- » Stiff goldenrod (*Solidago rigida*)
- » New England aster (*Symphyotrichum novae-angliae*)

SOUTHEAST REGION

For the Southeast region, I include the following states and areas: Alabama, Arkansas, Florida, Georgia, Louisiana, Mississippi, North Carolina, South Carolina, Tennessee, eastern Texas, Virginia, and Washington, D.C.

The Southeast region provides hot summer weather and mild winters. Because of its long growing season, you'll want to become familiar with the bloom times for different meadow plants; it's possible to have color for nine months of the year, if planned properly. Because of the hot weather during the summer months, your meadow may actually welcome having a bit of shade.

- » Butterfly weed (*Asclepias tuberosa*)
- » Partridge pea (*Chamaecrista fasciculata*)
- » Lanceleaf coreopsis (*Coreopsis lanceolata*)
- » Plains coreopsis (*Coreopsis tinctoria*)

- » Cosmos (*Cosmos bipinnatus*)
- » Chinese forget-me-not (*Cynoglossum amabile*)
- » Sweet William (*Dianthus barbatus*)
- » Purple coneflower (*Echinacea purpurea*)
- » Rattlesnake master (*Eryngium yuccifolium*)
- » Siberian wallflower (*Erysimum × marshallii*)
- » California poppy (*Eschscholzia californica*)
- » Indian blanket (*Gaillardia pulchella*)
- » Globe gilia (*Gilia capitata*)
- » Baby's breath (*Gypsophila elegans*)
- » Standing cypress (*Ipomopsis rubra*)
- » Rose mallow or tree mallow (*Lavatera trimestris*)
- » Shasta daisy (*Leucanthemum × superbum*)
- » Blazing star or gayfeather (*Liatris spicata*)
- » Scarlet flax (*Linum grandiflorum* var. *rubrum*)
- » Blue flax (Linum perenne)
- » Sweet alyssum (*Lobularia maritima*)
- » Wild lupine (*Lupinus perennis*)
- » Texas bluebonnet (*Lupinus texensis*)
- » Lemon mint (*Monarda citriodora*)
- » Large-flower evening primrose (*Oenothera glazioviana*)
- » Red poppy, Shirley poppy, or corn poppy (*Papaver rhoeas*)
- » Annual phlox (*Phlox drummondii*)
- » Mexican hat or prairie coneflower (*Ratibida columnifera*)
- » Clasping coneflower (*Rudbeckia amplexicaulis*)
- » Black-eyed Susan (*Rudbeckia hirta*)
- » Scarlet sage (*Salvia coccinea*)
- » Ohio spiderwort (*Tradescantia ohiensis*)

MIDWEST REGION

For the Midwest region, I typically include the following states and province: Illinois, Indiana, Iowa, Kansas, Kentucky, Michigan, Minnesota, Missouri, Nebraska, Ohio, Wisconsin, and Ontario. Like the Northeast, the Midwest region has a shorter growing season, but your meadow can still pack a punch of color and lots of variety year after year. By paying attention to frost dates, as well as weather trends and forecasts, you can stretch your growing season and enjoy your meadow as long as possible each season.

- » Eastern red columbine (*Aquilegia canadensis*)
- » Butterfly weed (*Asclepias tuberosa*)
- » Cornflower or bachelor's button (*Centaurea cyanus*)
- » Lanceleaf coreopsis (*Coreopsis lanceolata*)
- » Plains coreopsis (*Coreopsis tinctoria*)
- » Cosmos (*Cosmos bipinnatus*)
- » Sulphur cosmos (*Cosmos sulphureus*)
- » Purple prairie clover (*Dalea purpurea*)
- » Sweet William (*Dianthus barbatus*)
- » Pale purple coneflower (*Echinacea pallida*)
- » Purple coneflower (*Echinacea purpurea*)
- » Rattlesnake master (*Eryngium yuccifolium*)
- » Siberian wallflower (*Erysimum × marshallii*)
- » California poppy (*Eschscholzia californica*)
- » Blanketflower (*Gaillardia aristata*)
- » Indian blanket (*Gaillardia pulchella*)
- » Baby's breath (*Gypsophila elegans*)
- » Common sunflower (*Helianthus annuus*)
- » Oxeye sunflower (*Heliopsis helianthoides*)
- » Globe candytuft (*Iberis umbellata*)
- » Standing cypress (*Ipomopsis rubra*)
- » Shasta daisy (*Leucanthemum × superbum*)
- » Prairie blazing star (*Liatris pycnostachya*)
- » Scarlet flax (*Linum grandiflorum* var. *rubrum*)
- » Wild lupine (*Lupinus perennis*)
- » Prairie aster or tansy-leaf aster (*Machaeranthera tanacetifolia*)
- » Lemon mint (*Monarda citriodora*)
- » Baby blue eyes (*Nemophila menziesii*)
- » Large-flower evening primrose (*Oenothera glazioviana*)
- » Red poppy, Shirley poppy, or corn poppy (*Papaver rhoeas*)
- » Mexican hat or prairie coneflower (*Ratibida columnifera*)
- » Grey-head coneflower (*Ratibida pinnata*)
- » Clasping coneflower (*Rudbeckia amplexicaulis*)
- » Black-eyed Susan (*Rudbeckia hirta*)
- » Brown-eyed Susan (*Rudbeckia triloba*)
- » New England aster (*Symphyotrichum novae-angliae*)

127

Brown-eyed Susan

SOUTHWEST REGION

The Southwest region of the United States typically includes Arizona, southern California, New Mexico, southern Nevada, Oklahoma, and western Texas. This is a region that can present the most diverse weather conditions, depending on where you're located. Dry, hot summers; desert conditions; and cool winters are found in this region. It offers a long growing season, but is prone to drought; you'll need to provide your meadow with supplemental irrigation.

» Desert marigold (*Baileya multiradiata*)

» Cornflower or bachelor's button (*Centaurea cyanus*)

» Farewell-to-spring or godetia (*Clarkia amoena*)

» Elegant clarkia (*Clarkia unguiculata*)

» Chinese houses (*Collinsia heterophylla*)

» Lanceleaf coreopsis (*Coreopsis lanceolata*)

» Plains coreopsis (*Coreopsis tinctoria*)

» Cosmos (*Cosmos bipinnatus*)

» Sulphur cosmos (*Cosmos sulphureus*)

» African daisy (*Dimorphotheca sinuata*)

» Purple coneflower (*Echinacea purpurea*)

» Siberian wallflower (*Erysimum × marshallii*)

» California poppy (*Eschscholzia californica*)

» Mexican gold poppy (*Eschscholzia mexicana*)

» Indian blanket (*Gaillardia pulchella*)

» Bird's eyes (*Gilia tricolor*)

» Crown daisy or garland chrysanthemum (*Glebionis coronarium*)

» Baby's breath (*Gypsophila elegans*)

» Tidy tips (*Layia platyglossa*)

» Oxeye daisy (*Leucanthemum vulgare*)

» Toadflax or baby snapdragon (*Linaria maroccana*)

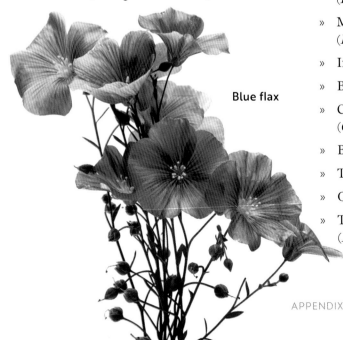

Blue flax

- » Scarlet flax
  (*Linum grandiflorum* var. *rubrum*)
- » Blue flax (*Linum perenne*)
- » Arizona lupine (*Lupinus arizonicus*)
- » Arroyo lupine (*Lupinus succulentus*)
- » Prairie aster or tansy-leaf aster
  (*Machaeranthera tanacetifolia*)
- » Linley's blazing star (*Mentzelia lindleyi*)
- » Five spot (*Nemophila maculata*)
- » Baby blue eyes (*Nemophila menziesii*)
- » Pale evening primrose
  (*Oenothera pallida*)
- » Showy pink evening primrose
  (*Oenothera speciosa*)
- » Rcd poppy, Shirley poppy, or corn
  poppy (*Papaver rhoeas*)
- » California bluebell
  (*Phacelia campanularia*)
- » Annual phlox (*Phlox drummondii*)
- » Mexican hat or prairie coneflower
  (*Ratibida columnifera*)
- » Black-eyed Susan (*Rudbeckia hirta*)
- » None-so-pretty or catchfly
  (*Silene armeria*)

WESTERN REGION

The Western region includes the following areas and states: Colorado, Idaho, Montana, northern Nevada, North Dakota, eastern Oregon, South Dakota, Utah, eastern Washington, and Wyoming. Spring rains and dry, warm summers can be found throughout this region. Cold winters with frosts and snow provide the perfect growing climate for establishing perennials. Amount of snow and winter temperatures are highly dependent on altitude.

- » Colorado blue columbine
  (*Aquilegia coerulea*)
- » Cornflower or bachelor's button
  (*Centaurea cyanus*)
- » Deerhorn clarkia (*Clarkia pulchella*)
- » Elegant clarkia (*Clarkia unguiculata*)
- » Rocky Mountain bee plant
  (*Cleome serrulata*)
- » Plains coreopsis (*Coreopsis tinctoria*)
- » Cosmos (*Cosmos bipinnatus*)
- » Sulphur cosmos (*Cosmos sulphureus*)
- » Purple prairie clover (*Dalea purpurea*)
- » Sweet William (*Dianthus barbatus*)

- » African daisy (*Dimorphotheca sinuata*)
- » Daisy fleabane (*Erigeron speciosus*)
- » Siberian wallflower (*Erysimum* × *marshallii*)
- » California poppy (*Eschscholzia californica*)
- » Blanketflower (*Gaillardia aristata*)
- » Indian blanket (*Gaillardia pulchella*)
- » Globe gilia (*Gilia capitata*)
- » Crown daisy or garland chrysanthemum (*Glebionis coronarium*)
- » Baby's breath (*Gypsophila elegans*)
- » Showy goldeneye (*Heliomeris multiflora*)
- » Tidy tips (*Layia platyglossa*)
- » Shasta daisy (*Leucanthemum* × *superbum*)
- » Mountain phlox (*Linanthus grandiflorus*)
- » Sweet alyssum (*Lobularia maritima*)
- » Arroyo lupine (*Lupinus succulentus*)
- » Prairie aster or tansy-leaf aster (*Machaeranthera tanacetifolia*)
- » Lemon mint (*Monarda citriodora*)
- » Pale evening primrose (*Oenothera pallida*)
- » Red poppy, Shirley poppy, or corn poppy (*Papaver rhoeas*)
- » Rocky Mountain penstemon (*Penstemon strictus*)
- » California bluebell (*Phacelia campanularia*)
- » Mexican hat or prairie coneflower (*Ratibida columnifera*)
- » Black-eyed Susan (*Rudbeckia hirta*)
- » None-so-pretty or catchfly (*Silene armeria*)
- » Smooth aster (*Symphyotrichum laevis*)

130

PACIFIC NORTHWEST REGION

The Pacific Northwest region can provide a year-round growing climate, depending on where you live. This region includes the following states and province: northern California, western Oregon, western Washington, and British Columbia. Mild winters and warm summers with rain present ideal conditions for your meadows. It's not unusual to have your annuals reseed, thanks to the mild winter conditions.

California poppy

- Common yarrow (*Achillea millefolium*)
- California yarrow (*Achillea millefolium* var. *californica*)
- Wild columbine (*Aquilegia vulgaris*)
- Cornflower or bachelor's button (*Centaurea cyanus*)
- Farewell-to-spring or godetia (*Clarkia amoena*)
- Elegant clarkia (*Clarkia unguiculata*)
- Chinese houses (*Collinsia heterophylla*)
- Lanceleaf coreopsis (*Coreopsis lanceolata*)
- Plains coreopsis (*Coreopsis tinctoria*)
- Rocket larkspur (*Delphinium ajacis*)
- Sweet William (*Dianthus barbatus*)
- Foxglove (*Digitalis purpurea*)
- Siberian wallflower (*Erysimum* × *marshallii*)
- California poppy (*Eschscholzia californica*)
- Blanketflower (*Gaillardia aristata*)
- Globe gilia (*Gilia capitata*)
- Bird's eyes (*Gilia tricolor*)
- Baby's breath (*Gypsophila elegans*)
- Globe candytuft (*Iberis umbellata*)
- Tidy tips (*Layia platyglossa*)

- Shasta daisy (*Leucanthemum* × *superbum*)
- Mountain phlox (*Linanthus grandiflorus*)
- Toadflax or baby snapdragon (*Linaria maroccana*)
- Scarlet flax (*Linum grandiflorum* var. *rubrum*)
- Sweet alyssum (*Lobularia maritima*)
- Sicklekeel lupine (*Lupinus albicaulis*)
- Arroyo lupine (*Lupinus succulentus*)
- Russell lupine (*Lupinus* × *regalis* Russell Group)
- Linley's blazing star (*Mentzelia lindleyi*)
- Five spot (*Nemophila maculata*)
- Baby blue eyes (*Nemophila menziesii*)
- Hooker's evening primrose (*Oenothera elata* subsp. *hookeri*)
- Large-flower evening primrose (*Oenothera glazioviana*)
- Red poppy, Shirley poppy, or corn poppy (*Papaver rhoeas*)
- California bluebell (*Phacelia campanularia*)
- Black-eyed Susan (*Rudbeckia hirta*)
- None-so-pretty or catchfly (*Silene armeria*)

GLOSSARY

ACID SOIL: Soil with a pH below 7.0.

ALKALINE SOIL: Soil with a pH above 7.0.

ANNUAL: A plant that completes its lifecycle in one year or less. It will grow, flower, produce and drop seed, then die.

BIENNIAL: A plant that completes its lifecycle in two years. It will develop green top growth in the first year. It will go dormant, then come back in the second year and flower, produce seed, and then die.

CLUMP FORMING: A plant that grows in small bunches or clumps. These plants are usually not aggressive.

COOL-SEASON GRASSES: These grow during the spring and fall when soil temperatures are cooler, and go dormant during warmer months.

EROSION: The weathering or removal of soil from the action of wind, rain, or other process.

FERTILIZER: A natural or synthetic substance that contains one or more nutrients to help promote plant growth.

GERMINATE: The process of a seed beginning to grow and sprout after emerging from dormancy.

HABITAT: The natural home or environment of a plant, animal, or other living organism.

HERBICIDE: A substance toxic to plants used to kill unwanted plant vegetation. Products such as Round-Up and Weed-Be-Gon are herbicides.

HOA: Home Owners Association. Sometimes they have special rules when it comes to installing and maintaining a meadow.

INVASIVE: A nonnative plant that negatively impacts habitat and ecosystems.

NATIVE: Of indigenous origin or growth. A plant that thrives naturally without human involvement and has been present in a region for many, many years.

NESTING BOX: A man-made structure to encourage and support nesting by birds and insects.

ORGANIC: Of or derived from living organisms; i.e. originating from plants or animals.

PERENNIAL: A plant that continues to grow and flower year after year.

PLUGS: Small plant starts grown in trays or cells, designed to be transplanted into larger containers or directly into the garden.

pH: This is the measure of hydrogen ion concentration indicating the acidity or alkalinity of a solution. Knowing the pH of your soil can be helpful in determining the right plants for your garden, since certain plants grow better in soil with a particular pH range.

SEED STRATIFICATION: The natural process of cold and moisture that can stimulate seed germination.

SUSTAINABLE: The enduring and continuous ability of an ecosystem to thrive and be productive.

WARM-SEASON GRASSES: Grasses that grow during the summer when soil temperatures are warmer and go dormant during fall and winter months.

RESOURCES

Gardens to Visit

I've been fortunate to have traveled across the United States and visited botanic gardens, national parks, Audubon centers, and private gardens from coast to coast. It's a never-ending journey and I continue to be inspired by the different shapes, sizes, textures, and meanings of the meadows and gardens I see. Here are some of my favorites.

The Atlanta Botanical Gardens

www.atlantabg.org

This 30-acre garden located next to Piedmont Park provides a diverse mix of gardens and unique plant collections. The conservation gardens are worth the visit, as is the amazing catwalk/garden canopy that makes it feel like you're walking in the trees.

Denver Botanic Gardens

www.botanicgardens.org

This 23-acre expanse includes more than 50 different types of gardens, from edible gardening to xeriscaping, and they seem to have a new exhibit every couple of months. Their website is also a great resource for gardeners; they are constantly updating and sharing new gardening information.

Lady Bird Johnson Wildflower Center

www.wildflower.org

This national treasure located in Austin, Texas, is a must-visit for any wildflower enthusiast. Founded by former first lady Claudia Alta Johnson and actress Helen Hayes back in 1982, this 279-acre property is the home to over 650 native Texas plant species.

The Los Angeles Arboretum and Botanic Garden

www.arboretum.org

This arboretum features 10 different theme gardens spread over 127 acres, with spectacular waterfalls and enormous diversity in plant species.

New England Wildflower Society Garden in the Woods

www.newenglandwild.org

This 45-acre garden has been a favorite of mine since my first visit back in 1991. Located in Framingham, Massachusetts, it offers a diverse mix of plantings and provides endless ideas and inspiration.

USDA Hardiness Zone Map

To find your USDA Hardiness Zone, go to the USDA website and enter your zip code. https://planthardiness.ars.usda.gov

Seed Sources

The following companies are reliable sources of pure seed, in the quantities needed for establishing a meadow garden.

American Meadows

www.americanmeadows.com

877-309-7333

Beauty Beyond Belief Wildflower Seed

www.bbbseed.com

303-530-1222

Ernst Conservation Seeds

www.ernstseed.com

800-873-3321

Outside Pride

www.outsidepride.com

800-670-4192

Prairie Moon Nursery

www.prairiemoon.com

866-417-8156

Prairie Nursery

www.prairienursery.com

800-476-9453

Reliable Sources of Native Plants

Bluestone Perennials

www.bluestoneperennials.com

800-852-5243

Dropseed Native Plant Nursery

www.dropseednursery.com
502-439-9033

High Country Gardens

www.highcountrygardens.com
800-925-9387

Ion Exchange

https://ionxchange.com
563-535-7231

Minnesota Native Landscapes

https://mnnativelandscapes.com
763-295-0010

North Creek Nurseries

www.northcreeknurseries.com
877-326-7584

For More Information

Growing a Greener World

www.growingagreenerworld.com
470-242-1982

Growing a Greener World is an award-winning TV show appearing on National Public Television that features organic gardening, green living, and farm-to-table food. Each episode focuses on compelling and inspirational people making a positive impact on the planet through gardening and shares DIY information that we can all use at home.

Habitat Network at the Cornell Lab of Ornithology

content.yardmap.org
800-843-2473

Habitat Network is a citizen science project designed to cultivate a richer understanding of wildlife habitat, for both professional scientists and people concerned with their local environments. They collect data by asking individuals across the country to literally draw maps of their backyards, parks, farms, favorite birding locations, schools, and gardens. They connect you with your landscape details and provide tools for you to make better decisions about how to manage landscapes sustainably.

Kids Gardening

https://kidsgardening.org
802-660-4604

KidsGardening has been a leading resource for school and youth gardening since 1982, providing garden grants, research, and curriculum. They create opportunities for kids to learn through the garden, engaging their natural curiosity and wonder by providing inspiration, know-how, networking opportunities, and additional educational resources.

Monarch Watch

www.monarchwatch.org
800-780-9986

Monarch Watch is a nonprofit education, conservation, and research program based at the University of Kansas that focuses on the monarch butterfly, its habitat, and its spectacular fall migration.

National Wildlife Federation

www.nwf.org
800-822-9919

National Wildlife Federation is a voice for wildlife, dedicated to protecting wildlife and habitat and inspiring the future generation of conservationists. Programs such as Butterfly Heroes and Garden for Wildlife are helping to restore habitat and wildlife populations across the United States.

PlantNative

www.plantnative.org
503-248-0104

PlantNative is dedicated to moving native plants and nature-scaping into mainstream landscaping practices. Its goal is to increase public awareness of native plants and related landscaping practices and to increase both the supply of and demand for native plants.

Pollinator Partnership

www.pollinator.org
415-362-1137

The Pollinator Partnership's mission is to promote the health of pollinators, critical to food and ecosystems, through conservation, education, and research. Signature initiatives include the NAPPC (North American Pollinator Protection Campaign), National Pollinator Week, and the Ecoregional Planting Guides.

USDA Natural Resources Conservation Service PLANTS Database

https://plants.sc.egov.vsda.gov

The PLANTS Database provides standardized information about the vascular plants, mosses, liverworts, hornworts, and lichens of the United States and its territories. It includes names, plant symbols, checklists, distributional data, species abstracts, characteristics, images, crop information, automated tools, onward web links, and references.

The Xerces Society

https://xerces.org
855-232-6639

The Xerces Society for Invertebrate Conservation is an international nonprofit organization that protects wildlife through the conservation of invertebrates and their habitats. They take their name from the now extinct Xerces Blue butterfly (*Glaucopsyche xerces*), the first butterfly known to go extinct in North America as a result of human activities.

INDEX

141

Grow Your Gardening Creativity
with More Books from Storey

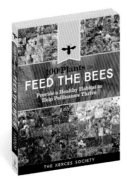

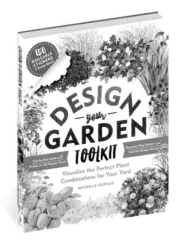

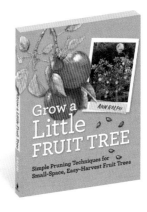

by The Xerces Society
When it comes to protecting our pollinators, you can make a difference! These 100 profiles of common flowers, herbs, shrubs, and trees that attract and nourish bees, butterflies, moths, and hummingbirds show you how.

by Michelle Gervais
Before picking up the trowel, pick up the stickers! Layer, arrange, and rearrange your perfect planting using 150 reusable cling stickers with beautiful botanically accurate illustrations, a fold-out design board, and an easy five-step design process.

by Ann Ralph
Grow your own apples, figs, plums, cherries, pears, apricots, and peaches in even the smallest backyard. Expert instruction for pruning a regular fruit tree down to a manageable size will make harvesting a snap.

Join the conversation. Share your experience with this book, learn more about Storey Publishing's authors, and read original essays and book excerpts at storey.com. Look for our books wherever quality books are sold or call 800-441-5700.